Cross-Cultural Advancements in Positive Psychology

Volume 14

Series Editor

Antonella Delle Fave, University of Milano, Milano, Italy

The aim of the Cross Cultural Advancements in Positive Psychology book series is to spread a universal and culture-fair perspective on good life promotion. The series will advance a deeper understanding of the cross-cultural differences in well-being conceptualization. A deeper understanding can affect psychological theories, interventions and social policies in various domains, from health to education, from work to leisure. Books in the series will investigate such issues as enhanced mobility of people across nations, ethnic conflicts and the challenges faced by traditional communities due to the pervasive spreading of modernization trends. New instruments and models will be proposed to identify the crucial components of well-being in the process of acculturation. This series will also explore dimensions and components of happiness that are currently overlooked because happiness research is grounded in the Western tradition, and these dimensions do not belong to the Western cultural frame of mind and values.

Andreas M. Krafft • Tharina Guse •
Alena Slezackova
Editors

Hope across cultures

Lessons from the International Hope Barometer

Springer

Editors
Andreas M. Krafft
Institute of Systemic Management
and Public Governance
Universty of St. Gallen
St. Gallen, Switzerland

Tharina Guse
Department of Psychology
University of Pretoria
Pretoria, South Africa

Alena Slezackova
Department of Medical Psychology and
Psychosomatics, Faculty of Medicine
Masaryk University
Brno, Czech Republic

ISSN 2210-5417 ISSN 2210-5425 (electronic)
Cross-Cultural Advancements in Positive Psychology
ISBN 978-3-031-24411-7 ISBN 978-3-031-24412-4 (eBook)
https://doi.org/10.1007/978-3-031-24412-4

This Springer imprint is published by the registered company Springer Nature Switzerland AG
The registered company address is: Gewerbestrasse 11, 6330 Cham, Switzerland

Preface

During the past few years, hope has received more and more attention from researchers in several disciplines. This book is not just an edited volume compiling unrelated contributions around the topic of hope. It is the result of many years of cooperative work performed by several researchers engaged in the Hope Barometer International Research Network. The Hope Barometer Research Program was created in 2009 as an annual cross-sectional survey that aimed at investigating the hopes and future expectations of the general population in several countries around the globe. Starting in Switzerland, the Hope Barometer expanded to an international research network bringing together researchers from universities in Australia, Colombia, Czechia, France, India, Israel, Italy, Malta, Nigeria, Poland, Portugal, South Africa, and Spain. Year after year, around 10,000 participants have been providing valuable insights for a deeper understanding of what and how people in different countries hope in daily life and, by doing so, experience the positive effects of a hopeful future orientation.

The universal and existential value as well as the culture-specific experiences and manifestations of hope can best be explored if we engage different scientific disciplines. Therefore, this book integrates the empirical results of the Hope Barometer with conceptual insights from positive psychology, philosophy, theology, futures studies, and risk management.

The Hope Barometer survey consists of a battery of validated scales, of which about half entail the core of the survey and the other half focus on a specific annual topic of interest. The main part of the survey that has been used consistently every year includes several items to assess future expectations in several life domains, the level of individual hopefulness, the targets and sources of hope, and variables to measure several dimensions of satisfaction and well-being. The other half of the survey has been selected each year based on two criteria: The first focus was dedicated to evaluating one particular element of the hope model that was developed following the transdisciplinary integration of insights from different disciplines. The second annual focus takes into consideration current social issues and challenges. In 2017, the special topics related to hope were about basic beliefs and assumptive worldviews, as well as about meaning in life, helping others, harmony in life, and volunteering. In 2018, we concentrated the study of hope on human values, subjective vitality, and flourishing. In 2019, the focus was on collective hope, long-term future trends, probable and desired future scenarios, and receiving and giving social support.

When we asked people in November 2019 about their expectations regarding long-term trends and future scenarios, we had no idea that in just a few months the largely gloomy prospects reported by the participants would become a painful reality. Due to the COVID-19 pandemic (and the war in the Ukraine), the world is no longer the same as it was a couple of years ago. Therefore, the surveys in 2020 and 2021 aimed at assessing the experiences of people during the COVID-19 pandemic, focusing especially on how they perceived the stressful situations, how they coped with the new realities, and how they could remain hopeful and by doing so grow psychologically.

While our research findings provided fundamental insights for a better understanding of the phenomenon of hope during the first years of the Hope Barometer, since 2020 the urgency and relevance of hope in times of crisis, full of uncertainty and profound changes, became apparent. In a time of social upheaval of all kinds, many people are asking themselves how things will and should continue in the future and what their own lives will look like. In many public interviews and lectures, we were able to share the knowledge of our cumulative work of more than ten years, and, thanks to it, provide encouragement and a hopeful view of the future. The positive feedback from all over the world has shown how profound the longing for the uplifting power of hope is. Hope is precisely not putting on rose-colored glasses. Hope means that we can and should wish for a better future for each of us, for our families, and for the world. Especially in times of crises, we can believe that a better future is possible, if we are able to trust in ourselves, in others, and in life, working together to achieve our more fervent wishes.

This book aims to reveal the importance of a hopeful attitude and of fundamental values and basic beliefs for the creation of a better future and to convey the conviction that everyone, no matter what the situation is, can hope for and contribute to this future. A better future can rarely be achieved by individuals alone, but almost exclusively in a community of hopers. One core message of the book is that hope is an essential part of life for every individual all over the globe and that each person can perceive and express hope in a very individual way. We trust that readers of this book will be encouraged to engage in activities and research to create personally meaningful futures.

Many people have contributed at one point or another to the creation of this book. First of all, we would like to thank the pioneers and members of the advisory board of the Hope Barometer Markus Baumgartner, Fritz Peyer-Müller, Andreas Walker, and Thomas Winkler and the "Stiftung Bildung und Forschung" for the continued support and encouragement over all these years. We also want to express our gratitude to all the reviewers who contributed to improve the quality of the individual chapters. Tharina Guse would like to thank the University of Pretoria for funding the South African data collection in 2019. Furthermore, we would like to thank Cameron Johnson for the valuable technical editing work on the manuscripts.

St. Gallen, Switzerland Andreas M. Krafft
Pretoria, South Africa Tharina Guse
Brno, Czech Republic Alena Slezackova

Contents

About the Editors

Andreas M. Krafft holds a doctoral degree in Management Sciences at the University of St. Gallen (Switzerland) with a special focus on organizational psychology, culture, and development. He has academic specializations in social psychology of organizations, work and health psychology, and positive psychology from the University of Zürich. Andreas is associate researcher for Futures Studies and lecturer at the Institute of Systemic Management and Public Governance at the University of St. Gallen. Furthermore, he teaches at the University of Zürich in the field of work and health, the Master of Applied Positive Psychology at the University of Lisbon, Portugal, and the Master of Futures Studies from the Free University Berlin. He is co-president of swissfuture, the Swiss Society for Futures Studies, and member of the executive board of SWIPPA (the Swiss Positive Psychology Association) and the DACH-PP (German-speaking Association of Positive Psychology). Since many years he leads the International Research Network of the Hope Barometer.

Tharina Guse is a counseling psychologist and obtained an MA (Counseling Psychology) degree from the Potchefstroom University (now North-West University) in 1989. She was in full time private practice for the next 15 years providing psychotherapy for children, adolescents, and adults. In 2003, she obtained her PhD (Psychology) from Potchefstroom University. She returned to academia in 2005 and joined the University of Johannesburg. Since April 2018 she is a professor and Head of the Department of Psychology at the University of Pretoria. Currently, she serves on the Professional Board for Psychology of the Health Professions Council of South Africa (HPCSA). She is also President of the recently founded South African Positive Psychology Association (SAPPA). Her research focuses on positive psychology in general and in particular on psychosocial well-being, positive psychology interventions, and psychological strengths such as hope and gratitude. Closely aligned with this broad focus she also conducts research on the application of hypnosis for the promotion of mental health and well-being.

Alena Slezackova is Associate Professor of Psychology and Vice Head of the Dept. of Psychology and Psychosomatics, Faculty of Medicine, Masaryk University, in Brno, Czech Republic. Her scientific interests include mainly hope, mental health, and well-being. She also has a special interest in the research and practice of mindfulness. Alena is a founder and director of the Czech Positive Psychology Centre (CPPC), a member of the Advisory Council of the International Positive Psychology Association (IPPA), and a member of the Executive Board of the European Network for Positive Psychology (ENPP). She has been a member of several international research projects, and she serves on the editorial boards of five academic psychological journals. Alena is the author of the first comprehensive monograph on positive psychology in the Czech language and dozens of scientific publications in positive psychology and health psychology.

Chapter 1
Introduction and Research Agenda

Andreas M. Krafft, Tharina Guse, and Alena Slezackova

Abstract This introductory chapter presents the antecedents and the purpose that originated the creation of this book on cross-cultural studies on hope. It sketches the existential and multifaceted nature of hope and points to the array of disciplines that, over many decades and even centuries, have studied the phenomenon of hope from various scientific perspectives and in different contexts. Based on the past focus and the current challenges in psychological research on hope, it pleads for an inter- and transdisciplinary approach to the study of hope in diverse cultural contexts. After briefly introducing a cultural perspective on hope, we present the purpose, development, and research focus of the Hope Barometer international research program. We highlight the necessity to conceptualize hope in a trans-disciplinary and culture-sensitive way and then formulate a number of fundamental research questions that guided the empirical studies reported in this book. Assessing hope across cultures requires the development of measures that, on the one hand, prevent bias in the general conceptualization of hope and, on the other hand, permit the analysis of several elements and dimensions of hope, such as different hope targets, sources, and activities. Hope and its various elements and dimensions are partly rooted in diverse culturally tinted worldviews and values, displaying different correlations and predictors of hope across cultures. A succinct overview of the structure and single chapters of the book aims to show up the overall logic that guided its outline.

A. M. Krafft (✉)
Institute of Systemic Management and Public Governance, University of St. Gallen, St. Gallen, Switzerland
e-mail: andreas.krafft@unisg.ch

T. Guse
Department of Psychology, University of Pretoria, Pretoria, South Africa

A. Slezackova
Department of Medical Psychology and Psychosomatics, Faculty of Medicine, Masaryk University, Brno, Czech Republic

A. M. Krafft et al. (eds.), *Hope across cultures*, Cross-Cultural Advancements in Positive Psychology 14, https://doi.org/10.1007/978-3-031-24412-4_1

1.1 Background

For many decades and even centuries, poets, philosophers, and scientists alike have been fascinated and inspired by the human phenomenon of hope. A huge number of theories and studies on hope have been conceived by numerous researchers from various different disciplines, with several philosophical and normative backgrounds anchored in specific historical and cultural environments. The range goes from the ancient Greeks and the myth of Pandora, through Christian theologians like Augustine and Thomas Aquinas, philosophers from different traditions such as the political and moral philosopher Hobbes and the empiricist and naturalist Hume, the Christian philosopher Kierkegaard, the moral philosopher and transcendental idealist of the Enlightenment Kant, the socialist and utopist Bloch, the Christian theologian Moltmann, the existentialist Marcel, the critical educator Freire, and the American pragmatists Dewey and Rorty (for an overview see Blöser, 2020 and Blöser & Stahl, 2017). More recently, many philosophers, theologians, psychologists, and scientists in the fields of futures studies, education, and nursing research have conducted valuable work on hope.

Hope seems to be an existential need in every life situation (Bloch, 1959; Marcel, 1951). Without hope we are unable to live in dignity and much less to experience a fulfilling life (Beck et al., 1990; McGeer, 2004). To hope is an existential feature of what it is to be human (Webb, 2007). Many authors have recognized hope as a fundamental condition for human flourishing (Callina et al., 2018; McCormick, 2017; Snow, 2019; Stitzlein, 2019). Hope is crucial in times of crises and in situations full of uncertainty and anxiety (Scioli & Biller, 2009). Hope appears to be an existential, universal, multifaceted yet simultaneously, to a certain degree, a mysterious and elusive phenomenon not easily studied in a scientific and systematic way (Marcel, 1951; Blöser, 2019). Further, hope contains many spheres and dimensions, ranging from concrete individual hopes to a general and fundamental feeling of hopefulness (Dufault & Martocchio, 1985; Shade, 2001).

As an example, the fundamental and existential nature of hope has been formulated by Václav Havel, former political dissident, and first democratically elected president of Czechoslovakia after communism and later the first president of the Czech Republic, in one of his letters from prison to his wife Olga:

> The more I think about it, the more I incline to the opinion that the most important thing of all is not to lose hope and faith in life itself. Anyone who does so is lost, regardless of what good fortune may befall him. On the other hand, those who do not lose it can never come to a bad end. This doesn't mean closing one's eyes to the horrors of the world—quite the contrary, in fact: only those who have not lost faith and hope can see the horrors of the world with genuine clarity. (Havel, 1989, p. 141).

Until now, beyond all the particular philosophies and theories, there is little consensus throughout all scientific disciplines about the general nature and definition of hope, which makes it very difficult to find common ground to integrate the current state of knowledge and research. What is certain is that hope is a very complex and multifaceted aspect of human experience. Since hope is an essential and existential part of life, people in different contexts and life situations may experience, understand, nurture, and express hope in many different ways. When thinking about the nature of hope, we have to be aware that in daily life, hope manifests itself in a great variety of forms. Just as there are many modes of feeling love or anxiety, there are numerous types of hope (Milona, 2019, 2020). For example, to hope for a cure from a chronic illness, to hope for one's children or to hope for the end of a war might differ from hoping for good weather during the weekend or to hope for a job promotion or from being hopeful about one's team winning the next match. How people hope is also related to how people face and deal with difficult and challenging situations (Kleist & Jansen, 2016), such as the unexpected pandemic in 2020 and 2021. There seem to exist many ways people can hope, reflecting different psychological processes and states, which can have diverse effects on their lives. When studying hope, researchers must therefore be open to acknowledging the multiplicity and plurality of hope aspects, processes, states, and practices (Green, 2019).

In this introductory chapter, we address the current challenges in the psychological research on hope, briefly describe the cultural perspective that guided our work and present the overall research program of the international network of the Hope Barometer. For several years, we have been working on how hope should be conceptualized and studied across cultures. Here we will pose the main questions that guided our empirical research and theory-building efforts. We discuss the fundamental issues about how to assess hope, highlight the importance of values and worldviews and explain how we analyze the meaning of hope across cultures. Finally, we give an overview of the general structure and the singular chapters of the book.

1.2 Current Research Challenges on Hope

During the last decades, scientists in several disciplines have developed a variety of concepts and models, focusing on single elements of hope. Several academics have investigated the nature and, above all, the positive qualities of hope in a variety of life situations, from early childhood (Erikson, 1959), through school and university (Marques et al., 2011), in times of illness and other hardships (Benzein et al., 2001; Herth, 2005), in the context of life crises (Beck et al., 1990) up to the moment of facing death (Eliott & Olver, 2002, 2007, 2009; Feudtner, 2005). Every philosopher and scientist dedicated to study hope has developed a special interest and a particular view on the phenomenon. Researchers developed particular views on hope based on their individual experience, education, and social context. This has resulted in a wide variety of conceptualizations, definitions, models, and operationalizations of hope and its different dimensions (Eliott, 2005). Hope has been characterized as an emotion, a cognitive process, an existential resource, a state of being, a disposition, a state of mind, an attitude, a social construct, a formed habit, a complex, multifaceted affective-cognitive-behavioural phenomenon, or, quite simply, a mystery (for an overview see Webb, 2007). For some, hope is primarily based on human agency and connected to people's individual goals, motivation, and cognitive capabilities (Snyder, 1994). For others, hope as a fundamental human emotion is mainly supported by social relationships (Fredrickson, 2004; McGeer, 2004). Others again see hope as basically related to a transcendent Higher Power and consider it to be a religious or human virtue (Pinsent, 2020; Snow, 2019). Some disciplines and authors centered their studies on the broader social and ecological environment (Hicks, 2012; Eckersley, 2002). To some extent, hope is linked to positive expectations about the future. However, it might also differ from future expectations (David et al., 2004) and be intimately tied to negative affect such as uncertainty and worries (Nordensvard, 2014).

Until now, psychologists, philosophers, theologians, and other scientists have not reached a consensus on the question of what hope really is (Miceli & Castelfranchi, 2010). Scioli (2020) pointed out that most theories of hope are either under-representations or over-definitions of the phenomenon under study. For example, Snyder's (1994) hope theory can be considered as being too limited in scope. This does not mean that the concepts of agency and pathways are wrong, but they are defining the concept and construct of hope too narrowly or, in some cases, even improperly. On the other hand, other theories tend to be too broad, including too many facets of hope, which describe several dimensions that in a certain context or situation might not be at the core of the concept and can but may not necessarily be present in every experience of hope (Bernardo, 2010; Scioli et al., 2011).

One major difficulty in psychological research on hope over the last decades has been the partial definition of hope based essentially on Western standards. Concerns were raised about hope theories that only focused on performance and self-mastery, overemphasizing individualism, neglecting the interpersonal and social aspects, and ignoring the quality of the many different targets and sources of hope (Scioli, 2020). Cognitive theories of hope, such as that of Stotland (1969) and Snyder (1994), conceptualize hope as an expectation of goal attainment with a high probability of success. Many authors consider that the individualist-cognitive goal-oriented approach reflects a cultural bias toward understanding hope as self-efficacy and outcome expectations. This makes hope very similar to other concepts describing positive future expectations, such as optimism, self-confidence, personal mastery, and perseverance in goal attainment, and does not capture the essential characteristics of hope (Aspinwall & Leaf, 2002; Braithwaite, 2004; Bruininks & Malle, 2005; Callina et al., 2018; Martin, 2011; Miceli & Castelfranchi, 2010; Scioli, 2020; Snow, 2019; Stitzlein, 2019; Tennen et al., 2002). Understanding hope as a high probability of achieving personal goals excludes the many other situations and possibilities of experiencing hope, with huge cultural and normative consequences of an oversimplifying individualistic bias (Scioli, 2020). By neglecting the interpersonal, societal, cultural, and normative dimensions of hope, psychological hope theories might have been promoting an egocentric conceptualization of well-being with no discussion about the quality and nature of hoped-for targets and ideals, which, according to several authors, could have serious undesired societal implications (Braithwaite, 2004; Te Riele, 2010; Webb, 2019).

While the constructs of will-power, personal mastery, and perseverance remain important to understanding hope, many authors are concerned because these aspects do not distinguish hope from other similar concepts. Moreover, hope does not always entail setting personal goals, and it is not always based on the efficacy of one's own capabilities. Most theories of hope highlight the fact that hope comes into play when the perceived probability of a wish or desire and the personal control are low (Bruininks & Malle, 2005; Meirav, 2008). Lazarus (1999), for example, argued that it would be wrong to equate hope with successful agency since people can also hope when they feel helpless. Hope is needed when people are confronted with the limits of their own capabilities and when future expectations are not positive anymore (McGeer, 2004; Shade, 2001). A sense of self-efficacy, competence, and control can facilitate the accomplishment of tasks and the achievement of goals, promoting hope, but they do not always encapsulate the essential elements of hope.

Surprisingly, for decades, psychologists have largely neglected the vast literature and empirical findings from other disciplines unraveling the distinct nature and the many facets and elements of hope. As Shweder et al. (2006) have underlined, it is problematic to take theories and measures developed in a certain cultural context or research discipline and uncritically consider them to be universal because they may include underlying assumptions that may not fit the general view of a certain concept. Therefore, we should avoid applying a certain theory of hope uncritically. A one-sided conceptualization of hope as a purely cognitive and individualistic phenomenon, without taking into consideration different cultural values and norms, while simultaneously ignoring alternative theories of hope (both in psychology and other disciplines such as philosophy, theology, sociology, education, and nursing research) has limited our psychological understanding of hope. What is required is a broad assessment of the nature of hope, including other disciplines, to provide a more balanced and differentiated view of hope.

Whereas several authors claim to have identified the central characteristics of hope, we have to be aware of the multiplicity of conceptualizations, dimensions, and elements, and acknowledge that each theory of hope captures something valuable about a particular aspect of its experience. The many conceptions of hope that have been developed by scientists from diverse disciplines can be seen as complementary and enriching. All these considerations reveal the necessity to integrate existing concepts and elements of hope from different research disciplines which each have highlighted a certain aspect or feature of hope in its own right (Callina et al., 2018). Because of its complexity and especially its relatedness to culture, hope research must be inter- and transdisciplinary, combining theories and research findings from psychology, philosophy, theology, and other disciplines into new concepts and models (Scioli, 2020). Our aim is thus to complement and enlarge the psychological conceptualization and research of hope and to test its different elements and dimensions through cross-cultural empirical studies.

1.3 The Cultural Perspective on Hope

Downey and Chang (2014) have noted that, in the field of positive psychology, hope and optimism have been studied in several countries, yet need to be further explored in order to be better understood within the context of culture. For Triandis (1997, p. 443), culture refers to a "shared set of beliefs, attitudes, norms, values, and behaviors organized around a central theme and found among speakers of one language, in one time period, and in one geographic region." This means that how people in different cultures think, feel, and act can differ in several ways (Suh et al., 2008). Culture influences the way we see ourselves, our own identity, and how we look at the world. It affects our fundamental understanding of the self and the meaning we give to our existence (Rasmussen & Lavish, 2014). Culture is a determinant of how we experience what happens in our lives and how we react to it (Teramoto Pedrotti & Edwards, 2014). The notion of the future and how people perceive the future is also shaped by culture (Kleist & Jansen, 2016). Further, culture affects, at least partially, what we judge as worthy and desirable and by doing so, what we might hope for, both for ourselves and for our environment. If people in a culture or region share some basic beliefs and values which are expressed through common practices that distinguish them from people in other cultures, it is to be assumed that hope could be experienced and would manifest itself differently in diverse cultures.

From a social constructionist perspective, hope is not only rooted in individual attributes but also in interpersonal discourses emerging from socialization and cultural characteristics (Averill et al., 1990; Averill & Sundararajan, 2005; Del Vecchio Good et al., 1990). Dominant and alternative worldviews about the conception and meaning of the world and a good life will affect people's desires and hopes as well as their ways of hoping. If hope is an existential phenomenon of our being-in-the-world (Billias, 2010), it always will be influenced by the larger frame of reference of the society and culture one is embedded in. Naderi Farsani and Abolghasemi (2008) proposed that beyond the universal predisposition to hope, culture is one of the most prominent variables in explaining and understanding what and how people hope. They further stated that people in different cultures with particular worldviews and belief systems will experience and manifest hope and the act of hoping differently. The authors argued that the phenomenon of hope and hoping is linked to meta-beliefs about what are valuable goals, about the nature of the world and existence in general, about the characteristics of human beings, and about standards of what is right and wrong behavior.

According to Webb, the many modes of hoping arise because "different individuals and social classes, at different historical junctures, embedded in different social relations, enjoying different opportunities and facing different constraints, will experience hope in different ways." (Webb, 2008, p. 25). From a cultural perspective, each society is characterized by a collective emotional orientation determining different modes of hoping, shaped by certain core ideas, social discourses, beliefs, myths, and collective memories at certain historical points, which are mediated by social institutions such as the education system, the media, art, etc. Different modes of hoping are based on different notions of the self and human agency, as well as particular orientations towards others and the world in general. Webb eloquently explained this by stating "that the characteristics of hope as a positive orientation toward an uncertain future good can vary immensely depending on the mode in which it is experienced. Thus, for example: hope can be active or passive; secure and trusting or restless and agitated; careful and realistic or ambitious and risky; resigned and accepting or passionate and critical; directed toward individual privatized goals or toward expansive social goals; directed toward a future that defies representation or a future given clear shape and form; apolitical or politically charged; a conservative force or a subversive one." (Webb, 2019, p. 131).

The different expressions of hope and modes of hoping can be distinguished based on what people hope for, on the sources of hope, on the cognitive-emotional processes and the activities people perform when hoping. The first question, often neglected by psychological hope theories, concerns the kind of hopes people embrace. During the past decades, two broader lines of research have evolved, focusing either on individual goals (e.g., health, academic or professional achievements, etc.), or on social goals (e.g., justice, sustainability, minority rights, etc.). Behind the numerous possible targets of hope, the fundamental question relates to what the hoping person considers to be worth hoping for, which includes a deeper sense of what a good life and a good society entails. The question that follows, is how people relate to these hopes emotionally, cognitively, and behaviorally. Moreover, hope is not only an individual mental and affective state but also a social and collective phenomenon.

One major issue that has scarcely been studied until now is to what extent hope can be characterized as a universal phenomenon across the world and to what extent different people in different cultures have diverse understandings and experiences of hope. Comparative studies have revealed that hope manifests and works differently across societies and social groups (Averill et al., 1990; Shin et al., 2013). People in different cultures might have particular conceptions of hope, adopt certain targets of hope as preferable or worthwhile and experience distinct sources of hope as valuable. However, some aspects and elements of hope might be similar across many cultures. Other aspects might be of special interest or value in some cultures but not in others. Individuals can differ in many elements and experiences of hope but share some universal patterns. Whereas some aspects of hope are more or less similar across cultures, other elements might be distinctive for a certain culture or region in a particular epoch of its history.

Until now, we know very little about how people in different cultures value and experience hope, what they hope for and what they do to support their hopes. All these concepts may be experienced differently in varied cultural contexts and thus cannot be researched or applied without consideration of the cultural environment. Therefore, we have to be aware of the cultural context in which hope is perceived, fostered, and expressed. For our research purposes and the studies reported in this book, we understand hope as a universal human phenomenon with culture and group-specific manifestations that make hope vary across nations. Especially the central dimensions of hope, e.g., the individual-cognitive, the socio-emotional, and the spiritual-religious, may vary from one culture to another. On the one hand, hope is part of our human core; on the other hand, the way it is experienced and how it manifests in certain moments, at a particular time, in the context of a specific culture or social group, emerges as the result of a process of social and cultural mediation (Webb, 2007).

1.4 The Hope Barometer International Research Program

The studies in this book on cross-cultural perspectives on hope are rooted in the discipline of Positive Psychology. Since its beginnings, researchers in Positive Psychology have been very attentive to studying the philosophical groundings of human virtues and character strengths (Peterson & Seligman, 2004), positive emotions (Fredrickson, 1998), and well-being (Ryan et al., 2013). Following this attitude and approach, the scope of the current book will be inter- and transdisciplinary since it attempts to integrate theories, conceptual models, methods, and empirical findings from several disciplines. We still know very little about the similarities and differences in the cultural factors and manifestations of hope. Therefore, to open the horizon to many aspects of human nature, we start by exploring and broadening our understanding of hope giving an overview of different philosophies and theories relevant to the cross-cultural study of hope. These are of interest since every concept and theory reflects and can be seen as an expression of certain cultural values and worldviews.

1.4.1 Defining and Studying Hope Across Cultures

The Hope Barometer is an annual international cross-sectional survey with the objective of contributing to the general understanding of hope through empirical studies from a cross-cultural perspective. The methodology of the Hope Barometer research program takes an inter- and transdisciplinary approach, drawing on scientific insights and research findings from the fields of philosophy, theology, psychology, futures studies, nursing research, and risk management. Our aim is to investigate areas of hope that have been scarcely researched until now. Therefore, before comparing hope across cultures, we first have to clarify the concept of hope, its elements and components and discuss the basic assumptions behind the current theories and research measures derived from them. We will discuss how scientists and researchers in psychology and other disciplines conceptualize and measure hope. We have to evaluate the theories of hope and their implicit assumptions in order to acquire a deeper and more differentiated understanding of this complex and multifaceted phenomenon. On this bases, we can develop an integrated model of hope that will serve as a guide for the empirical studies and the structure of this book.

There is still a vast need of empirical research and theory building in relation to the nature and experience of hope as well as its dimensions and sources. A main research goal is to understand how people hope, what people hope for, and what sources and conditions help people to maintain hope. It is our task as researchers to reflect on and investigate how hope manifests in different contexts and situations and which factors relate to a sense of hopefulness (Lazarus, 1999; McGeer, 2004). We want to open the horizon to acknowledge alternative conceptualizations of hope but, above all, to understand how people understand and experience hope for themselves, without imposing pre-established definitions. In order to understand how people experience hope in different contexts and situations, it has to be studied not only "top-down" but also from the "bottom-up" (Barilan, 2012; Shin et al., 2013).

We understand hope as a human universal that can be experienced and expressed in different ways (Webb, 2007). Thus, there will always exist a tension between being interested in studying cultural differences and at the same time trying to discover the universal features of hope. Consequently, our studies will have implications for the general theoretical understanding of the phenomenon of hope, the way we measure and assess hope as well as the detection of culture specific dimensions or variations of hope, in addition to universal characteristics or features across cultures. Our aim in this book is therefore twofold: On the one hand we want to achieve a better understanding of how people in different countries experience and express hope. People in different cultures might have distinct ways of thinking, feeling, and behaving in relation to what and how they hope. Beyond identifying the characteristics of individual cultures, it will be of value to recognize common patterns that might be relevant with regard to a better understanding of the basic conceptualization and nature of hope in general. The question is first and foremost about how people in different world regions and throughout different cultures experience the universal phenomenon of hope. On this basis, we want to discover which core values, assumptions, thoughts, attitudes, and behaviors contribute the most to cultivating a hopeful view of the future.

Based on the above-mentioned topics and issues, we can define a list of general research questions:

1. Is hope always and everywhere exclusively a cognitive and individual phenomenon, or are there also other dimensions such as the socio-emotional and the religious-spiritual domains of importance?
2. How do different concepts and measures of hope function in different countries? What and how do we have to measure in order to understand better the nature and quality of hope?
3. What are the differences between samples from different countries regarding the basic elements of hope? Has hope the same contents and meaning in different cultures?
4. How can differences in mean levels of hope across countries be explained? Why do people in different countries maintain higher or lower levels of hope?
5. Are there specific worldviews and values that nurture and support hope among people in different countries?

6. What are the most valued targets of hope for different people? How does culture affect the domains people might choose to hope for because they are especially important to them?
7. Which factors affect the way people hope? What are the main activities that people perform in order to fulfil their hopes? What are the most important sources of hope?
8. What are universal aspects of hope as well as unique elements that influence the way hope is perceived and experienced in diverse countries?
9. What are similar and what are culture specific correlates and predictors of hope in different countries?

1.4.2 Assessing Hope Across Cultures

A central question in hope research is how to assess hope across countries and cultures. When studying the phenomenon of hope, we have to clarify what and how to measure, since different methods will provide different kind of results. In this sense, one major challenge is how to operationalize the construct of hope to allow cross-cultural comparisons without biasing the research with our own values and theories. For example, Snyder's Dispositional Hope Scale (Snyder et al., 1991) taps into nearly the same concepts as Schwarzer and Jerusalem's (1995) Self-Efficacy Scale. Perceived self-efficacy has been defined as an optimistic self-belief that a person can perform difficult tasks, achieve goals or cope with adversity in various life domains. Similarly, to Snyder's hope concept, perceived self-efficacy is related to individual goal-setting, personal engagement, persistence in the face of obstacles and recovery from setbacks, and being considered as resilience and positive resource factor.

Another approach is to ask people about their subjective estimation of their level of hope in an unbiased and direct manner, without imposing a pre-defined understanding about what hope should be or entail. Levels of general hope can be compared across countries if we use a measure of hope that is neutral to the culturally tinted pre-conceptions and definitions researchers from different disciplines and world regions might have. For this, we needed a short, reliable, and comprehensive measure to capture hope as perceived by the people without imposing a certain theoretical concept or pre-defined dimensions. Such a measure should avoid as far as possible any individual bias and could then be connected it to many different elements, dimensions, and life domains. One important task in the Hope Barometer research program was, therefore, to develop the Perceived Hope Scale as a short measure for assessing hope in a direct and unbiased manner (Marujo et al., 2021; Krafft et al., 2019, 2020; Slezáčková et al., 2020).

One aim of the cross-cultural study of hope is to compare mean levels of hope across samples of different countries and to explore the main factors associated with their variance. A major issue for comparing mean values of samples from different nations was to assess the assumption of measurement invariance across languages and countries. The task is to evaluate whether the meaning of a construct such as hope and the way in which this construct is measured is the same across different groups (Chen, 2007). This was done in several studies with good psychometric results.

The results presented in this book show that throughout the investigated countries, there are significant differences between the levels of general hope related to one's personal life. The level of hope seems to be associated with a variety of individual, social and cultural factors. Diener et al. (2009) have proposed that in certain countries, such as in Latin America, people maintain cultural norms and values that result in a positive disposition towards life that is relative stable independently from concrete economic, political, or even individual situations. Some national differences in hope can be explained by these cultural factors influencing positivity through the fundamental tendency to see life and the future in positive terms.

Beyond the general measure of hopefulness in one's life, our aim is to investigate cross-cultural issues regarding the nature and expressions of hope by applying alternative measures to assess different elements of hope. Averill and his colleagues suggested that the experience of hope may differ with regard to the kind of targets a person may hope for and the kind of actions the person will perform to attain his/her hopes (Averill et al., 1990; Averill & Sundararajan, 2005). In order to explore the several elements of hope and inspired by the work of Averill et al. (1990) and Staats and Stassen (1985), three pools of items have been developed to assess (1) the targets of hope in the form of personal wishes, (2) the sources of hope people turn to or count on, and (3) the activities performed to attain the targets people hope-for (Krafft & Walker, 2018).

The targets of hope belong to things people wish or desire in different domains of their lives: Personal achievements, interpersonal relationships, materialistic targets, hedonistic pursuits, health-related outcomes, altruistic motives, and religious/spiritual experiences. The second instrument consists of hope sources from which people expect to obtain hope. A central question in this regard is whether hope is a purely individual trait or rather a social phenomenon. The items were formulated taking into consideration sources of hope from different domains: individual capabilities, social support, personal experiences, religious faith, etc. The purpose of the third instrument is to gain a better knowledge of what kind of actions people undertake to see their hopes fulfilled. Here again, the items belong to distinct domains of action: cognitive, social, religious, etc. In our studies, these three scales have been used to explore the nomological network of hope as perceived by people, relating them to the values and worldviews of hope, and comparing them with other concepts of hope.

Hope is a complex phenomenon that integrates cognition, emotions, values, and behavior. However, not every dimension of hope is equally relevant in all nations, cultures, or social groups. The question is, how do the experiences and contents of hope differ across nations? Do people put a different emphasis on some components of hope than on others? The importance of different dimensions of hope (cognitive, emotional, motivational, spiritual, etc.) may also vary across social groups. Close relationships are not only an asset that nurtures hope, but they could be a constitutive component of the very nature of what hope is, in terms of what people experience when they feel hopeful, of what people hope for, of the most important sources of hope and of the activities people perform to see their hopes fulfilled. The studies in this book disclose that there are many similarities but also significant differences across countries with respect to the targets of hope that are considered most desirable, as well as to the most appreciated sources of hope and the activities people perform in order to get their hopes fulfilled.

1.4.3 Values and Worldviews of Hope Across Cultures

Culture involves implicit or explicit assumptions about what is good and right, including certain common ideas, believes and values. If culture "can be thought of as a specific way to view the world based on a socially constructed set of beliefs, values, and norms" (Rasmussen & Lavish, 2014), then it will also affect the way we think and feel about the future. Worldviews and value orientations might be important when attempting to understand the nature and the elements of hope. Different dimensions, targets, and sources of hope can be related to cultural values and norms. For example, personal hopes might be guided by personal worldviews and values. The particular values dominant in one or more countries, such as tolerance, care, creativity, power, or performance, can have an influence on the types of hopes and on the sources of hope. Whereas in one context, personal goals and achievements are more valued, in another environment the emphasis could be more on positive relationships to other people. Some individuals rely on the social support of family members and close friends. Other persons ground their hope on their personal capabilities and experiences and still others on their faith in a transcendent Higher Power.

The nature and level of hope can differ along with different worldviews in terms of judgements attitudes about the nature and meaning of the world as well as in terms of images and judgements of oneself. The question is how cultural norms and values influence the phenomenon and experience of hope. A central question of the research presented in this book is therefore: How are values and worldviews related to people's hopes, to the sources of hope, and to people's activities to fulfill their hopes? By considering how personal and culturally accepted values and worldviews affect visions of the future, hopes and fears, we can develop a much richer and broader understanding of hope and by doing so open new fields of theory building and research.

1.4.4 Correlates and Predictors of Hope Across Cultures

If people in several nations differ with regard to their levels of hope, the question is which factors contribute to these differences and what are similarities and distinctive characteristics in the cultural dimensions related to hope. One important question in our studies is therefore related to the correlates and predictors of hope across different nations. The predictors of hope can vary across societies and groups, depending on salient norms and values. Some basic assumptions and values may correlate with general hope similarly in several countries. In other cases, the correlations between basic assumptions, values, personal hopes, and the general level of hope could be influenced by culture-specific norms. For example, there could be differences between individualist and collectivist countries. In some countries, factors such as self-efficacy, self-worth, and self-control might be stronger predictors of hope, while in other countries, social relationships could have a relatively higher weight. In some countries, religious and spiritual experiences and values will have a stronger connection with hope than in others.

Throughout the book, we want to assess which determinants of hope are rather universal and which are culture specific. With this, we can start to study the cultural aspects of how people in different countries experience and price hope in their lives. Several studies will report about the commonalities but also interesting differences between countries. One major finding is that there are several predictors of hope in common to most people but also significant differences of effect sizes across countries. For example, self-worth correlates positively with hope across all countries but with different intensity. Furthermore, the association between perceived hope and dispositional hope was more robust in some countries than in others. The factors that are more strongly related to hope will give us an indication of the nature and the different dimensions of the phenomenon.

1.5 Structure and Chapters of the Book

The book comprises ten chapters. The introductory Chap. 2 sets the theoretical and conceptual basis for the cross-cultural studies of hope presented in the following contributions. Chapters. 3, 4, 5, and 6 are dedicated to studying and evaluating the single elements of the hope concept at the individual and societal levels developed in the theoretical chapter. The studies include and compare data from several countries of the Hope Barometer research network and aim to find commonalities and differences between cultures. Chapters 7 and 8 aim to deepen these findings by relating hope to other well-being variables and comparing the results of selected countries with some similar and some individual characteristics concerning historical and cultural backgrounds. Chapter 9 contains studies reporting on how people in several countries coped with stress during the COVID-19 pandemic, putting a particular emphasis on the role and nature of hope and personal growth. The concluding

Chap. 10 summarizes, integrates, and discusses the findings of the previous contributions in a comprehensive way and derives new topics and questions for further research on hope from a cross-cultural perspective.

Chapter 2 is dedicated to laying the grounds for the empirical cross-cultural research program of the Hope Barometer, providing the individual elements and the structure for the studies presented in the book. The chapter starts by giving a brief overview of some of the most relevant theories on hope in psychology, philosophy, and theology integrating them into six main dimensions of hope as cognition, as affect, as agency, as a social phenomenon, as a virtue, and from a religious perspective. Based on the similarities and complementary views of the different conceptualizations of hope, a basic culture-sensitive transdisciplinary concept of hope is presented. The definition of hope in this book seeks to explain the universal features of hope that allows integration of singular dimensions and cultural manifestations as needed. Throughout this book, we understand hope as composed of a wish or desire for a relevant outcome coupled with the belief that its realization is possible (although not necessarily probable or likely) together with the trust in the availability of internal or external resources to make it happen. All three domains are directed and related to different levels such as the individual, the closer social environment, the broader social context, up to the world, and the natural environment at large.

Chapter 3 on "Values and Targets of Hope" presents the empirical study related to the first element of the hope concept described in Chap. 2. The first domain of hope addresses the wishes and desires as well as the fundamental values directed to certain goals or state of affairs. The central elements in this hope domain are the targets of hope. What people hope for is generally connected to their values and interests, to their normative judgements, to what they consider to be desirable for a good life for themselves and for their closer environment. Based on data collected with the Hope Barometer in November 2018 ($N = 5832$) in German- and French-speaking Switzerland, Spain, Portugal, and the Czech Republic, the study analyzes the commonalities and possible cultural differences in the levels of perceived hope, in individual hope targets, and in the effects of particular human value orientations on hope. The findings indicate that hope is not determined by the wealth of a nation (e.g., in terms of GDP) but by personal and collective characteristics, to a certain extent influenced by basic human values. Beyond common features across cultures, this study reveals subtle cultural differences worth to be further investigated in future studies.

In Chap. 4 entitled "Long-term Future Expectations and Collective Hope", a further facet of the wish/desire domain of the general hope concept is explored. The purpose of the chapter is to draw attention to the phenomenon of collective hope defined as the shared desire for a better future not only for oneself, but for the entire social community, with the belief that a better future for all is possible but not necessarily guaranteed or even likely, and the trust in the human capacity to cooperate and support each other towards the realization of a better world despite current struggles and challenges. In this chapter, the authors combine Positive Psychology with the discipline of humanistic Futures Studies. The interdisciplinary approach was termed "Positive Futures". The main purpose is to combine individual future prospects with visions of the good life in a better world and thus to support people in developing a more fundamental hope for happiness and fulfillment. The empirical study with data collected in November 2019 analyzes the subjective expectations of long-term social trends as well as the likelihood and desirability of global scenarios in 12 countries (Australia, Colombia, Czechia, India, Israel, Italy, Nigeria, Poland, Portugal, South Africa, Spain, and Switzerland, $N = 10{,}665$). In today's society, two almost opposite phenomena seem to shape people's lives. On the one hand, a general lack of perspective becomes apparent with regard to social and global developments. We live in a time in which most people, especially in Europe, assume that the future will be worse than the present. On the other hand, most people are rather optimistic with regard to their own future. Positive and negative outlooks in personal and global areas can have an effect on one's own social well-being, characterized by an assessment of the society in which one lives and by one's own role within that society. Thinking about alternative and desired futures can offer people new sources of purpose, meaning, and orientation in life. Images of a better world can give them inspiration and hope. For this, they first need a realistic picture of the good life and of a better world as well as long-term visions for the individual and for society at large.

Chapter 5 on "Worldviews and Basic Beliefs of Hope" concentrates on the second domain of the hope concept, which is the belief in the possibility of fulfillment of a valued wish or desire. According to the widely accepted philosophical notion backed by empirical evidence from psychological studies, hope is distinct from optimism in such a way that the hoping person must believe in an even slight possibility of the attainment of a certain wish, whereas to be optimistic it has to be retained as rather or highly probable. The belief in the possibility or not of the desired outcome is largely of subjective nature and will depend on individual and collective worldviews and beliefs. These beliefs serve as theories to anticipate the future and guide the way people interpret new experiences, especially when a person is confronted with a stressful situation or the feeling of despair. Based on data collected in 2017 in German- and French-speaking Switzerland, Germany, Israel, South Africa, Poland, and Czechia ($N = 6548$), the study in this chapter analyzes the basic assumptions and worldviews of people concerning their perception of the world as good or bad, the meaningfulness of the world, beliefs about oneself, religious faith as well as the pro-social attitude of helping others and correlates them with the general level of perceived hope. Beyond universal patterns, the study supports the idea that certain basic beliefs have distinct effects on perceived hope in different countries and that people in several cultural contexts sustain and perceive hope in different ways.

Chapter 6 on "Trust, Social Support and Hope Resources" deals with the third domain of the hope concept, focusing on forms and expressions of trust related to personal, social, and other resources that encourage people to believe in the realization of the hoped-for outcomes. Following insights from Risk Management the chapter makes the basic distinction between trust and confidence. Trust is a relational phenomenon characterized by uncertainty and vulnerability, supported by shared values such as benevolence, integrity, fairness, and caring. On the other hand, confidence is a reason-based subjective assessment of high probability expectations, which fits the concept of optimism. Self-confidence embraces the belief in individual achievements, persistence, resilience, self-awareness, knowledge, experience, and personal success, all attributes closely related to the definition of dispositional hope. Two studies analyze the multiple sources and activities of hope in different countries using data collected in 2018 and 2019. Study one comprises 12 countries—Australia, Colombia, Czechia, India, Israel, Italy, Nigeria, Poland, Portugal, South Africa, Spain, and Switzerland (N = 10,193)—and aims to analyze several personal and external hope sources with a specific focus on social support, religiosity, and the feeling of luck in relation to hope. Study two was performed with eight samples from seven countries—German- and French-speaking Switzerland, France, Spain, Portugal, Czechia, Poland, and South Africa (N = 6245)—centering on the assessment of several hope activities and their effects on perceived hope. The findings highlight the importance of external factors of hope, demonstrate the differential nature of perceived and dispositional hope, and show significant differences between countries.

Chapter 7 entitled"Hope and mental health among Czech and Polish adults in a macrosocial perspective and religiosity context" presents the outcomes of the empirical study exploring the role of hope in the context of depression and anxiety, positive mental health, and loneliness. It also focuses on exploring the age- and religion-related differences between the respondents from the two Central European countries, which both underwent a significant socio-political change in the late 1980s, share similar cultures and languages, but they significantly differ in other areas such as religiosity. The sample consisted of 526 Czech and 481 Polish adults who completed the Hope Barometer questionnaire. The results showed that both samples demonstrated similar patterns in predictors of positive mental health. However, significant differences were observed in positive and negative indicators of mental health. The obtained results are discussed within a broader framework of life experiences on the micro- and macro-level in the context of Central European countries that recently underwent macrosocial transitions.

Chapter 8 "Hope and flourishing": A cross-cultural examination between Spanish and South African samples" explores the commonalities and differences in hope between a Spanish (N = 206) and South African (N = 100) sample based on data collected with the Hope Barometer in November 2018. The chapter further investigates similarities and differences in the sources of hope between the two samples, as reflected in the activities that people engage in to fulfil their hopes and to attain the hoped-for targets (hope activities). The authors also examine these activities as predictors of hope. Finally, they explore the role of sociodemographic indicators as predictors of hope and flourishing. The results indicated that South African participants had higher levels of hope than the Spanish sample. There were also differences and commonalities in terms of endorsement of specific hope activities. These findings highlight the need to conduct more cross-cultural research on hope and pave the way for further cross-cultural understanding of this important human resource.

Chapter 9 "Mastering the COVID-19 Pandemic Crisis—From Anxiety to Hope" addresses the question of how people in different countries perceived and dealt with the COVID-19 pandemic crisis. The studies in this chapter report selected results of the Hope Barometer survey during the pandemic years of 2020 and 2021, analyzing and comparing data from Australia, Czechia, France, India, Italy, Nigeria, Poland, Portugal, South Africa, Spain, and Switzerland. Relating to cross-sectional data collected in November 2019 ($N = 9092$), November 2020 ($N = 9536$), and November 2021 ($N = 9093$), the central aim of the studies is to investigate the culture-specific choices of different coping styles as well as the perception of stress, hope (as the counterpart of anxiety), well-being, and personal growth. The findings highlight the importance of trust in other people as well as in a transcendent Higher Power for solving existing problems, overcoming concrete difficulties, and, by doing so, mastering the crisis successfully, which is predominant in collectivistic societies.

Chapter 10, "Beacons of Hope in a Challenging World", serves to conclude the findings reported across the various chapters and to highlight salient aspects thereof. It further provides an example of implementation of the proposed hope model in an educational context. Finally, we propose a future research agenda and suggestions for practice.

References

Aspinwall, L. G., & Leaf, S. L. (2002). In search of the unique aspects of hope: Pinning our hopes on positive emotions, future-oriented thinking, hard times, and other people. *Psychological Inquiry, 13*(4), 276–288.

Averill, J. R., Catlin, G., & Chon, K. K. (1990). *Rules of hope: Recent research in psychology*. Springer.

Averill, J. R., & Sundararajan, L. (2005). Hope as rhetoric: Cultural narratives of wishing and coping. In J. Eliott (Ed.), *Interdisciplinary perspectives on hope* (pp. 133–165). Nova Science.

Barilan, Y. M. (2012). From hope in palliative care to hope as a virtue and a life skill. *Philosophy, Psychiatry, & Psychology, 19*(3), 165–181.

Beck, A. T., Brown, G., Berchick, R. J., Stewart, B. L., & Steer, R. A. (1990). Relationship between hopelessness and ultimate suicide: A replication with psychiatric patients. *American Journal of Psychiatry, 147*, 190–195. https://doi.org/10.1176/foc.4.2.291

Benzein, E., Norberg, A., & Saveman, B. I. (2001). The meaning of the lived experience of hope in patients with cancer in palliative home care. *Palliative Medicine, 15*(2), 117–126. https://doi.org/10.1191/026921601675617254

Bernardo, A. B. I. (2010). Extending hope theory: Internal and external locus of trait hope. *Personality and Individual Differences, 49*, 944–949. https://doi.org/10.1016/j.paid.2010.07.036

Billias, N. (2010). Hope as a moral virtue. In J. McDonald & A. M. Stephenson (Eds.), *The resilience of hope* (pp. 17–27). Brill Rodopi. https://doi.org/10.1163/9789042030237_003

Bloch, E. (1959). *The principle of Hope* (N. Plaice, S. Plaice, P. Knight, Trans., 3 volumes), The MIT Press.

Blöser, C. (2019). Hope as an irreducible concept. *Ratio, 32*(3), 205–214. https://doi.org/10.1111/rati.12236

Blöser, C. (2020). Enlightenment views of hope. In S. van den Heuvel (Ed.), *Historical and multidisciplinary perspectives on hope* (pp. 61–76). Springer. https://doi.org/10.1007/978-3-030-46489-9_4

Blöser, C., & Stahl, T. (2017). Hope. In E. Zalta (Ed.), *Stanford Encyclopedia of Philosophy. Online version.*

Braithwaite, V. (2004). The hope process and social inclusion. *The Annals of the American Academy of Political and Social Science, 592*(1), 128–151. https://doi.org/10.1177/0002716203262096

Bruininks, P., & Malle, B. F. (2005). Distinguishing hope from optimism and related affective states. *Motivation and Emotion, 29*(4), 324–352. https://doi.org/10.1007/s11031-006-9010-4

Callina, K. S., Snow, N., & Murray, E. D. (2018). The history of philosophical and psychological perspectives on hope: Toward defining hope for the science of positive human development. In M. W. Gallagher & S. J. Lopez (Eds.), *The Oxford handbook of hope* (pp. 9–26).

Chen, F. F. (2007). Sensitivity of goodness of fit indexes to lack of measurement invariance. *Structural Equation Modeling: A Multidisciplinary Journal, 14*(3), 464–504. https://doi.org/10.1080/10705510701301834

David, D., Montgomery, G. H., Stan, R., DiLorenzo, T., & Erblich, J. (2004). Discrimination between hopes and expectancies for nonvolitional outcomes: Psychological phenomenon or artifact? *Personality and Individual Differences, 36*(8), 1945–1952. https://doi.org/10.1016/j.paid.2003.08.013

Del Vecchio Good, M. J., Good, B. J., Schaffer, C., & Lind, S. E. (1990). American oncology and the discourse on hope. *Culture, Medicine and Psychiatry, 14*(1), 59–79. https://doi.org/10.1007/BF00046704

Diener, E., Diener, M., & Diener, C. (2009). Factors predicting the subjective well-being of nations. In E. Diener (Ed.), *Culture and well-being* (pp. 43–70). Springer. https://doi.org/10.1007/978-90-481-2352-0_3

Downey, C. A., & Chang, E. C. (2014). History of cultural context in positive psychology: We finally come to the start of the journey. In J. Teramoto Pedrotti & L. M. Edwards (Eds.), *Perspectives on the intersection of multiculturalism and positive psychology* (pp. 3–16). Springer. https://doi.org/10.1007/978-94-017-8654-6_1

Dufault, K., & Martocchio, B. C. (1985). Hope: Its spheres and dimensions. *The Nursing Clinics of North America, 20*(2), 379–391.

Eckersley, R. (2002). Future visions, social realities, and private lives: Young people and their personal well-being. In J. Gidley, N. Ingwersen, & S. Inayatullah (Eds.), *Youth futures: Comparative research and transformative visions* (pp. 31–42). Greenwood Publishing Group.

Eliott, J. A. (2005). What have we done with hope? A brief history. In J. Eliott (Ed.), *Interdisciplinary perspectives on hope* (pp. 3–45). Nova Science.

Eliott, J., & Olver, I. N. (2002). The discursive properties of "hope": A qualitative analysis of cancer patients' speech. *Qualitative Health Research, 12*(2), 173–193. https://doi.org/10.1177/104973230201200204

Eliott, J. A., & Olver, I. N. (2007). Hope and hoping in the talk of dying cancer patients. *Social Science and Medicine, 64*(1), 138–149. https://doi.org/10.1016/j.socscimed.2006.08.029

Eliott, J. A., & Olver, I. N. (2009). Hope, life, and death: A qualitative analysis of dying cancer patients' talk about hope. *Death Studies, 33*(7), 609–638. https://doi.org/10.1080/07481180903011982

Erikson, E. H. (1959). *Identity and the life cycle: Selected papers*. International Universities Press.

Feudtner, C. (2005). Hope and the prospects of healing at the end of life. *Journal of Alternative & Complementary Medicine, 11*(Supplement 1), 23–30. https://doi.org/10.1089/acm.2005.11.s-23

Fredrickson, B. L. (1998). What good are positive emotions? *Review of General Psychology, 2*(3), 300–318. https://doi.org/10.1037/1089-2680.2.3.300

Fredrickson, B. L. (2004). The broaden-and-build theory of positive emotions. *Philosophical Transactions-Royal Society of London Series B Biological Sciences, 359*(1449), 1367–1378. https://doi.org/10.1098/rstb.2004.1512

Green, R. M. (2019). *Theories of hope—Exploring alternative affective dimensions of human experience*. Lexington Books.

Havel, V. (1989). *Letters to Olga*. (Paul Wilson, Trans.). Henry Holt.

Herth, K. (2005). State of the science of hope in nursing practice: Hope, the nurse, and the patient. In J. A. Eliott (Ed.), *Interdisciplinary perspectives on hope* (pp. 169–211). Nova Science Publishers.

Hicks, D. (2012). The future only arrives when things look dangerous: Reflections on futures education in the UK. *Futures, 44*(1), 4–13. https://doi.org/10.1016/j.futures.2011.08.002

Kleist, N., & Jansen, S. (2016). Introduction: Hope over time—Crisis, immobility and future-making. *History and Anthropology, 27*(4), 373–392. https://doi.org/10.1080/02757206.2016.1207636

Krafft, A. M., Guse, T., & Maree, D. (2020). Distinguishing perceived hope and dispositional optimism: Theoretical foundations and empirical findings beyond future expectancies and cognition. *Journal of Well-Being Assessment, 4*(3), 217–243. https://doi.org/10.1007/s41543-020-00030-4

Krafft, A. M., Martin-Krumm, C., & Fenouillet, F. (2019). Adaptation, further elaboration, and validation of a scale to measure hope as perceived by people: Discriminant value and predictive utility vis-à-vis dispositional hope. *Assessment, 26*(8), 1594–1609. https://doi.org/10.1177/1073191117700724

Krafft, A. M., & Walker, A. M. (2018). Exploring the concept and experience of Hope–Theoretical and methodological foundations. In A. Krafft, P. Perrig-Chiello, & A. Walker (Eds.), *Hope for a good life* (pp. 3–19). Springer. https://doi.org/10.1007/978-3-319-78470-0_1

Lazarus, R. S. (1999). Hope: An emotion and a vital coping resource against despair. *Social Research, 66*(2), 653–678.

Marcel, G. (1951). *Homo Viator: Introduction to a metaphysic of hope*. St. Augustine's Press.

Marques, S. C., Lopez, S. J., & Pais-Ribeiro, J. L. (2011). Building hope for the future: A program to foster strengths in middle-school students. *Journal of Happiness Studies, 12*(1), 139–152. https://doi.org/10.1007/s10902-009-9180-3

Martin, A. M. (2011). Hopes and dreams. *Philosophy and Phenomenological Research, 83*(1), 148–173. https://doi.org/10.1111/j.1933-1592.2010.00422.x

Marujo, H. Á., Velez, M. J., Gonçalves, S. P., Neto, L. M., Krafft, A. M., & Casais, M. (2021). The value of hope: Validation of the perceived hope scale in the Portuguese population. *Current Psychology*, 1–9. https://doi.org/10.1007/s12144-021-02115-6

McCormick, M. S. (2017). Rational hope. *Philosophical Explorations, 20*(supp 1), 127–141. https://doi.org/10.1080/13869795.2017.1287298

McGeer, V. (2004). The art of good hope. *The Annals of the American Academy of Political and Social Science, 592*(1), 100–127. https://doi.org/10.1177/0002716203261781

Meirav, A. (2008). Distinguishing between hope and despair. In W. Bauman (Ed.), *Hope: Global interdisciplinary perspectives* (pp. 11–16). Inter-Disciplinary Press.

Miceli, M., & Castelfranchi, C. (2010). Hope: The power of wish and possibility. *Theory & Psychology, 20*(2), 251–276. https://doi.org/10.1177/0959354309354393

Milona, M. (2019). Finding hope. *Canadian Journal of Philosophy, 49*(5), 710–729.

Milona, M. (2020). Philosophy of hope. In S. van den Heuvel (Ed.), *Historical and multidisciplinary perspectives on Hope* (pp. 99–116). Springer. https://doi.org/10.1007/978-3-030-46489-9_6

Naderi Farsani, S., & Abolghasemi, M. J. (2008). An investigation on the possibility of mutual understanding in a pluralistic world. In W. Bauman (Ed.), *Hope: Global interdisciplinary perspectives, Papers presented at the 3rd global conference Hope: Probing the boundaries* (pp. 111–130). Inter-Disciplinary Press.

Nordensvard, J. (2014). Dystopia and disutopia: Hope and hopelessness in German pupils' future narratives. *Journal of Educational Change, 15*(4), 443–465. https://doi.org/10.1007/s10833-014-9237-x

Peterson, C., & Seligman, M. E. (2004). *Character strengths and virtues: A handbook and classification*. Oxford University Press.

Pinsent, A. (2020). Hope as a virtue in the middle ages. In S. van den Heuvel (Ed.), *Historical and multidisciplinary perspectives on hope* (pp. 47–60). Springer. https://doi.org/10.1007/978-3-030-46489-9_3

Rasmussen, H. N., & Lavish, L. (2014). Broad definitions of culture in the field of multicultural psychology. In J. Teramoto Pedrotti & L. M. Edwards (Eds.), *Perspectives on the intersection of multiculturalism and positive psychology* (pp. 17–30). Springer. https://doi.org/10.1007/978-94-017-8654-6_2

Ryan, R. M., Huta, V., & Deci, E. L. (2013). Living well: A self-determination theory perspective on eudaimonia. In A. Delle Fave (Ed.), *The exploration of happiness: Present and future perspectives* (pp. 117–139). Springer. https://doi.org/10.1007/s10902-006-9023-4

Schwarzer, R., & Jerusalem, M. (1995). Generalized self-efficacy scale. In J. Weinman, S. Wright, & M. Johnston (Eds.), *Measures in health psychology: A user's portfolio. Causal and control beliefs* (pp. 35–37). NFER-Nelson.

Scioli, A. (2020). The psychology of hope: A diagnostic and prescriptive account. In S. van den Heuvel (Ed.), *Historical and multidisciplinary perspectives on hope* (pp. 137–163). Springer. https://doi.org/10.1007/978-3-030-46489-9_8

Scioli, A., & Biller, H. (2009). *Hope in the age of anxiety*. Oxford University Press.

Scioli, A., Ricci, M., Nyugen, T., & Scioli, E. R. (2011). Hope: Its nature and measurement. *Psychology of Religion and Spirituality, 3*(2), 78–97. https://doi.org/10.1037/a0020903

Shade, P. (2001). *Habits of hope–a pragmatic theory*. Vanderbilt University Press.

Shin, S. H., De Pretto, L., & Simpson, A. (2013). What does hope mean to people? The lay construct of Hope under achievement-oriented settings in Australia, Italy and South Korea. In G. Karabin (Ed.), *Hope in all directions* (pp. 197–212). Brill Publishers. https://doi.org/10.1163/9781848882591_018

Shweder, R. A., Goodnow, J. J., Hatano, G., LeVine, R. A., Markus, H. R., & Miller, P. J. (2006). The cultural psychology of development: One mind, many mentalities. In R. Lerner (Ed.), *Handbook of child psychology: Theoretical models and human development* (Vol. 1, pp. 716–792). Wiley.

Slezáčková, A., Prošek, T., Malatincová, T., & Krafft, A. M. (2020). Psychometrické vlastnosti české verze Škály prožívané naděje: faktorová struktura a vnitřní konzistence. *Československá psychologie/Czechoslovak Psychology, 64*(3), 288–305.

Snow, N. (2019). Is hope a moral virtue? In C. Blöser & T. Stahl (Eds.), *The moral psychology of hope* (pp. 171–187). Rowman & Littlefield.

Snyder, C. R. (1994). *The psychology of hope: You can get there from here*. Simon & Schuster.

Snyder, C. R., Harris, C., Anderson, J. R., Holleran, S. A., Irving, L. M., Sigmon, S. T., & Harney, P. (1991). The will and the ways: Development and validation of an individual-differences measure of hope. *Journal of Personality and Social Psychology, 60*(4), 570–585. https://doi.org/10.1037/0022-3514.60.4.570

Staats, S. R., & Stassen, M. A. (1985). Hope: An affective cognition. *Social Indicators Research, 17*(3), 235–242. https://doi.org/10.1007/BF00319312

Stitzlein, S. (2019). Pragmatist hope. In C. Blöser & T. Stahl (Eds.), *The moral psychology of hope* (pp. 93–112). Rowman & Littlefield.

Stotland, E. (1969). *The psychology of hope*. Jossey-Bass.

Suh, E. M., Diener, E. D., & Updegraff, J. A. (2008). From culture to priming conditions: Self-construal influences on life satisfaction judgments. *Journal of Cross-Cultural Psychology, 39*(1), 3–15. https://doi.org/10.1177/0022022107311769

Te Riele, K. (2010). Philosophy of hope: Concepts and applications for working with marginalized youth. *Journal of Youth Studies, 13*(1), 35–46. https://doi.org/10.1080/13676260903173496

Tennen, H., Affleck, G., & Tennen, R. (2002). Clipped feathers: The theory and measurement of hope. *Psychological Inquiry, 13*(4), 311–317.

Teramoto Pedrotti, J., & Edwards, L. M. (2014). Introduction. In J. T. Pedrotti & L. M. Edwards (Eds.), *Perspectives on the intersection of multiculturalism and positive psychology* (pp. xv–xviii). Springer.

Triandis, H. C. (1997). Cross-cultural perspectives on personality. In R. Hogan, J. Johnson, & S. Briggs (Eds.), *Handbook of personality psychology* (pp. 439–464). Academic Press.

Webb, D. (2007). Modes of hoping. *History of the Human Sciences, 20*(3), 65–83. https://doi.org/10.1177/0952695107079335

Webb, D. (2008). Modes of hoping and the utopian impulse. In W. Bauman (Ed.), *Hope: Global interdisciplinary perspectives* (pp. 25–38). Inter-Disciplinary Press.

Webb, D. (2019). Education and the construction of Hope. In R. Green (Ed.), *Theories of Hope: Exploring alternative affective dimensions of human experience* (pp. 131–153). Rowman & Littlefield.

Andreas Krafft holds a doctoral degree in Management Sciences at the University of St. Gallen (Switzerland) with special focus on Organizational Psychology, Culture and Development. He has academic specializations in Social Psychology of Organizations, Work and Health Psychology as well as Positive Psychology from the University of Zürich. Andreas is associate researcher for Futures Studies and lecturer at the Institute of Systemic Management and Public Governance at the University of St. Gallen. Furthermore, he teaches at the University of Zürich in the field of Work and Health, at the Master of Applied Positive Psychology at the University of Lisbon, Portugal, as well as at the Master of Futures Studies from the Free University Berlin. He is co-president of swissfuture, the Swiss Society for Futures Studies, member of the executive board of SWIPPA (the Swiss Positive Psychology Association) and of the DACH-PP (German speaking Association of Positive Psychology). Since many years he leads the International Research Network of the Hope Barometer.

Tharina Guse is a counselling psychologist and obtained an MA (Counselling Psychology) degree from the Potchefstroom University (now North-West University) in 1989. She was in full-time private practice for the next 15 years providing psychotherapy for children, adolescents and adults. In 2003 she obtained her PhD (Psychology) from Potchefstroom University. She returned to academia in 2005 and joined the University of Johannesburg. Since April 2018 she is a professor and Head of the Department of Psychology at the University of Pretoria. Currently she serves on the Professional Board for Psychology of the Health Professions Council of South Africa (HPCSA). She is also President of the recently founded South African Positive Psychology Association (SAPPA). Her research focuses are on positive psychology in general and in particular on psycho-social well-being, positive psychology interventions and psychological strengths such as hope and gratitude. Closely aligned with this broad focus she also conducts research on the application of hypnosis for the promotion of mental health and well-being.

Alena Slezackova, Ph.D., is an Associate Professor of Psychology and a Vice Head of the Dept. of Psychology and Psychosomatics, Faculty of Medicine, Masaryk University, in Brno, Czech Republic. Her scientific interests include mainly hope, mental health, and well-being. She also has a special interest in the research and practice of mindfulness. Alena is a founder and director of the Czech Positive Psychology Centre (CPPC), a member of the Advisory Council of the International Positive Psychology Association (IPPA), and a member of the Executive Board of the European Network for Positive Psychology (ENPP). She has been a member of several international research projects, and she serves on the editorial boards of five academic psychological journals. Alena is the author of the first comprehensive monograph on positive psychology in the Czech language and dozens of scientific publications in positive psychology and health psychology.

Chapter 2
Theoretical Foundations and a Transdisciplinary Concept of Hope

Andreas M. Krafft, Tharina Guse, and Alena Slezackova

Abstract The current chapter has the primary purpose of laying the theoretical grounds on which the cross-cultural empirical research program of the Hope Barometer between 2017 and 2021 was developed and executed. The two main goals of this chapter correspond to the inter- and transdisciplinary methodology applied in our work. The first goal is to give a brief interdisciplinary overview of psychological, philosophical, and theological theories presenting different perspectives from which the existential phenomenon of hope has been studied. Following previous research, hope will be examined along six general dimensions, which highlight the nature of hope as cognition, as affect, as behavior, as a social phenomenon, as a virtue, and from a religious perspective. Based on the similarities and complementary views of these different conceptualizations of hope, a basic transdisciplinary concept or model of hope will be presented. The proposed concept should do justice to the essence of hope, taking into account the diversity of situations in which people might hope and being sensitive to different cultural backgrounds. Our conceptualization of hope contains three fundamental elements, which are (1) a wish or desire for a valuable good, (2) the belief that the realization of this wish is possible but uncertain or even unlikely, and (3) the trust in the availability of current or future internal and external resources which can facilitate the fulfillment of the hoped-for good in the face of obstacles and setbacks. We understand wish, belief, and trust as the universal elements in the process of hoping. In concrete situations and different cultural contexts, these three elements can assume different forms and characteristics related to those mentioned above cognitive, affective, behavioral, social, religious, and

A. M. Krafft (✉)
Institute of Systemic Management and Public Governance, University of St. Gallen, St. Gallen, Switzerland
e-mail: andreas.krafft@unisg.ch

T. Guse
Department of Psychology, University of Pretoria, Pretoria, South Africa

A. Slezackova
Department of Medical Psychology and Psychosomatics, Faculty of Medicine, Masaryk University, Brno, Czech Republic

A. M. Krafft et al. (eds.), *Hope across cultures*, Cross-Cultural Advancements in Positive Psychology 14, https://doi.org/10.1007/978-3-031-24412-4_2

value dimensions. The singular elements and dimensions serve as the core research domains, which will be elaborated on in detail in the following chapters of the book.

2.1 Introduction

During the past decades, hope research has evolved in many different and sometimes opposite directions. In a very fundamental way, current hope theories can be traced back to basic philosophical and theological works rooted in specific cultural, religious, and scientific paradigms or worldviews (Eliott, 2005; Kleist & Jansen, 2016). Different theories emerged, conceptualizing hope either as a cognitive process (Snyder, 2002; Stotland, 1969), as an emotion (Lazarus, 1999; Nussbaum, 2019; Stockdale, 2019), or as a virtue (Barilan, 2012a; Billias, 2010; Kadlac, 2015; Moellendorf, 2006; Snow, 2013, 2018, 2019b). Two major paradigms are called "agency" and "receptivity" theories of hope. Receptivity theories maintain that hope is instilled from sources external to the individual, e.g., from a transcendent Higher Power, and then empowers the hoping person (Lear, 2006; Marcel, 1951). On the other hand, agency theories can be divided into two strands: the individualistic (Snyder, 2002) and the interpersonal approaches (McGeer, 2004). Other theories of hope are centered on social relationships and highlight the collective character of hope (Braithwaite, 2004; Cobb & Green, 2017). In healthcare studies, supportive relationships with family and peers have been recognized as the most important factors in sustaining hope in patients (Olsman, 2020; Stockdale, 2019). Several authors have highlighted the multidimensional character of hope, integrating cognitive, emotional, relational, behavioral, existential, and transcendent elements in its definition (Dufault & Martocchio, 1985; Farran et al., 1995; Scioli & Biller, 2009).

Contemporary philosophers have found a first common ground for the conceptualization of hope. The so-called standard account or orthodox definition of hope ascertains that hope involves at least two basic elements: (1) A wish or desire for a valued good or outcome (we only hope for what is important to us); and (2) The belief that the realization of what we desire is possible but not certain (Day, 1969; Meirav, 2009). Furthermore, there is a (more or less) common understanding among contemporary hope philosophers that these two fundamental elements of the standard definition (desire and possibility) can be considered as necessary but not sufficient conditions to explain the phenomenon of hope (Downie, 1963). Two persons in the same situation (for example, two patients diagnosed with cancer) could hold a certain desire (to be cured) and could believe that there is little possibility of occurrence (e.g., if the cure prognoses are about 20%), but whereas one of them can remain hopeful, the second capitulates and gives up hope (Martin, 2013). This example shows that, at least in critical cases, some additional factor is necessary to help distinguish the hopeful attitude of the first person from the defeated stance of the other.

Several authors have proposed different explanations giving account for this missing factor: The "license" to act or incorporation argument (Martin, 2013), the cognitive resolve process (Pettit, 2004), the energy of mental imaging (Bovens, 1999), the external factor account (Meirav, 2009), and in numerous cases an attitude of fundamental or substantial trust (Braithwaite, 2004; Erikson, 1959; McGeer, 2008; Tennen et al., 2002). Each of these concepts has provided a valuable contribution for a better understanding of the multifaceted phenomenon of hope and will be presented in the coming sections of this chapter.

It is further relevant to distinguish between the general disposition or attitude of hopefulness, on the one hand, and singular hopes directed towards particular ends in concrete situations, on the other (Calhoun, 2018; Dufault & Martocchio, 1985; Shade, 2001). The general attitude of hope has been conceptualized as a character trait or virtuous disposition whose target is not a specific goal but the good life in general (Shade, 2001). Otherwise, particular hopes embrace certain wishes or desires focused on more or less concrete hoped-for ends. Calhoun (2018) has referred to the former as basal hopefulness and the latter as practical or intentional hope and conceptualized basal hope in terms of mood and intentional hope in terms of emotions. Whereas emotions are directed towards something, moods are a general orientation to the world. Therefore, basal hopefulness is a kind of hope in the present and for the present, which extends into the future (Snow, 2019a). From a theological point of view, Christian denominations, as well as Buddhist and Hinduist traditions, draw the fundamental distinction between ordinary, secular, or mundane hopes, which are characterized as passions, and transcendent, authentic, or radical hope, which is based on the will for the good and related to the Divine (Dunlap, 2019; Jeffrey, 2019; Krafft & Choubisa, 2018; Lear, 2006; Pinsent, 2020).

The present chapter has two primary objectives. The first aim is to give a succinct overview of the most dominant theories and concepts of hope in psychology, philosophy, and theology. The second aim is to present a conceptualization or model of hope that has guided the empirical research program of the Hope Barometer between 2017 and 2021. The essential elements of this conceptualization of hope integrate the psychological, philosophical, and theological theories in such a way that they can be applied to different kinds of situations and hopes, in different circumstances and in a culturally sensitive way. The singular elements of the hope model are briefly presented in this chapter and will be further elaborated on in the specific chapters of the book.

2.2 Basic Dimensions of Hope

To present the theoretical foundations not only in a multi- but also in an inter- and transdisciplinary manner, we decided to introduce the relevant psychological, philosophical, and theological theories relating them to six basic dimensions of hope, which are the cognitive, the affective, the behavioral, the social, the spiritual (religious or transcendental), and the existential (hope as a virtue).

2.2.1 The Cognitive Dimension of Hope

Theories related to the cognitive and rational dimension of hope can be traced back to philosophers in Ancient Greece, who were very ambivalent about hope. Remember Pandora's myth, where hope was brought to the earth in a jar together with all evils but remained at the bottom of the jar. Was hope the worse of all evils as Nietzsche interpreted it? Or is it there to relieve humanity from pain? For Plato and Aristotle, hope was seen as a passion of desire. In their eyes, hope generally lacked rational grounds and was, therefore, at least in part, considered to be blind, unreliable, and dangerous. Only such future expectations based on firm evidence, knowledge, and reason, in which case the hoped-for ends could be regarded as probable or likely and as an expression of confidence, were considered to be good hopes (Cairns, 2019; Gravlee, 2020). Because of its ambiguous nature, neither Plato nor Aristoteles considered hope explicitly as a human virtue. On the one hand, hope seems to contradict other virtues, such as courage and wisdom, because it leads people to be overconfident and pretentious, ignore the risks of an endeavor, and overlook concrete facts. However, on the other hand, hope is part of the act of deliberating about the future and a facet of high-mindedness. In this case, hope motivates and supports people to become more virtuous and to develop their own agency in order to live a flourishing human life (Gravlee, 2000).

Traditional psychological theories of hope (Snyder, 1994; Stotland, 1969) have been focused on individual goals, willpower, and personal capabilities to overcome obstacles. Similar to ancient Greeks, these theories view hope as a cognitive process based on concrete evidence, high probability estimations, and positive expectations of goal attainment. From this point of view, high-hope people are more optimistic, have the perception of control, display higher levels of self-esteem, rely on their own capabilities, and are more competitive. Low-hope people, instead, perceive a low likelihood of achieving their goals and have a higher sense of uncertainty (Snyder et al., 1998).

An alternative view on the cognitive character of hope has been developed by Pettit (2004), who differentiates between superficial and substantial hope. According to Pettit, substantial hope can be distinguished from superficial hope because it involves a cognitive resolve, which means that a hoping person will act as if the hoped-for end is likely to occur, even if the probability of its occurrence and the control a person can exert are perceived to be low. This argument is different from the cognitive approach in psychology, since it highlights how people can remain motivated to believe and act in situations of great uncertainty. Substantial hope, in Pettit's view, occurs when the hoping person considers that the likelihood of attaining a desired end is low. Especially in situations where the hoped-for ends are beyond the control of the individual, cognitive resolve is a self-motivating attitude that encourages those who otherwise would be low-hopers (Callina et al., 2018). This is by no means an act of self-deception, as the ancient Greeks or philosophers like Spinoza, Schopenhauer and Nietzsche would have interpreted it. It is an attitude, as Marcel (1951) described it, of believing beyond negative evidence. This holds not only for the individual but also for social and collective hopes. In the context of collective hope, cognitive resolve is the conviction that people who share common hopes will collaborate and be successful in their undertakings, despite discouraging evidence, but based on energizing desires and feelings and the belief and trust in others (Pettit, 2004).

2.2.2 *The Affective Dimension of Hope*

Philosophers in the seventeenth and eighteenth centuries like Descartes, Hobbes, and Hume considered hope to be a passion of the soul embracing desires and emotions that motivate people to act (Blöser, 2020). In its quality as a passion, hope leads to volition, and volition to motion, i.e., to a motivation to act in order to fulfill one's desires. Similarly, many modern philosophers conceptualized hope as an emotional stance or affective attitude related to specific desires, perceptions, and feelings that motivate the person who hopes to act (Bloch, 1959/1986; Calhoun, 2018; Ratcliffe, 2013; Walker, 2006).

According to Bloch (1959/1986), hope is the most human of all affects, since it is not entirely involuntary but emerges in combination with the capacity of anticipation of a potential future state. Bloch developed his Principle of Hope to counter Heidegger's phenomenological philosophy of worries and anxiety. For Heidegger, the essence of human existence as being-in-the-world was characterized by worries and the fundamental feeling or mood of anxiety. Bloch's Principle of Hope suggests that the same can be said for hope as the existential feeling of finding oneself in the world (Ratcliffe, 2013). In a similar way, Calhoun (2018) suggests that hope is a kind of meta-emotion in terms of a mood or general affective state she calls basal hope, which is critical for engaging oneself in the world. This kind of basal hope exists even in the absence of concrete hopes.

Hope seems especially indicated to be described with Nussbaum's (2003, 2004) concept of "eudaimonic judgment", because it addresses beliefs and evaluations involved in emotions related to things, people, and situations that we consider central to our (mutual) flourishing. Nussbaum has convincingly exposed that emotions are shaped by the evaluation of their objects in terms of beliefs and judgments related to their importance for our (and others') well-being. This means that beliefs are constituent parts of our emotions, integrating cognitive and affective elements. From this point of view, it can be deduced that hope is characterized as an emotional experience embracing beliefs about what we consider central to our well-being and the well-being of others (Nussbaum, 2019).

Fredrickson (1998, 2004) considers hope as one of the ten most frequently experienced positive emotions in daily life, which is especially relevant in challenging situations. The effect of hope, as a positive emotion, is that it broadens the mindset, nurturing psychological, social, and even physical resources to cope with adversity. A further effect of hope as a positive emotion is that it transforms the individual for the better. While certain emotions such as a good mood and pleasure nourish hedonic happiness, hope can be considered a part of the eudaimonic domain of flourishing and, therefore, as a virtue that is connected to inner personal growth, meaning in life, and the relationship with others (Cohn & Fredrickson, 2009). Because of this broadening and growth effect, hopeful people tend to display a more altruistic and generative behavior by helping others, taking a long-term view of things, instead of satisfying short-term needs, thinking beyond the struggles of the present moment, and adopting moral values such as friendship, gratitude, generativity, selflessness, kindness, and inclusiveness towards strangers (Cohn & Fredrickson, 2006).

When focusing on the affective quality of hope, we must recognize that feelings like anxiety and sadness that arise during dire experiences such as an illness or war are not at all incompatible with hope. Since uncertainty is a constitutive element of hope that causes anxiety, worry, and fear, these feelings are, to a greater or lesser degree, part of and at the same time the opposite of hope (Nussbaum, 2019; Stockdale, 2019). One can feel miserable about what is occurring in the world and still, or because of that, embrace a deep hope for betterment (Milona, 2019).

2.2.3 Agency and the Behavioral Dimension of Hope

Most psychologists and philosophers agree that hope is closely related to a fundamental sense of agency. However, many of them also recognize that our hopes exceed our capabilities as agents in several situations (McGeer, 2004; Pettit, 2004). According to Snyder's hope theory (1994, 2002), agency refers to the willpower and motivation needed to implement certain pathways in order to achieve personal goals. Willpower is related to the confidence in one's own abilities to achieve the things in life that seem important to oneself. Snyder speaks of agency as purposeful mental energy and determination, which are necessary to follow specific and sometimes novel pathways. Agential hope consists of the conviction "I can do this!" (Snyder, 2002, p. 251). Mental energy comes from the thought "I am not going to be stopped". This willpower is also of great importance when things do not go the way we want them to and when new ways have to be tried again and again with commitment, perseverance, and persistence. Closely related to agency is therefore the belief that when facing obstacles and setbacks, one will be able to find several ways to achieve one's goals, an attitude which is called pathways thinking. This can be understood as a kind of coping competence based on mental flexibility and creativity.

From a broader philosophical standpoint, several authors have proposed that Snyder's hope theory in reality describes concepts such as tenacity, perseverance, or self-confidence and that his theory could be called for example "theory of successful goal pursuit" instead of hope (Snow, 2019a, p. 8, see for similar arguments Aspinwall & Leaf, 2002; Callina et al., 2018; Scioli, 2020). An alternative perspective on agency, willpower, and the connection to hope has been proposed by McGeer (2004). According to her, good (responsive) hope must be distinguished from two detrimental forms of hoping she describes as wishful and willful hope. Wishful hope is derived from the commonly known concept of wishful thinking, which expresses a relatively passive, disengaged, and unrealistic form of hoping. Willful hope, on the other hand, expresses an over-reliance on the individual's own powers and capabilities. Willful hopers, as defined by McGeer, suffer from ego-anxiety solipsism, making them unreflective, self-deceived, and sometimes unscrupulous, showing little care for others who they mistreat as means to their ends. Basically, good hope must always be located, as Thomas Aquinas also stated, between the extremes of helplessness or despair and presumption (Pinsent, 2020). Good hope, as will be presented more in detail in the following sections, is a socially responsive hope that acknowledges the limitations of our individual agency and, at the same time, helps to scaffold the development of an interpersonal and collective sense of agency taking into account not only current capabilities but also future potentialities of oneself and others.

Similarly, several philosophers have developed a substantial conception of agency, personal identity, and selfhood in relation to hope (Blöser & Stahl, 2017b; Martin, 2013; McGeer, 2004; Shade, 2001). These authors distinguish between the "agentic" quality of hope and the idea of successful agency, which is not necessarily a characteristic feature of hope (Miceli & Castelfranchi, 2010). On the one hand, all our actions, everything we do, are consciously or unconsciously connected with the hope for success (Dalferth, 2016). Thus, hope is closely linked to our ability to act. It provides the practical reason for and is the impulse behind all purposive actions. For Martin (2013), to hope well is to embrace a desire and the belief in its possibility and to use this desire and this belief as justification for engaging in meaningful activities. Because we wish and believe, we act.

Moreover, the hope towards personal ideals and values plays a fundamental role in the construction of our sense of selfhood and practical identity, a conception that can be traced back to Kierkegaard's and also Marcel's philosophical works (Fremstedal, 2019; Blöser & Stahl, 2017b). When feeling hopeless and despaired, the person not only renounces his or her hopes but in a deeper sense, also gives up his/her own agency and selfhood. In order to keep one's own self and identity, a person needs to believe and hope for a better future. For Kierkegaard, this is ultimately possible when the person can believe and trust in a benevolent and omnipotent God and therefore believes that a better future is possible (Fremstedal, 2019). In a more secular form, Blöser and Stahl (2017b) argued that hoping in a fundamental way is constitutive to a person's practical identity, i.e., defining who the person is. For example, it is constitutive to our self-understanding as parents to hope for our children since we desire their well-being and are ready to help them in whatever way is possible. In order to be able to sustain this identity as (good) parents, it is necessary not to cease hoping for them (see also Nussbaum, 2019).

2.2.4 The Social Dimension of Hope and Agency

Several authors in psychology and philosophy went beyond the individualistic conception of agency and developed an interpersonal theory of agency and hope. From a developmental perspective, Erikson (1959) explained the very first emergence of hope in the infant's vulnerability and struggling between the feelings of basic anxiety and basic trust in the encounter with a caring person. According to Erikson, hope is the earliest and the most indispensable virtue of every human being, deeply anchored in trust, love, and care. At this first stage, hope is eminently emotional and relational and the fundament for the future development of willpower, purpose, competence, identity, social attachment, generativity, and wisdom. For McGeer (2004), the art of good hope consists of a "responsive hope" that, at its core, requires the social emotion of care. This kind of sound hope involves an emotional sensitivity that nurtures hopeful energy in the wake of difficulties and disappointments. Substantial hope displays an affective state or attitude towards others, enabling substantial trust in uncertain situations (McGeer, 2008).

In her conceptualization of hope and agency, McGeer (2004) proposes a social account of hope as a fundamental force in fostering and developing human agency. Besides being the driving force to act, hope arises when confronted with the limitations of our own agency (see also Shade, 2001). In this sense, "hope signifies our recognition that what we desire is beyond our current (or sole) capacity to bring about—and in the limiting case, it is beyond our capacity: "We hope for something that could not be in any way affected by our efforts to bring it about" (McGeer, 2004, p. 103). However, these limitations or the incapacity to act, must not mean at all, that we are giving up our agency. Precisely in such situations is where the power and energy of hope come to bear. From this perspective, "... hoping is a matter, not only of recognizing but also of actively engaging with our own current limitations in affecting the future we want to inhabit. It is, in other words, a way of actively confronting, exploring, and sometimes patiently biding our limitations as agents, rather than crumbling in the face of their reality." (2004, p. 104). Therefore, she suggests, "that hope is the energy and direction we are able to give, not just toward making the world as we want it to be but also toward the regulation and development of our own agency. [...] To hope well is thus to do more than focus on hoped-for ends; it is crucial to take a reflective and developmental stance toward our own capacities as agents—hence, it is to experience ourselves as agents of potential as well as agents in fact." (2004, p. 105). Therefore, in order to expand our agency, we must learn to hope, since the energy of hope infuses human agency. To be a hoping agent means orienting our attention and thoughts on our hopes, even when we feel unable to bring about our hoped-for ends.

But what is it that nourishes our hope when facing our limitations and, by doing so, helps us to expand and develop our agency? It is the care, trust, and hope other persons show towards us. Good hope, according to McGeer (2004), is therefore an emotional responsive and scaffolding hope. From this point of view, hope is both, an integral part of our agency and, in its essence, a social phenomenon. Our agency is by and large supported by others, who care for us, believe in us, and motivate us by supporting our hopes. At the same time, we have to be responsive to their care and support in order to be able to nurture our capacity to hope. This fundamental capacity to hope, even when influencing the hoped-for outcome is not possible, makes the agent feel stronger (McCormick, 2017). If we do this reciprocally, we can build a community of good and flourishing hopers, who jointly support their hopes, infuse the energy of substantial hope into each other and support one another in the development of one's own agency. At this point, the essential role of trust becomes evident. By trusting in the care and support of others and, at the same time, placing our hope and trust in them, we automatically extend our mutually intertwined agencies (Martin, 2019).

2.2.5 The Religious and Spiritual Dimension of Hope

Because of its existential and transcendental character, hope is, in one way or another, a central element in the many theological traditions. Already in the Jewish Torah and Psalms hope is directed toward something positive. For the Jewish people, the concept of hope is based on the understanding of Yahweh as savior and redeemer in times of need. The Jewish understanding of hope is characterized above all by faith and trust in God in challenging times. God, Yahweh, is the savior and helper and at the same time the goal of hope. In the Psalms, the believer is repeatedly affirmed that God, in spite of all suffering and hardships, means well with man, that He wants only the best for him, and he will always protect and support him (Bietenhard et al., 1989; Nebe & Goetzmann, 1997). On the one hand, hope refers to earthly existence and is based on the graces that people have received from God and have been recorded in the form of stories. This includes the hope for health, family, well-being, and peace, proven by the covenant with Noah after the Flood, the assurance of the Promised Land to Abraham and the liberation from Egyptian oppression. God defends his people against their enemies and lets manna rain down from heaven so that they do not starve.

On the other hand, Jewish hope refers to future salvation, to liberation from all the tribulations of life, to life after death, and to a new and just world of God through the coming of the promised Messiah (Bietenhard et al., 1989). Jewish hope is an imperative for the believer and is largely linked to patience. The believer is exhorted to hope. Especially in difficult times the believer is urged to wait patiently and persevere in the certainty that sooner or later the fulfillment of the promise and the eagerly awaited liberation will come. Although this enduring patience suggests a certain passivity, it is rather an active hoping in prayer.

In the Christian faith, hope is one of the three theological virtues, besides faith and charity. Whereas in Aristotelian philosophy virtues are acquired by practice and habituation, in Christian theology, virtues are infused by and received from God as a gift. This is because the theological virtues can only be rooted in God's love, benevolence, omnipotence, and grace (Pinsent, 2020). This means that in a supreme sense, we are not able to hope for ourselves but need the assistance of God. In the Christian tradition, hope is not directed to what is likely to occur but to what sometimes seems to be impossible but becomes possible in the eyes of the believer thanks to the grace and omnipotence of God (Jeffrey, 2019). Since for God everything is possible, to hope in this way is an absolute or fundamental hope, transcending any kind of facts, evidence, or reality. Especially in apparently hopeless situations the Judeo-Christian hope is a hope against all human hopelessness, i.e., where there is nothing more to be expected from a human point of view, the believer puts his faith and trust in God.

Moreover, to hope in the Christian sense is not only to be hopeful with regard to a certain wish or desire but also to hope for the right ends, which basically means to hope for more kindness, goodness, and ultimately for a reunion with God Himself (Jeffrey, 2019). Therefore, the three theological virtues of charity, faith, and hope are closely intertwined and must emerge as a unity. Someone can only hope properly when he/she has faith in God, believes in His unconditional and eternal love, and wants to do good. In so far as it is a hope in a benevolent God, hope is an eminently relational, interpersonal, and social phenomenon guided by the charity as an orientation and love for others (Elliot, 2020; Marcel, 1951). It is rationality and the capabilities of the individual that are at the forefront, but faith in God and trust, care, and harmonious social relationships with other persons.

The only requirement behind this fundamental hope lies in the human will to yearn for God and consequently to long for moral goodness (Elliot, 2020). In Christian terms, only this theological hope in and for God can finally be defined as virtuous (Blöser & Stahl, 2017a). At the same time, as Marcel (1951) manifested, it is this hope that guides the individual toward the fullness of his/her existence here on earth. According to Pieper, Christian hope combines the two virtues of magnanimity and humility: "Magnanimity directs this hope to its true possibilities; humility, with its gaze fixed on the infinite distance between man and God, reveals the limitations of these possibilities and preserves them from sham realization and for true realization." (Pieper, 1997, p. 102).

In a similar sense, Muslim hope is anchored in the belief in Allah and is the opposite of despair, which is the consequence of disbelief and atheism (Osmani, 2008). Hope in the Islamic tradition must also be grounded in the wish for good deeds. According to Laila (2008), Muslim hope has several dimensions, such as social justice, economic equality and financial security, political brotherhood, scientific reason/truth, and spiritual salvation.

In the Buddhist tradition, ordinary hopes rooted in earthly desires and material goods are the origin of all suffering and, therefore, the greatest obstacle to enlightenment. Buddhist hope, instead, aims to liberate oneself and others from suffering (McDonald, 2008). Dunlap (2019) proposes a Buddhist conception of hope focused on three fundamental values: Love for the present moment and Buddhist practice herein, feeling gratitude for everything that exists and expressing compassion for all beings.

Krafft and Choubisa (2018) elaborated on the concept of hope in the Indian psychology context. The Indian psychology roots go back to thousands of years of

Indian traditions, thoughts, Vedic texts such as the Upanishads and later Bhagavad Gita, and the practices of yoga and meditation (Rao & Paranjpe, 2016). Interpreters of the ancient scriptures presented two opposite kinds of hope, differentiated by the targets they are directed to: Materialistic and egoistic hopes are of ephemeral, illusive, and detrimental nature. Sublime hope, instead, aims to achieve liberation and self-realization. Therefore, in order to live a healthy, harmonious, happy, and fulfilling life, hope should be directed to existential aspects in life and have a transformative effect on the individual. The law of Karma (of cause and effect) compels us to hope for the good and never for something evil. Finally, the scope of hope is located at the individual and collective levels to lift the human race to a higher level of evolution.

Religiosity and spirituality have often been recognized as significant roots of hope, particularly in the face of illness, suffering, and death, (Del Vecchio Good et al., 1990; Dyson et al., 1997; Saleh & Brockopp, 2001; Knapp et al., 2011). Several studies have demonstrated the positive associations between religiosity, health, and hope (Galek et al., 2005; Lima et al., 2013; Matthews et al., 1999; Meireles et al., 2015; Schneider & Mannell, 2006; Taylor, 2003). A hope based on religious faith is relevant when the possibility of achieving a goal is low or seems impossible. Faith in God is the foundation for being able to hope for the best even in supposedly hopeless situations and against all (medical) expectations. In times when normal life is challenged, many people seek meaning and comfort in God or superior power. The connection to God and the belief in the unity of body, soul, and spirit gives the believer support and helps him to find new hope (Espinha & Lima, 2012; Hendricks-Ferguson, 2008). In secular terms, this kind of spiritual or religious hope can be related to the idea of "living in hope", instead of "hoping for something", focusing away from future-oriented hopes and centering on the meaning of life in the present (Benzein et al., 2001; Parker-Oliver, 2002). This kind of hope in the present for the present is oriented to the inner self and aims at living a fulfilling life in connection to other people and, for some people, to a transcendent higher power.

2.2.6 *Hope as a Virtue*

Because of its existential character and importance, several authors have conceptualized hope not as a theological and externally infused but as a secular virtue in the Aristotelian sense. Kadlac (2015) suggests that hope is a virtue because it (1) promotes a more realistic view of the future (other than optimism and pessimism), (2) encourages oneself to engage in the fulfillment of hoped-for ends, and (3) develops more solidarity towards others. Similarly, Snow (2013, 2018, 2019b) describes hope as a moral, intellectual, and civic virtue directed to a good life. Hope can be a moral virtue if a person hopes for moral ends and engage him/herself practically to attain them (Billias, 2010; Snow, 2019b). Therefore, to recognize if hope is a moral virtue, we have to evaluate the values, contents, and targets people hope for.

Furthermore, hope can also be an intellectual virtue (Snow, 2013). According to Zagzebski (1996, 2003), to be intellectually virtuous requires not only the capacity to acquire existing knowledge and discover the truth but to develop new forms of knowledge in an original and inventive way that will help the person to flourish. In Bloch's (1959/1986) terms, we can hope for things that do not exist yet but are a real future possibility we can (virtuously) believe in. In this respect, to hope virtuously is to be open to future possibilities beyond existing facts and knowledge. According to Kretz (2019), for example, humanity needs to develop moral imagination if it wants to transform ecological despair into hope for a sustainable future. In this sense, hope can also be a social, political, and civic virtue if it manifests itself as collective hope for a better and flourishing society (Cobb & Green, 2017; Moellendorf, 2006; Snow, 2018).

Common to all theological and philosophical conceptualizations is that hope is a virtue insofar as it promotes human (individual and social) flourishing, especially in challenging times when facing suffering, anxiety, and despair. For this reason, Peterson and Seligman (2004) included hope in their handbook and classification of character strengths common across cultures as belonging to the virtue of transcendence. For the initiators of positive psychology, hope belongs to the virtue of transcendence because it goes beyond one's own knowledge and coping capabilities and allows us to build connections to something bigger than ourselves that provides us with meaning, purpose, and basic beliefs. In their categorization, hope is linked to other character strengths such as gratitude, appreciation of beauty and excellence, humor, and spirituality. As a transcendent character strength, hope is related to values that provide a moral framework that keeps the person committed to the expectation and pursuit of goodness (Krafft & Walker, 2018).

2.3 Towards a Transdisciplinary and Culture Sensitive Concept of Hope

Backed by the existing psychological, philosophical, and theological theories of hope, we would now like to propose a transdisciplinary conceptualization of hope that contains its basic elements and, at the same time, avoids, as recommended by Scioli (2020), under- or over-conceptualizing the phenomena. These fundamental elements should address the essence of hope and, at the same time, be broad enough to be applied in as many situations as possible, at many different levels (individual, interpersonal and social/collective), and in different cultural contexts. We understand hope as composed of a wish or desire for a valued outcome or state of affairs together with the belief that its realization is possible (although uncertain and not necessarily likely) and the trust in the (existing or future) availability of some internal or external resources that could facilitate its realization, especially when confronting obstacles and setbacks. The willpower to act and persist is a consequence of the nature and importance of the desired good and the intensity of the belief and trust held by the person who hopes.

The three essential components of hope are, therefore:

1. A wish or desire, which could be the longing for a good life in general, or a certain state of affairs (peace), an event (that something happens), a circumstance (a happy family), or a goal (something that I want to achieve). Hope can but must not necessarily involve a concrete goal or personal achievement, for example, when people hope for peace or the well-being of other persons. However, wishes and desires express values for which people commit themselves (Blöser & Stahl, 2017b). Furthermore, values (as well as virtues) are infused with emotions (Erikson, 1959; Lazarus, 1999; Schwartz, 1994). To hope for something always includes a (conscious or unconscious) motive (the reason to hope), and every motive is related to some underlying emotion (Nussbaum, 2004; Zagzebski, 2008).
2. The belief in the possibility of its realization. Although the realization of the wish is uncertain, it must not be considered impossible. The second element in this basic definition of hope is the belief that the realization of the desired good is regarded as possible and, at the same time, uncertain and difficult. Neither an expected high probability of its fulfillment nor personal control over the hoped-for outcome are conditions for hope (Bruininks & Malle, 2005). The belief in the possibility of a particular outcome or state of affairs is largely of subjective nature and only in part (and sometimes not at all) determined by evidence.
3. The third element is trust in the existence or future availability of resources that can make hope happen. A fundamental prerequisite of trust is the uncertainty regarding the outcome and our own capabilities (Miceli & Castelfranchi, 2010). Trust can be focused on internal resources related to personal strengths, talents and capabilities or it can be related to external resources such as the trust in another person (family members, teachers, doctors, etc.), the trust in institutions (science, technology, the government) or the trust in a transcendental Higher Power.

This concept of hope has the advantage that it can be applied at two distinct levels of abstraction, which in the literature are known as the level of specific hopes and the level of general or fundamental hopefulness (Calhoun, 2018; Dufault & Martocchio, 1985; Godfrey, 1987; Shade, 2001): (1) Specific hopes are directed to concrete outcomes (goals, events, circumstances) connected with the belief in the possibility of their fulfillment and linked to particular resources for their realization; (2) Fundamental hope is usually oriented to a good life in general, it might be based on the overall belief in the goodness of the world and relies on a basic trust in one's own capabilities or some external power, fortune or fate. Figure 2.1 presents the elements of the hope concept in a graphical way.

In the following sections, we will further elaborate on these three basic elements of hope by connecting them to the different dimensions presented in the first part of

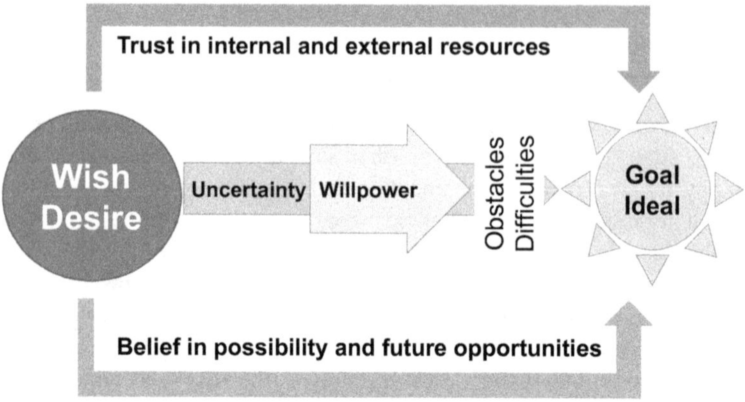

Fig. 2.1 Elements of the hope concept

this chapter and by additionally integrating the first reflections regarding cultural aspects, which will be explained more in detail in the following chapters of the book.

2.3.1 *Individual and Collective Wishes and Hoped-for Ends*

If the first element of hope is about one's wishes and desires, it must be related to what people value and what they want to happen because it is important to them. Different people in different circumstances may hope for different things: health, a good job, a happy family, fame, and so on (Burke, 2012; Shin et al., 2013). Shade (2001) described the process of hoping as the development and coordination of attitudes, activities, and habits in light of certain hoped-for ends. Since hope is a strong motivator for action, the first task must be to pay attention to the quality and value of the targets of hope. However, as we have already seen, some hopes can be achieved by our own efforts and other hopes are beyond our capabilities. One central question is how far the objects, targets, and state of affairs people hope for may influence the way people hope, the sources of hope people draw on, the actions people undertake, as well as the thoughts and feelings related to hope (Olsman, 2020).

In general terms, Chae (2019) speaks about "meaningful hope" when the aim of one's hope is of intrinsic value. We hope for something only when what we hope for has meaning and value for us. Individuals tend to grade their hopes according to their relative value, creating a rank order or hierarchy of hopes (Schwartz & Bardi, 2001; Shade, 2001). Therefore, the formulation of hoped-for ends and the conscious assessment of the desirability of certain hopes are of utmost importance (Shade, 2001). Sometimes, our more fervent hopes define the person we are or would like to be, becoming part of our identity and sense of self (Blöser & Stahl, 2017b). For Bovens (1999), hope has an intrinsic value through the epistemic capacity and energy of mental imaging, which is much more than just imagining a future state of affairs. In the mental anticipation of a future event, hope is associated with positive feelings and increases the knowledge of oneself and the world connected to our love for others and ourselves. Mental imaging also serves to develop guiding ideals in collective and utopian hopes. All this will engender new hopes, since "as I come to have such insights, I will set new constitutive hopes that I am more likely to realize because they are more in line with what I truly stand for, with my skills or with the limitations of my surroundings." (Bovens, 1999, p. 673).

These insights can lead to the general idea that hoping for certain things will probably affect how people in different circumstances and environments might hope (Averill et al., 1990). People can hold various types of hopes, such as material goods, personal achievements, hedonic pursuits, interpersonal relationships, and altruistic motives (Averill & Sundararajan, 2005), which might also have an effect on the quality of the general perception of hope. It might not be the same to hope for the achievement of a specific career goal, to hope for a happy partnership, or to hope for more religious and spiritual experiences.

Different dimensions and targets of hope can be related to culturally transmitted worldviews, values, and norms. Wong et al. (2006, p. 1) highlight that "in many important ways, cultures are the expressions of human nature in all its complexity and duality—fears and hopes, cravings and aspirations, selfishness and generosity, cruelty and compassion." Culture embraces implicit or explicit assumptions about what is good and right, including certain common ideas, wishes, and behaviors. If culture can be thought of as a specific way to view the world based on a socially constructed set of beliefs, values, and norms (Rasmussen & Lavish, 2014), then it will also affect how we think and feel about the future. The particular values dominant in one or more countries, such as tolerance, care, creativity, power, or performance, can influence the types of hopes people assume.

Therefore, people in different societies and cultures can coincide or differ with regard to what is most relevant to them in terms of personal desires, wishes, and targets of hope. Singelis et al. (1995), for example, distinguished between individualist and collectivist cultures based on the type of goals that people have. People in individualistic societies tend to hold and pursue more self-centered goals that reflect personal wishes, whereas people in more collectivist cultures are more inclined to cherish goals related to the desires and wishes of the family and a closer social environment, including good social relationships, to be in harmony with their environment and to support others (Triandis, 1997). In one case, the focus is on the accomplishment of one's own wishes and desires, personal success, and on novel experiences. Goals have to be achieved by one's own efforts. In the other case, people appreciate tolerance, respect, and care for others. Common projects and endeavors are more valued than the own wishes and goals and individual performance (Eid & Diener, 2009).

One recurrent topic in philosophy and theology is whether people hope for the right ends. In his book Principle of Hope, Bloch (1959/1986) urges us not only to hope well but above all, to be attentive to hope for the right things. To hope well, people should pay special attention to the quality of their wishes and desires. One common concern in ancient Greek as well as in Christian, Buddhist, and Hinduist concepts, is that virtuous hope must be guided towards a morally good end, which must be the direction in which our desires and actions should be oriented (Gravlee, 2020). Hope can be a moral virtue if one hopes for morally worthy ends which help people and communities to flourish (Snow, 2019b).

One central question is what should be considered a good and flourishing human life? Most religious traditions distinguish between two kinds of hopes, the theological or spiritual hope and the mundane or earthly hope (Jeffrey, 2019). Whereas mundane hopes are motivated by pleasures and worldly desires, authentic hope is the aspiration of expecting and doing good and hoping not only for oneself but also for others (Elliot, 2020; Fremstedal, 2019; Marcel, 1951; Michener, 2020). As far as earthly hopes like wealth, status, power, and pleasures are detached from theological hope, they represent human passions or appetites that can lead men in the wrong direction [probably the willful mode of hoping in McGeer's, 2004 terms], away from the supreme good of eternal happiness. The nature of theological hope is interpersonal, social, and transcendental rather than directed to concrete objects. Aristotle holds a similar standpoint when he recommends not to invest oneself in hedonic pleasures but to live a eudaimonic life, which means a virtuous life according to one's good spirit. However, earthly hopes, although of secondary nature, can be aligned with the supreme hope (Pinsent, 2020).

For example, the ultimate purpose of Christian and Muslim hope is guided by the desire of personal union with God. The theologically virtuous hope should be focused on goods and ends that, through charity and love, brings the individual, the community, and humanity closer to redemption and salvation. Human flourishing can best take place within a community of hopers that believe in a benevolent and almighty God and support each other with generosity and kindness (Pinsent, 2020). Ultimately, theological hope is about wishing, believing, and trusting that good will triumph over evil and that individual and social happiness will overrule suffering (Lerner, 2019). Earthly endeavors and goods should always be oriented towards this supreme aim.

A similar, although more secular, standpoint concerning hope is represented by pragmatist philosophy and meliorism (Stitzlein, 2019). According to pragmatist philosophers, hope should be motivated by the desire to improve the world together. Collective hope is based on shared visions for a desired social change and the commitment to shared values and goals a community of people endorses and engages for because they believe in the possibility of their realization (Braithwaite, 2004). The rationality of idealistic hopes lies in the motivation, attention, and feelings they release toward socio-political ends (Milona, 2019). Our ideals for a better world should guide our actions (Rorty, 1999).

2.3.2 Basic, Cultural, and Collective Beliefs

The second domain of the hope concept presented here refers to the belief in the possibility of fulfilling a meaningful wish or desire. In the classical cognitive psychological theories, we hope when we believe, based on experience or evidence, that what we desire is likely to occur (Snyder, 1994; Stotland, 1969). Furthermore, hope is rooted in the belief in one's own capabilities to overcome obstacles and setbacks. However, according to widely accepted philosophical concepts supported by empirical evidence from psychological studies, hope is distinct from future expectations in the sense that hope is related to the belief in an even small possibility of the attainment of a certain wish, whereas optimism retains it as highly probable (Bruininks & Malle, 2005; Krafft et al., 2021; Milona, 2020a, 2020b; Scioli et al., 1997). For Pettit (2004), substantial hope is characterized by the belief in the possibility of the attainment of the desired outcome with a low level of confidence.

One proposed difference between hope and future expectations refers to the idea that whereas future expectancies (on which the concepts of dispositional optimism and dispositional hope are based) are grounded on rational considerations, the perception of hope is basically related to personal beliefs and worldviews (Leung et al., 2009). However, a recurrent question is whether hope can be distinguished from wishful thinking based on how justified or unjustified these underlying beliefs are. Wishful thinking, has been argued, occurs when a person desires something that he or she regards as possible but in reality it must be deemed impossible (Milona, 2019). Since the attribution made in terms of possible/impossible is primarily a subjective judgement, the question is whether a clear distinction between true and false beliefs and, therefore, between hope and wishful thinking is possible (Martin, 2011). Consider, for example, Barack Obama as a little boy having the dream of one day becoming president of the United States: Would this dream at that time be classified as hope or wishful thinking? Hundred years ago, most people would have considered the possibility of traveling to the moon impossible. In past epochs, the abolishment of slavery, the equality of rights for men and women or the marriage of homosexual couples must have been contemplated as impossible. Today they are, or at least are becoming, a reality in many countries. Most of us would deem recovery from a so-called incurable disease impossible, although affected people who believed in that possibility were already healed (Hamilton, 2008; Spiro, 1998).

In order to hope, it is relevant to believe in the possibility of its realization, independently of this belief is justified or not. The belief in the possibility of a certain event is not based on evidence and objective facts, but it is mainly of subjective nature. This means that, as philosophers and psychologists already know, beliefs can be justified by the quality of their underlying emotions and values (Nussbaum, 2003, 2004; Stockdale, 2019; Walker, 2006). This entails that to hope and, therefore, to believe for a certain outcome, can be meaningful based on the emotions and values that bring this hope about (McDonald, 2008). Hope can have a practical and sometimes even a life-sustaining value for an individual or group of individuals, beyond the question of whether a particular belief is correct or appropriate or not

(McCormick, 2017). As we have already seen, hope exists when the belief in the possibility of a certain good is taken as a license or right to engage oneself in whatever mental (e.g., patient waiting) or practical (e.g., performance of tasks) deeds are possible (Martin, 2013). In order to sustain our practical identity and selfhood, we sometimes are compelled to believe in our dreams and wishes (Blöser & Stahl, 2017a, 2017b). The same urge appears when hoping for a loved person's well-being, healing, success, or flourishing (Marcel, 1951).

Since the future does not exist and we cannot have knowledge about the future, it is basically a domain of beliefs (Slaughter, 1993). Hope is always linked to uncertainty, which gives the reason to believe that the future is always open to new possibilities (Bloch, 1959/1986). To hope is to be open to the future and to believe how things could be instead of how they currently are. As Fromm (1968) once said, hope requires the belief in the yet-unproven. This belief enables the emergence of transformative hope, which, according to Webb (2013, 2019), is not about collecting evidence but about developing a utopian vision of the future supported by the belief in the socially instilled human capacity to improve the world by changing the status quo. To hold a belief that permits the individual to hope despite negative evidence is neither a sign of self-deception nor an illusion or delusion of how things seem to be. Radical hope, according to Lear (2006), is rooted in the belief that, especially in times of trials, the future will hold new possibilities which we are not able to imagine or think about yet.

According to Meirav (2008, 2009), in order to understand the true nature of hope, we must recognize that hope is always related to some external factor beyond our own resources or agency. The external factor account comprises the belief that the hoped-for good is possible but uncertain and arduous and not entirely within one's control (Miceli & Castelfranchi, 2010). This external factor can be another person or group of individuals, like our own family, it could be related to social institutions such as the government or employers, but it can also be the belief in fate, luck, or a transcendent higher power. What is central is that, to be hope-sustaining, the external factor must be conceived as being in favor of one's values, interests and wishes. "If one views the external factor as good, then one hopes for the prospect: "If one views it as not good, then one despairs for it" (Meirav, 2009, p. 230). Hope is rational and appropriate as far as one believes in the goodness of the external factor. It is important to point out that to believe and rely on external forces is not necessarily a sign of passivity, disengagement, or wishful thinking, but can be experienced as expanding and empowering one's own agency, commitment, and willingness to act (Shade, 2001).

According to Janoff-Bulman (1989, 1992), people maintain basic unquestioned beliefs about themselves and the world. In a broader sense, beliefs are constitutive elements of worldviews, i.e., assumptions about the nature, quality, and meaningfulness of what and how the world is, why it is as it is and how it should be. These basic beliefs are theories or narratives that guide our thoughts, emotions, and behaviors, especially in anticipating or expecting what will happen in the future (Janoff-Bulman, 1989, 1992). Basic beliefs also serve as theories to anticipate the future and guide the way people interpret new situations (Kelly, 1955). These worldviews are especially important when a person is confronted with a stressful situation or the experience of despair. For example, basic beliefs concern the quality and basic character of human nature as good or evil and of the world as just or unjust (Lerner, 1980). Hope is therefore very much influenced by basic beliefs, assumptions and attitudes that guide our perceptions about the world and ourselves as well as our behavior (Clifton et al., 2019; Ibrahim, 1984; Janoff-Bulman, 1992; Koltko-Rivera, 2004).

From a cultural perspective, individual and social hopes emerge through shared beliefs, which at a specific time and place in history are constitutive of collective worldviews (Naderi & Abolghasemi, 2008). Cultural beliefs about how things are and how they could and should be, are constituent of the individual's perception and volition (Miller, 1999). For example, people in Western cultures tend to believe in the importance of personal responsibility, control, and merit. In other, more collectivistic cultures, a meaningful world is one governed by social relationships or religious beliefs (Robitschek et al., 2014; Triandis, 1997). The quality and role of these basic cultural beliefs can greatly impact the quality and the sources of individual and collective hope.

For example, returning to the ancient Greeks, people in those times believed in a cyclical repetition of painful events and in the prevalence of suffering without the possibility of progress. The (bad) fortune of men and women depended on factors beyond the control of the individual, mainly because they believed in capricious, unpredictable, and sometimes even cruel gods and goddesses (Blöser & Stahl, 2019; Gravlee, 2020).Within such a belief system, future expectations were mainly bleak. The future was considered a matter of irreversible fate instead of human will, and individual hopes were conceived as foolish and harmful illusions (Cairns, 2019; Miceli & Castelfranchi, 2010).

To the contrary, in the Christian and Muslim traditions, hope is considered a Divine gift. Hope is grounded in the belief of God's / Allah's absolute goodness and power (Lerner, 2019; Miceli & Castelfranchi, 2010). This means that hope is always hope in God. For Marcel (1951) our existence is entrenched in a spiritual order in which the most important thing is to build a bond of love with other people. In Islam, accordingly, true hope can only be rooted in the belief in Allah and in His mercy and forgiveness. In this sense, religious hope is a hope rooted in what we cannot know or see and therefore we must believe in (Jeffrey, 2019). Remarkably, when to believe takes the quality of religious faith, the uncertainty attached to hope converts into certainty. Therefore, faith is the assurance of things hoped for because everything good comes from God's power and mercy (Pinsent, 2020).

Nevertheless, this does not mean that religious hope is a passive hope. The faith in God conveys the belief that the individual is entitled, empowered, and assisted by God to do whatever is necessary in order to achieve the hoped-for good. To do so is a matter of our power of will (Elliot, 2020). For Moltmann (2021) (like for Kant), humanity has the mission to work for the promised world by changing our own lives as well as the existing circumstances on earth for the better. From a Muslim perspective, hope becomes a trait when the believer expresses his or her faith in Allah not only in thoughts and words but especially in deeds of kindness, helpfulness, and compassion (Osmani, 2008). However, this is only possible with God's support. In the Buddhist and Hinduist tradition, people believe that liberation and enlightenment must be acquired by one's own efforts, discipline, and practice (e.g., meditation), but that this path is open and achievable if based on gratitude, compassion, and detachment from superfluous earthly desires (Dunlap, 2019; McDonald, 2008).

From a secular point of view, pragmatist hope is anchored in the conviction that it is justified to believe in life's benevolence and that through joint efforts we may constantly make the world a better place (Blöser & Stahl, 2017a). Rorty (1982) claims that hope for a better world does not require any foundation at all, that certain hopes may even be unjustifiable, and that to be able to hope we do not need a rational argument. The only thing we need is the belief in the possibility that "unnecessary human suffering can be decreased, and human happiness thereby increased" (Rorty, 2002, p. 154). As Rorty says, hope is "the ability to believe that the future will be unspecifiably different from, and unspecifiably freer than, the past" (Rorty, 1999, p. 120) which is the condition for social progress. Collective hope is not only characterized by shared ideals and visions but also by common beliefs in a brighter future and in the power of collective action and mutual care. From the point of view of ecological hope, Northcott (2020) urges us to believe in the restoration capacity of nature so that we also can assume that our endeavors to protect the natural environment are not in vain.

These examples also show that beliefs and desires can influence each other. The meaning, value, and importance of a certain desire will influence the belief or even conviction that this desire is at least possible. There seems to exist a reciprocal influence between belief and desire: If one believes that the fulfillment of an important wish is possible, one desires it even more fervently, and vice-versa, the importance of a desire can affect the belief in its possibility (Milona, 2019). On the contrary, the belief in the impossibility or difficulty of a wish or desire might steer the individual to a passive attitude towards it or even fully renounce it. The belief in the impossibility of the desired outcome produces apathy, frustration, and even depression (Beck et al., 1990; Farran et al., 1995). What seems important to emphasize is that the emotional state of hopelessness can be transformed, on the one hand, by underscoring the importance of the wished-for end and, on the other hand, by changing the beliefs, evaluations, and judgements of the individual. Sometimes it is only a matter of reframing the problem and looking at it from another perspective.

In sum, hope is significantly associated with the belief in one's dignity and self-worth but beyond that with the belief in the benevolence of the world and of people in general. Some people might believe mainly in what they can see, in evidence and hard facts. Other people believe in external forces they cannot explain, such as luck and fortune. Hope is connected with the propensity the person has to believe in the goodness of the world, in a positive future, in favorable development of life in general, in the social support one receives and in the appreciation of one's own capabilities. People with different worldviews and beliefs may hope differently. People in individualistic cultures may hope differently than people in collectivistic cultures. Higher levels of hopefulness might sometimes be rooted in the belief in one's capabilities and in some cases in the belief in a benevolent higher power. Religious and spiritual individuals may hope differently than people indifferent or distant to religious beliefs and practices.

2.3.3 Trust and Sources of Hope

We have seen that hope comprises a wish or desire and the belief in the possibility of its realization but that these two elements are not sufficient to explain the phenomenon of hope and that a third factor is still needed to understand why people in uncertain situations adopt either a hopeful or a hopeless attitude. Most authors agree that hope does not coincide with positive expectations about a probable outcome and that a constitutive element of hope is uncertainty, both about the realization of the hoped-for end as well as the own self-efficacy (Miceli & Castelfranchi, 2010). Therefore, hope and negative expectations can coexist and do not contradict each other (David et al., 2004, 2006; Leung et al., 2009; Montgomery et al., 2003). But then, what gives people the power to believe in healing, despite an unfavorable prognosis? What strengthens the belief in a positive outcome despite all negative evidence? Some authors focus on people's own capabilities (Snyder, 1994), others refer to the importance of social support from family members or close friends (Scioli & Biller, 2009), still others highlight the faith in a benevolent higher power (Scioli, 2007) to whom one can revert when facing critical life situations.

Based on Erikson's (1959) and Marcel's (1951) original works, many authors recommended including trust as a unique and distinctive element of hope. They proposed a relational approach to hope, which recognizes that hope is rooted in relationships of trust between individuals (Barilan, 2012b; Braithwaite, 2004; Callina et al., 2018; Cobb & Green, 2017; Godfrey, 1987; Kadlac, 2015; Martin, 2019; McCormick, 2017; McGeer, 2004; Olsman, 2020; Rorty, 1999; Shade, 2001; Tennen et al., 2002). According to these authors, human flourishing takes place within a community of people who hope and act collectively for a common future. Through trusting relationships to other people, we can extend our agencies and produce a better future together. This is what collective hope is all about.

Therefore, the third element in our conceptualization of hope focuses on forms and expressions of trust related to resources that encourage people to believe in the realization of the hoped-for outcomes in circumstances of uncertainty. Trust is the ability to transcend current conditions and courageously be open to new and unknown social and technological solutions. In hoping, we experience the world as open to its possibilities and its development and trust the power of our others' actions (Webb, 2007, 2008). To trust is to see the future as a realm of new possibilities. We trust our children, for example, not because of their current abilities and behaviors but due to their potential to learn and grow (McGeer, 2008). We not only believe that they will be capable of solving their problems, but also trust that they will do so. Fundamental or radical hope is about trusting that the unexpected, things we cannot foresee but wish and believe in, can occur (Lear, 2006).

Again, two extreme positions can be traced back to the ancient Greek and the Christian philosophical traditions, which had an immense impact on the culture and people of their times. In the Greek philosophy "elpis" had different connotations but basically denoted the prediction or anticipation of a future state of affairs. Due to the unreliable nature of the gods and goddesses, most philosophers considered elpis as irrational optimism and haughty self-confidence (Cairns, 2019). Ignoring hard facts and lack of experience makes people hope for the better, which in reality is nothing other than wishful thinking (Blöser & Stahl, 2017a). This lack of trust in the grounds and conditions for a better future was adopted by philosophers of the twentieth century like Schopenhauer (1918/2010) and Nietzsche (1885/2006), who believed in the impossibility of progress to overcome evil and pain on earth.

Precisely the opposite is represented by the Christian virtue of hope, which is anchored in the faith and trust in a benevolent God as the elementary source of hope. Christian hope is not based on knowledge but on faith in those things we do not see and do not understand. Through faith in God, hope escapes the realm of fear and despair related to uncertainty and adopts the quality of certainty and conviction that only can be explained by God's love and mercy (van Vliet, 2020). Based on this faith in God, Christian hope evolves and expands into interpersonal trust in other human beings (Jeffrey, 2019; Marcel, 1951). The opposite of hope is not only despair, a lack of faith in God, but also the presumption of trusting only oneself rather than relating to and trusting other people and God (Pinsent, 2020).

To trust others is, as Marcel (1951) pointed out, to be open to the other. In Heidegger's (1953/2010) philosophy, man is thrown back on himself in a world that is inhospitable for him. In contrast to Heidegger, for Marcel human existence is not embedded in a threatening world, but rather in a personal community of concrete relationships with other people. For Marcel, the question is how man can break through loneliness in a technocratic and materialistic world and regain meaning to lead a happy and fulfilling life. This hope is an interpersonal and self-transcendent phenomenon. Marcel sees the very essence of existence and hope in the relationship with other people and contrasts this with a philosophy of fear and despair. True hope must be directed towards someone else to escape the temptation to destroy oneself in despair. In a living relationship with someone else the suffering and desperate person ceases to be an object, he or she becomes a subject and is thus restored to his or her being and dignity. Hope at its best is not only a hope for me but a hope for something that unites us. It presupposes that we share life. Therefore, for Marcel, every fundamental "I hope" is in fact an "I hope for you". At the same time, hope is essentially for-us, i.e., hope for all members of our community. The resulting formula of true hope is "I hope in thee for us".

At the bottom of the interpersonal and social account of hope is a relational understanding of the self. Whereas people in individualistic cultures see the self as an isolated entity, people in collectivistic cultures view the self mainly in relation to others. According to Triandis (1997), the interdependent (relational) conceptualization of the self is characterized by the conviction that the self cannot be separated from others or from the social context. In individualistic cultures, on the contrary, the individual is defined by an independent self in search of self-actualization. Trust in the face of uncertainty implies a sense of vulnerability when hoping. The recognition and acceptance of our own vulnerability and the conviction that human flourishing is only possible within a community of people who care for each other is what makes solidarity a vital element of hope (Kadlac, 2015). When we trust, we expose ourselves to the possibility of being disappointed.

In Erikson's developmental psychology, hope is the first human virtue that must be developed in early childhood out of the tension between existential fear and fundamental trust in the caregivers. McGeer (2004, 2008) recognized in hopeful trust the key force in the development of one's own and others' agencies. According to McGeer (2008), substantial trust and substantial hope can go far beyond existing evidence and current capabilities. They are the driving force for the transcendence of our limits and the development of new competencies in collaboration with others. Therefore, substantial hope is based on trust in the availability of resources that sometimes are at hand and sometimes are not accessible yet but could be available in the future. For McGeer (2004), good hope is therefore a responsive hope characterized by mutual care and support. Trust and hope are therefore linked to humility, patience, and persistence (Shade, 2001). When we trust others we recognize our limitations with modesty and the need for support and care. Trust is also the requirement for persistence and perseverance, not only in keeping our active commitment towards our hopes but also in being able to wait until better conditions arrive patiently.

In a similar sense, and following the work of Earle and Siegrist (2006), we must distinguish between the concepts of trust and confidence. Whereas confidence is defined as a reason-based assessment of a high probability of achieving a goal, fitting the concepts of optimism and dispositional hope, trust is basically a relational phenomenon supported by social attachment and characterized by shared values such as benevolence, integrity, fairness, and caring. Perceived hope, as we understand it, is related to trust rather than with confidence since if one is confident, there is no need to hope (Miceli & Castelfranchi, 2010). Trust relates to the interdependency with another person and therefore with vulnerability, uncertainty, and faith. To the contrary, self-confidence (White, 2009) is characterized by the belief in individual achievements, persistence, resilience, self-awareness, knowledge, experience, and personal success, all attributes closely related to the definition of Snyder's (1994) dispositional hope.

Pragmatist philosophers highlight our dependency on others, and the necessity to trust that others will also hope and engage themselves for the common cause, especially regarding social and collective hope, e.g., for peace, justice, or a sustainable society, (Stitzlein, 2019). Trust has been identified as the most fundamental condition for the willingness to develop a shared vision of the future and to cooperate in promoting social change (Braithwaite, 2004). Furthermore, political hope needs public trust in social and democratic institutions (Huber, 2021; Moellendorf, 2006; Stahl, 2019). Northcott (2020) also encourages us to trust nature and all living creatures to cooperate with them and create a network of ecological practices to enact a sustainable future.

In sum, trust is at the core of most sources of hope: Trust in our current and future abilities, trust in family members and friends who are ready to support us emotionally and instrumentally, trust in the broader community and in social and political institutions, and trust in a Divine Power always present and on our side. People in different countries or belonging to different social groups can vary in what they consider to be sources of hope (Averill et al., 1990; Averill & Sundararajan, 2005). People in collectivistic cultures may rely more on the emotional and instrumental support of their family members and closest friends. Very religious people might put their hope on a benevolent Higher Power. In individualistic societies, hope is based on the notion of autonomy, independence, and self-efficacy, relying mainly on oneself, on one's capabilities and commitment. However, sometimes there is little that one can do to contribute to the fulfillment of one's hopes.

2.4 Conclusion

The primary purpose of this chapter was to lay the theoretical foundation and present a basic universal conceptualization of hope which would allow a differentiated and culture-sensitive study of the phenomenon. In order to make justice to numerous modes of hoping, we adopted an inter- and transdisciplinary approach. During the past decades and even centuries, hope theory and research in psychology, philosophy, and theology evolved in different, sometimes opposite directions, illuminating various facets of the existential, pervasive, and mysterious phenomenon of hope. Although each school and concept can be rooted in specific religious, cultural, and scientific worldviews, there seems to exist a common core underlying all or at least most of the concrete experiences. The main endeavor is thus twofold. Firstly, to distinguish universal features of hope common to a great variety of situations and cultural contexts in which hope comes to bear and to distinguish them from other concepts such as optimism and self-confidence. The second main focus is to identify several forms in which the universal features of hope manifest themselves in different experiences and environments.

Based on traditional theories and recent research, we proposed a transdisciplinary concept of hope that could integrate many aspects and dimensions related to a diversity of intra- and interpersonal processes. We conceptualized hope as composed by three basic elements which are a wish or desire for a valuable good, the belief that the realization of the hope-for good is possible but uncertain or even unlikely, and the trust in the availability of existing or future, either internal or external, resources that could foster its fulfillment. These three elements—wish, belief, and trust—seem to have a universal character that manifests itself in a variety of forms. Different people in different circumstances hope for different ends, believe in different things, and trust various sources of hope. From individual hopes for personal endeavors, through interpersonal hope from and for people we love, to collective hope for a better world, we must recognize and study the many targets, beliefs, and sources of hope and their effects on people's general level of hopefulness. With this theoretical approach and conceptualization of hope, we intend to set the foundations for a differentiated, culturally responsive, and transdisciplinary empirical research agenda. The subsequent chapters will present the first theoretical and empirical findings of the Hope Barometer program and generate new questions for further research.

References

Aspinwall, L. G., & Leaf, S. L. (2002). In search of the unique aspects of hope: Pinning our hopes on positive emotions, future-oriented thinking, hard times, and other people. *Psychological Inquiry, 13*(4), 276–288.

Averill, J. R., Catlin, G., & Chon, K. K. (1990). *Rules of hope: Recent research in psychology*. Springer.

Averill, J. R., & Sundararajan, L. (2005). Hope as rhetoric: Cultural narratives of wishing and coping. In J. Eliott (Ed.), *Interdisciplinary perspectives on hope* (pp. 133–165). Nova Science.

Barilan, Y. M. (2012a). From hope in palliative care to hope as a virtue and a life skill. *Philosophy, Psychiatry, & Psychology, 19*(3), 165–181.

Barilan, Y. M. (2012b). Hope and friendship: Being and having. *Philosophy, Psychiatry, & Psychology, 19*(3), 191–195.

Beck, A. T., Brown, G., Berchick, R. J., Stewart, B. L., & Steer, R. A. (1990). Relationship between hopelessness and ultimate suicide: A replication with psychiatric patients. *American Journal of Psychiatry, 147*, 190–195. https://doi.org/10.1176/foc.4.2.291

Benzein, E., Norberg, A., & Saveman, B. I. (2001). The meaning of the lived experience of hope in patients with cancer in palliative home care. *Palliative Medicine, 15*(2), 117–126. https://doi.org/10.1191/026921601675617254

Bietenhard, H., Stock, K., & Lochmann, J. M. (1989). Hoffnung. In E. Fahlbusch, J. M. Lochmann, & L. Vischer (Eds.), *Evangelisches Kirchenlexikon. Internationale theologische Enzyklopädie*. (Bd. 2, 3. Aufl.) (pp. 543–550). Vandenhoeck & Ruprecht.

Billias, N. (2010). Hope as a moral virtue. In J. McDonald & A. M. Stephenson (Eds.), *The resilience of hope* (pp. 17–27). Brill Publishers.

Bloch, E. (1959/1986). *The principle of hope* (Vol. 3, N. Plaice, S. Plaice, & P. Knight, Trans.). The MIT Press.

Blöser, C. (2020). Enlightenment views of hope. In S. van den Heuvel (Ed.), *Historical and multidisciplinary perspectives on hope* (pp. 61–76). Springer. https://doi.org/10.1007/978-3-030-46489-9_4

Blöser, C., & Stahl, T. (2017a). Hope. In E. Zalta (Ed.), *Stanford encyclopedia of philosophy.*, Online version. Center for the Study of Language and Information.

Blöser, C., & Stahl, T. (2017b). Fundamental hope and practical identity. *Philosophical Papers, 46*(3), 345–371. https://doi.org/10.1080/05568641.2017.1400918

Blöser, C., & Stahl, T. (2019). The moral psychology of hope–An introduction. In C. Blöser & T. Stahl (Eds.), *The moral psychology of hope* (pp. 1–11). Rowman & Littlefield.

Bovens, L. (1999). The value of hope. *Philosophy and Phenomenological Research, 59*(3), 667–681.

Braithwaite, V. (2004). The hope process and social inclusion. *The Annals of the American Academy of Political and Social Science, 592*(1), 128–151. https://doi.org/10.1177/0002716203262096

Bruininks, P., & Malle, B. F. (2005). Distinguishing hope from optimism and related affective states. *Motivation and Emotion, 29*(4), 324–352. https://doi.org/10.1007/s11031-006-9010-4
Burke, P. (2012). Does Hope have a history? *Estudos Avançados, 26*(75), 207–218. https://doi.org/10.1590/S0103-40142012000200014
Cairns, D. (2019). Hope in archaic and classical Greek. In C. Blöser & T. Stahl (Eds.), *The moral psychology of hope* (pp. 15–35). Rowman & Littlefield.
Calhoun, C. (2018). *Doing valuable time: The present, the future, and meaningful living*. Oxford University Press.
Callina, K. S., Snow, N., & Murray, E. D. (2018). The history of philosophical and psychological perspectives on hope: Toward defining hope for the science of positive human development. In M. W. Gallagher & S. J. Lopez (Eds.), *The Oxford handbook of hope* (pp. 9–26). Academic Press.
Chae, L. A. (2019). Hoping for peace. *Australasian Journal of Philosophy, 98*(2), 211–221. https://doi.org/10.1080/00048402.2019.1611893
Clifton, J. D., Baker, J. D., Park, C. L., Yaden, D. B., Clifton, A. B., Terni, P., Miller, J. L., Zeng, G., Giorgi, S., Schwartz, H. A., & Seligman, M. E. (2019). Primal world beliefs. *Psychological Assessment, 31*(1), 82–99.
Cobb, A. D., & Green, A. (2017). The theological virtue of hope as a social virtue. *Journal of Analytic Theology, 5*, 230–250.
Cohn, M. A., & Fredrickson, B. L. (2006). Beyond the moment, beyond the self: Shared ground between selective investment theory and the broaden-and-build theory of positive emotions. *Psychological Inquiry, 17*(1), 39–44.
Cohn, M. A., & Fredrickson, B. L. (2009). Positive emotions. In S. Lopez & C. R. Snyder (Eds.), *Oxford handbook of positive psychology* (Vol. 2, pp. 13–24). Oxford University Press.
Dalferth, I. U. (2016). *Hoffnung*. de Gruyter.
David, D., Montgomery, G., & DiLorenzo, T. (2006). Response expectancy versus response hope in predicting distress. A brief research report. *Erdelyi Pszichologiai Szemle, 1*, 1–13.
David, D., Montgomery, G. H., Stan, R., DiLorenzo, T., & Erblich, J. (2004). Discrimination between hopes and expectancies for nonvolitional outcomes: Psychological phenomenon or artifact? *Personality and Individual Differences, 36*(8), 1945–1952. https://doi.org/10.1016/j.paid.2003.08.013
Day, J. P. (1969). Hope. *American Philosophical Quarterly, 6*(2), 89–102.
Del Vecchio Good, M. J., Good, B. J., Schaffer, C., & Lind, S. E. (1990). American oncology and the discourse on hope. *Culture, Medicine and Psychiatry, 14*(1), 59–79. https://doi.org/10.1007/BF00046704
Downie, R. S. (1963). Hope. *Philosophy and Phenomenological Research, 24*(2), 248–251.
Dufault, K., & Martocchio, B. C. (1985). Hope: Its spheres and dimensions. *The Nursing Clinics of North America, 20*(2), 379–391.
Dunlap, R. (2019). A Zen Buddhist conception of hope in enlightenment. In C. Blöser & T. Stahl (Eds.), *The moral psychology of Hope* (pp. 209–226). Rowman & Littlefield.
Dyson, J., Cobb, M., & Forman, D. (1997). The meaning of spirituality: A literature review. *Journal of Advanced Nursing, 26*(6), 1183–1188. https://doi.org/10.1046/j.1365-2648.1997.00446.x
Earle, T. C., & Siegrist, M. (2006). Morality information, performance information, and the distinction between trust and confidence. *Journal of Applied Social Psychology, 36*(2), 383–416. https://doi.org/10.1111/j.0021-9029.2006.00012.x
Eid, M., & Diener, E. (2009). Norms for experiencing emotions in different cultures: Inter-and intranational differences. In E. Diener (Ed.), *Culture and well-being* (pp. 169–202). Springer. https://doi.org/10.1007/978-90-481-2352-0_9
Eliott, J. A. (2005). What have we done with hope? A brief history. In J. A. Eliott (Ed.), *Interdisciplinary perspectives on hope* (pp. 3–45). Nova Science Publishers.
Elliot, D. (2020). Hope in theology. In S. van den Heuvel (Ed.), *Historical and multidisciplinary perspectives on hope* (pp. 117–136). Springer. https://doi.org/10.1007/978-3-030-46489-9_7
Erikson, E. H. (1959). *Identity and the life cycle: Selected papers*. International Universities Press.

Espinha, D. C. M., & Lima, R. A. G. D. (2012). Spiritual dimension of children and adolescents with cancer: An integrative review. *Acta Paulista de Enfermagem, 25*(SPE1), 161–165. https://doi.org/10.1590/S0103-21002012000800025

Farran, C. J., Herth, K. A., & Popovich, J. M. (1995). *Hope and hopelessness: Critical clinical constructs*. Sage.

Fredrickson, B. L. (1998). What good are positive emotions? *Review of General Psychology, 2*(3), 300–318. https://doi.org/10.1037/1089-2680.2.3.300

Fredrickson, B. L. (2004). The broaden-and-build theory of positive emotions. *Philosophical Transactions-Royal Society of London Series B Biological Sciences, 359*(1449), 1367–1378. https://doi.org/10.1098/rstb.2004.1512

Fremstedal, R. (2019). Kierkegaard on hope as essential to selfhood. In C. Blöser & T. Stahl (Eds.), *The moral psychology of hope* (pp. 75–92). Rowman & Littlefield.

Fromm, E. (1968). *The revolution of hope: Toward a humanized technology*. Harper & Row.

Galek, K., Flannelly, K. J., Vane, A., & Galek, R. M. (2005). Assessing a patient's spiritual needs: A comprehensive instrument. *Holistic Nursing Practice, 19*(2), 62–69.

Godfrey, J. J. (1987). *A philosophy of human hope*. Martinus Nijhoff.

Gravlee, G. S. (2000). Aristotle on hope. *Journal of the History of Philosophy, 38*(4), 461–477. https://doi.org/10.1353/hph.2005.0029

Gravlee, G. S. (2020). Hope in ancient Greek philosophy. In S. van den Heuvel (Ed.), *Historical and multidisciplinary perspectives on hope* (pp. 3–23). Springer. https://doi.org/10.1007/978-3-030-46489-9_1

Hamilton, A. J. (2008). *The scalpel and the soul: Encounters with surgery, the supernatural, and the healing power of hope*. Penguin.

Heidegger, M. (1953/2010). *Being and time*. Suny Press.

Hendricks-Ferguson, V. (2008). Hope and spiritual well-being in adolescents with cancer. *Western Journal of Nursing Research, 30*(3), 385–401. https://doi.org/10.1177/0193945907303045

Huber, J. (2021). Defying democratic despair: A Kantian account of hope in politics. *European Journal of Political Theory, 20*(4), 719–738. https://doi.org/10.1177/1474885119847308

Ibrahim, F. A. (1984). Cross-cultural counseling and psychotherapy: An existential-psychological approach. *International Journal for the Advancement of Counselling, 7*(3), 159–169. https://doi.org/10.1007/BF00116188

Janoff-Bulman, R. (1989). Assumptive worlds and the stress of traumatic events: Applications of the schema construct. *Social Cognition, 7*(2), 113–136. https://doi.org/10.1521/soco.1989.7.2.113

Janoff-Bulman, R. (1992). *Shattered assumptions: Towards a new psychology of trauma*. Free Press.

Jeffrey, A. (2019). Hope in christianity. In C. Blöser & T. Stahl (Eds.), *The moral psychology of hope* (pp. 37–55).

Kadlac, A. (2015). The virtue of hope. *Ethical Theory and Moral Practice, 18*(2), 337–354. https://doi.org/10.1007/s10677-014-9521-0

Kelly, G. A. (1955). The psychology of personal constructs. In G. A. Kelly (Ed.), *A theory of personality* (Vol. 1). WW Norton and Company.

Kleist, N., & Jansen, S. (2016). Introduction: Hope over time—Crisis, immobility and future-making. *History and Anthropology, 27*(4), 373–392. https://doi.org/10.1080/02757206.2016.1207636

Knapp, C., Madden, V., Wang, H., Curtis, C., Sloyer, P., & Shenkman, E. (2011). Spirituality of parents of children in palliative care. *Journal of Palliative Medicine, 14*(4), 437–443. https://doi.org/10.1089/jpm.2010.0387

Koltko-Rivera, M. E. (2004). The psychology of worldviews. *Review of General Psychology, 8*(1), 3–58. https://doi.org/10.1037/1089-2680.8.1.3

Krafft, A. M., & Choubisa, R. (2018). Hope in the Indian psychology context: Philosophical foundations and empirical findings. In A. M. Krafft, P. Perrig-Chiello, & A. M. Walker

(Eds.), *Hope for a good life* (pp. 131–163). Springer. https://doi.org/10.1007/978-3-319-78470-0_7

Krafft, A. M., Guse, T., & Maree, D. (2021). Distinguishing perceived hope and dispositional optimism: Theoretical foundations and empirical findings beyond future expectancies and cognition. *Journal of Well-Being Assessment, 4*(3), 217–243. https://doi.org/10.1007/s41543-020-00030-4

Krafft, A. M., & Walker, A. M. (2018). Exploring the concept and experience of hope–theoretical and methodological foundations. In A. Krafft, P. Perrig-Chiello, & A. Walker (Eds.), *Hope for a good life* (pp. 3–19). Springer. https://doi.org/10.1007/978-3-319-78470-0_1

Kretz, L. (2019). Hope, the environment and moral imagination. In R. Green (Ed.), *Theories of hope: Exploring alternative affective dimensions of human experience* (pp. 155–176). Lexington Books.

Laila, T. (2008). The phenomenology of hope. In W. Bauman (Ed.), *Hope: Global interdisciplinary perspectives* (pp. 91–97). Inter-Disciplinary Press.

Lazarus, R. S. (1999). Hope: An emotion and a vital coping resource against despair. *Social Research, 66*(2), 653–678.

Lear, J. (2006). *Radical hope: Ethics in the face of cultural devastation*. Harvard University Press.

Lerner, M. J. (1980). *The belief in a just world–A fundamental delusion*. Springer. https://doi.org/10.1007/978-1-4899-0448-5_2

Lerner, A. (2019). Redemptive transgressions: The dialectical evolution of hope and freedom in the west. In R. Green (Ed.), *Theories of hope: Exploring alternative affective dimensions of human experience* (pp. 71–93). Lexington Books.

Leung, K. K., Silvius, J. L., Pimlott, N., Dalziel, W., & Drummond, N. (2009). Why health expectations and hopes are different: The development of a conceptual model. *Health Expectations, 12*(4), 347–360. https://doi.org/10.1111/j.1369-7625.2009.00570.x

Lima, N. N. R., do Nascimento, V. B., de Carvalho, S. M., Neto, M. L., Moreira, M. M., Brasil, A. Q., Celestino Junior, F. T., de Oliveira, G. F., & Reis, A. O. (2013). Spirituality in childhood cancer care. *Neuropsychiatric Disease and Treatment, 9*, 1539–1544.

Marcel, G. (1951). *Homo Viator: Introduction to a metaphysic of hope*. St. Augustines Press.

Martin, A. M. (2011). Hopes and dreams. *Philosophy and Phenomenological Research, 83*(1), 148–173. https://doi.org/10.1111/j.1933-1592.2010.00422.x

Martin, A. M. (2013). *How we hope–A moral psychology*. Princeton University Press. https://doi.org/10.1515/9781400848706

Martin, A. (2019). Interpersonal hope. In C. Blöser & T. Stahl (Eds.), *The moral psychology of hope* (pp. 229–248). Rowman & Littlefield.

Matthews, D. A., McCollough, M. E., Swyers, J. P., Milano, M. G., Larson, D. B., & Koenig, H. G. (1999). Religious commitment and health status. *Archives of Family Medicine, 8*(6), 476–482.

McCormick, M. S. (2017). Rational hope. *Philosophical Explorations, 20*(supp 1), 127–141. https://doi.org/10.1080/13869795.2017.1287298

McDonald, J. E. (2008). The spirit of hope and its near enemy indifference: A phenomenological continuum. In W. Bauman (Ed.), *Hope: Global interdisciplinary perspectives* (pp. 39–49). Inter-Disciplinary Press.

McGeer, V. (2004). The art of good hope. *The Annals of the American Academy of Political and Social Science, 592*(1), 100–127. https://doi.org/10.1177/0002716203261781

McGeer, V. (2008). Trust, hope and empowerment. *Australasian Journal of Philosophy, 86*(2), 237–254. https://doi.org/10.1080/00048400801886413

Meirav, A. (2008). Distinguishing between Hope and despair. In W. Bauman (Ed.), *Hope: Global interdisciplinary perspectives* (pp. 11–16). Inter-Disciplinary Press.

Meirav, A. (2009). The nature of hope. *Ratio, 22*(2), 216–233. https://doi.org/10.1111/j.1467-9329.2009.00427.x

Meireles, C. B., Maia, L. C., Miná, V. A. L., Novais, M. D. S. M. C., Peixoto, J. A. C., Cartaxo, M. A. B. S., Ferreira de Lima, J. M., Vieria dos Santos, F. A., de Matos Cassiano, C. J., Pinheiro,

P. G., & Neto, M. L. R. (2015). Influence of spirituality in pediatric cancer management: A systematic review. *International Archives of Medicine, 8*, 1–13. https://doi.org/10.3823/1634

Miceli, M., & Castelfranchi, C. (2010). Hope: The power of wish and possibility. *Theory & Psychology, 20*(2), 251–276. https://doi.org/10.1177/0959354309354393

Michener, R. T. (2020). Post-Kantian to postmodern considerations of (theological) hope. In S. van den Heuvel (Ed.), *Historical and multidisciplinary perspectives on hope* (pp. 77–95). Springer. https://doi.org/10.1007/978-3-030-46489-9_5

Miller, J. G. (1999). Cultural psychology: Implications for basic psychological theory. *Psychological Science, 10*, 85–91. https://doi.org/10.1111/1467-9280.00113

Milona, M. (2019). Finding hope. *Canadian Journal of Philosophy, 49*(5), 710–729. https://doi.org/10.1080/00455091.2018.1435612

Milona, M. (2020a). Philosophy of hope. In S. van den Heuvel (Ed.), *Historical and multidisciplinary perspectives on hope* (pp. 99–116). Springer. https://doi.org/10.1007/978-3-030-46489-9_6

Milona, M. (2020b). *Hope and optimism*. John Templet on Foundation. https://www.templeton.org/wp-content/uploads/2020/10/JTF-Hope-O. . .PDF file

Moellendorf, D. (2006). Hope as a political virtue. *Philosophical Papers, 35*(3), 413–433.

Moltmann, J. (2021). *Theology of hope: For the 21st century*. SCM Press.

Montgomery, G. H., David, D., DiLorenzo, T., & Erblich, J. (2003). Is hoping the same as expecting? Discrimination between hopes and response expectancies for nonvolitional outcomes. *Personality and Individual Differences, 35*(2), 399–409. https://doi.org/10.1016/S0191-8869(02)00202-7

Naderi, F. S., & Abolghasemi, M. (2008). Is hope culture bound? In W. Bauman (Ed.), *Hope: Global interdisciplinary perspectives* (pp. 111–130). Inter-Disciplinary Press.

Nebe, G., & Goetzmann, J. (1997). Hoffnung/Furcht/Sorge. In L. Coenen & K. Haacker (Eds.), *Theologisches Begriffslexikon*. (Bd. 1) (pp. 993–1015). Brockhaus.

Nietzsche, F. (1885/2006). In A. del Caro & R. B. Pippin (Eds.), *Thus spoke Zarathustra*. Cambridge University Press.

Northcott, M. S. (2020). Ecological hope. In S. van den Heuvel (Ed.), *Historical and multidisciplinary perspectives on hope* (pp. 215–238). Springer.

Nussbaum, M. C. (2003). *Upheavals of thought: The intelligence of emotions*. Cambridge University Press.

Nussbaum, M. (2004). Emotions as judgments of value and importance. In R. Solomon (Ed.), *Thinking about feeling: Contemporary philosophers on emotions* (pp. 183–204). Oxford University Press.

Nussbaum, M. C. (2019). *The monarchy of fear: A philosopher looks at our political crisis*. Simon & Schuster.

Olsman, E. (2020). Hope in health care: A synthesis of review studies. In S. van den Heuvel (Ed.), *Historical and multidisciplinary perspectives on hope* (pp. 197–214). Springer. https://doi.org/10.1007/978-3-030-46489-9_11

Osmani, N. M. (2008). In W. Bauman (Ed.), *Phenomenology of hope and despair: A Qur'anic perspective* (pp. 191–202). Inter-Disciplinary Press.

Parker-Oliver, D. (2002). Redefining hope for the terminally ill. *American Journal of Hospice and Palliative Medicine, 19*(2), 115–120. https://doi.org/10.1177/104990910201900210

Peterson, C., & Seligman, M. E. (2004). *Character strengths and virtues: A handbook and classification*. Oxford University Press.

Pettit, P. (2004). Hope and its place in mind. *The Annals of the American Academy of Political and Social Science, 592*(1), 152–165. https://doi.org/10.1177/0002716203261798

Pieper, J. (1997). *Faith, hope, love* (p. 102). Ignatius Press.

Pinsent, A. (2020). Hope as a virtue in the middle ages. In S. van den Heuvel (Ed.), *Historical and multidisciplinary perspectives on hope* (pp. 47–60). Springer. https://doi.org/10.1007/978-3-030-46489-9_3

Rao, K. R., & Paranjpe, A. C. (2016). *Psychology in the Indian tradition*. Springer. https://doi.org/10.1007/978-81-322-2440-2_7

Rasmussen, H. N., & Lavish, L. (2014). Broad definitions of culture in the field of multicultural psychology. In J. T. Pedrotti & L. M. Edwards (Eds.), *Perspectives on the intersection of multiculturalism and positive psychology* (pp. 17–30). Springer. https://doi.org/10.1007/978-94-017-8654-6_2

Ratcliffe, M. (2013). What is it to lose hope? *Phenomenology and the Cognitive Sciences, 12*(4), 597–614. https://doi.org/10.1007/s11097-011-9215-1

Robitschek, C., Sirles, D., & Hardin, E. E. (2014). Cognitive constructs in the context of positive psychology. In J. Teramoto Pedrotti & L. M. Edwards (Eds.), *Perspectives on the intersection of multiculturalism and positive psychology* (pp. 75–91). Springer. https://doi.org/10.1007/978-94-017-8654-6_6

Rorty, R. (1982). *Consequences of pragmatism*. University of Minnesota Press.

Rorty, R. (1999). *Philosophy and social hope*. Penguin Books.

Rorty, R. (2002). Hope and the future. *Peace Review, 14*(2), 149–155. https://doi.org/10.1080/10402650220140166

Saleh, U. S., & Brockopp, D. Y. (2001). Hope among patients with cancer hospitalized for bone marrow transplantation: A phenomenologic study. *Cancer Nursing, 24*(4), 308–314.

Schneider, M. A., & Mannell, R. C. (2006). Beacon in the storm: An exploration of the spirituality and faith of parents whose children have cancer. *Issues in Comprehensive Pediatric Nursing, 29*(1), 3–24. https://doi.org/10.1080/01460860500523731

Schopenhauer, A. (1918/2010), *The world as will and representation*. (Vol. I, J. Norman, A. Welchman, C. Janaway, Eds.). Cambridge University Press.

Schwartz, S. H. (1994). Are there universal aspects in the structure and contents of human values? *Journal of Social Issues, 50*(4), 19–45. https://doi.org/10.1111/j.1540-4560.1994.tb01196.x

Schwartz, S. H., & Bardi, A. (2001). Value hierarchies across cultures: Taking a similarities perspective. *Journal of Cross-Cultural Psychology, 32*(3), 268–290. https://doi.org/10.1177/0022022101032003002

Scioli, A. (2007). Hope and spirituality in the age of anxiety. In R. J. Estes (Ed.), *Advancing quality of life in a turbulent world* (pp. 135–150). Springer. https://doi.org/10.1007/978-1-4020-5110-4_9

Scioli, A. (2020). The psychology of hope: A diagnostic and prescriptive account. In S. van den Heuvel (Ed.), *Historical and multidisciplinary perspectives on hope* (pp. 137–163). Springer. https://doi.org/10.1007/978-3-030-46489-9_8

Scioli, A., & Biller, H. (2009). *Hope in the age of anxiety*. Oxford University Press.

Scioli, A., Chamberlin, C. M., Samor, C. M., Lapointe, A. B., Campbell, T. L., Macleod, A. R., & McLenon, J. (1997). A prospective study of hope, optimism, and health. *Psychological Reports, 81*(3), 723–733. https://doi.org/10.2466/pr0.1997.81.3.723

Shade, P. (2001). *Habits of hope–A pragmatic theory*. Vanderbilt University Press.

Shin, S. H., De Pretto, L., & Simpson, A. (2013). What does hope mean to people? The lay construct of hope under achievement-oriented settings in Australia, Italy and South Korea. In G. Karabin (Ed.), *Hope in all directions* (pp. 197–212). Brill Publishers. https://doi.org/10.1163/9781848882591_018

Singelis, T. M., Triandis, H. C., Bhawuk, D. P., & Gelfand, M. J. (1995). Horizontal and vertical dimensions of individualism and collectivism: A theoretical and measurement refinement. *Cross-Cultural Research, 29*(3), 240–275. https://doi.org/10.1177/106939719502900302

Slaughter, R. A. (1993). The substantive knowledge base of futures studies. *Futures–Guildford, 25*(3), 227–233.

Snow, N. (2013). Hope as an intellectual virtue. In M. Austin (Ed.), *Virtues in action–New essays in applied virtues ethics* (pp. 153–170). Palgrave Macmillan.

Snow, N. E. (2018). Hope as a democratic civic virtue. *Metaphilosophy, 49*(3), 407–427. https://doi.org/10.1111/meta.12299

Snow, N. (2019a). Faces of hope. In R. Green (Ed.), *Theories of hope: Exploring alternative affective dimensions of human experience* (Vol. 2018, pp. 5–23). Rowman & Littlefield.

Snow, N. (2019b). Is hope a moral virtue? In C. Blöser & T. Stahl (Eds.), *The Moral Psychology of Hope* (pp. 171–187).

Snyder, C. R. (1994). *The psychology of hope: You can get there from here*. Simon & Schuster.

Snyder, C. R. (2002). Hope theory: Rainbows in the mind. *Psychological Inquiry, 13*(4), 249–275. https://doi.org/10.1207/S15327965PLI1304_01

Snyder, C. R., LaPointe, A. B., Jeffrey Crowson, J., & Early, S. (1998). Preferences of high-and low-hope people for self-referential input. *Cognition & Emotion, 12*(6), 807–823. https://doi.org/10.1080/026999398379448

Spiro, H. M. (1998). *The power of hope: A doctor's perspective*. Yale University Press.

Stahl, T. (2019). Political hope and cooperative community. In C. Blöser & T. Stahl (Eds.), *The moral psychology of hope* (pp. 265–283). Rowman & Littlefield.

Stitzlein, S. (2019). Pragmatist hope. In C. Blöser & T. Stahl (Eds.), *The moral psychology of hope* (pp. 93–112). Rowman & Littlefield.

Stockdale, K. (2019). Emotional hope. In C. Blöser & T. Stahl (Eds.), *The moral psychology of hope* (pp. 93–112). Rowman & Littlefield.

Stotland, E. (1969). *The psychology of hope*. Jossey-Bass.

Taylor, E. J. (2003). Spiritual needs of patients with cancer and family caregivers. *Cancer Nursing, 26*(4), 260–266.

Tennen, H., Affleck, G., & Tennen, R. (2002). Clipped feathers: The theory and measurement of hope. *Psychological Inquiry, 13*(4), 311–317.

Triandis, H. C. (1997). Cross-cultural perspectives on personality. In R. Hogan, J. Johnson, & S. Briggs (Eds.), *Handbook of personality psychology* (pp. 439–464). Academic Press.

van Vliet, J. (2020). An ontology of human flourishing: Economic development and epistemologies of faith, hope, and love. In S. van den Heuvel (Ed.), *Historical and multidisciplinary perspectives on hope* (pp. 239–261). Springer. https://doi.org/10.1007/978-3-030-46489-9_13

Walker, M. U. (2006). *Moral repair: Reconstructing moral relations after wrongdoing*. Cambridge University Press.

Webb, D. (2007). Modes of hoping. *History of the Human Sciences, 20*(3), 65–83.

Webb, D. (2008). In W. Bauman (Ed.), *Modes of hoping and the utopian impulse* (pp. 25–38). Inter-Disciplinary Press.

Webb, D. (2013). Pedagogies of hope. *Studies in Philosophy and Education, 32*(4), 397–414. https://doi.org/10.1007/s11217-012-9336-1

Webb, D. (2019). Education and the construction of Hope. In R. Green (Ed.), *Theories of hope: Exploring alternative affective dimensions of human experience* (pp. 131–153). Rowman & Littlefield.

White, K. A. (2009). Self-confidence: A concept analysis. *Nursing Forum, 44*, 103–114. https://doi.org/10.1111/j.1744-6198.2009.00133.x

Wong, P. T. P., Wong, L. C. J., & Scott, C. (2006). The positive psychology of transformation: Beyond stress and coping. In P. T. P. Wong & L. C. J. Wong (Eds.), *Handbook of multicultural perspectives on stress and coping*. Springer.

Zagzebski, L. (1996). *Virtues of the mind: An inquiry into the nature of virtue and the ethical foundations of knowledge*. Cambridge University Press.

Zagzebski, L. (2003). The search for the source of epistemic good. *Metaphilosophy, 34*(1–2), 12–28. https://doi.org/10.1111/1467-9973.00257

Zagzebski, L. (2008). Virtues of the mind, selections. In E. Sosa, J. Kim, J. Fantl, & M. McGrath (Eds.), *Epistemology: An anthology* (pp. 442–453). Blackwell Publishing.

Andreas Krafft holds a doctoral degree in Management Sciences at the University of St. Gallen (Switzerland) with special focus on Organizational Psychology, Culture and Development. He has academic specializations in Social Psychology of Organizations, Work and Health Psychology as well as Positive Psychology from the University of Zürich. Andreas is associate researcher for Futures Studies and lecturer at the Institute of Systemic Management and Public Governance at the University of St. Gallen. Furthermore, he teaches at the University of Zürich in the field of Work and Health, at the Master of Applied Positive Psychology at the University of Lisbon, Portugal, as well as at the Master of Futures Studies from the Free University Berlin. He is co-president of swissfuture, the Swiss Society for Futures Studies, member of the executive board of SWIPPA (the Swiss Positive Psychology Association) and of the DACH-PP (German speaking Association of Positive Psychology). Since many years he leads the International Research Network of the Hope Barometer.

Tharina Guse is a counselling psychologist and obtained an MA (Counselling Psychology) degree from the Potchefstroom University (now North-West University) in 1989. She was in full-time private practice for the next 15 years providing psychotherapy for children, adolescents and adults. In 2003 she obtained her PhD (Psychology) from Potchefstroom University. She returned to academia in 2005 and joined the University of Johannesburg. Since April 2018 she is a professor and Head of the Department of Psychology at the University of Pretoria. Currently she serves on the Professional Board for Psychology of the Health Professions Council of South Africa (HPCSA). She is also President of the recently founded South African Positive Psychology Association (SAPPA). Her research focuses are on positive psychology in general and in particular on psycho-social well-being, positive psychology interventions and psychological strengths such as hope and gratitude. Closely aligned with this broad focus she also conducts research on the application of hypnosis for the promotion of mental health and well-being.

Alena Slezackova, Ph.D., is an Associate Professor of Psychology and a Vice Head of the Dept. of Psychology and Psychosomatics, Faculty of Medicine, Masaryk University, in Brno, Czech Republic. Her scientific interests include mainly hope, mental health, and well-being. She also has a special interest in the research and practice of mindfulness. Alena is a founder and director of the Czech Positive Psychology Centre (CPPC), a member of the Advisory Council of the International Positive Psychology Association (IPPA), and a member of the Executive Board of the European Network for Positive Psychology (ENPP). She has been a member of several international research projects, and she serves on the editorial boards of five academic psychological journals. Alena is the author of the first comprehensive monograph on positive psychology in the Czech language and dozens of scientific publications in positive psychology and health psychology.

Chapter 3
Values and Targets of Hope

Andreas M. Krafft, Alena Slezackova, Helena Águeda Marujo, and Valle Flores-Lucas

Abstract The current chapter is dedicated to evaluate the first element of the proposed hope concept, examining the role of human values in the general perception of hope and in the adoption of significant targets of hope across different cultures. The study employed the value model of Shalom Schwartz and elaborated conceptual connections to the phenomenon of hope. Based on data collected with the Hope Barometer in November 2018 ($N = 5832$) in German and French speaking Switzerland, Spain, Portugal and the Czech Republic, this study analyzes the commonalities and possible cultural differences in the levels of perceived hope, in individual hope targets, and in the effects of particular human value orientations on hope. Our findings indicate that hope is not determined by the wealth of a nation (e.g., in terms of GDP) but by personal and collective characteristics, to a certain extent influenced by basic human values. The results disclose the almost universal significance of self-transcendence and openness to change, as well as the relevance of tradition and achievement in relation to a hopeful attitude and to central prosocial and altruistic targets of hope. Beyond common features across cultures, this study reveals subtle cultural differences worth to be further investigated in future studies.

A. M. Krafft (✉)
Institute of Systemic Management and Public Governance, University of St. Gallen, St. Gallen, Switzerland
e-mail: andreas.krafft@unisg.ch

A. Slezackova
Department of Medical Psychology and Psychosomatics, Faculty of Medicine, Masaryk University, Brno, Czech Republic

H. Á. Marujo
Instituto Superior de Ciências Sociais e Politicas, University of Lisbon, Lisbon, Portugal

V. Flores-Lucas
Department of Psychology, University of Valladolid, Valladolid, Spain

A. M. Krafft et al. (eds.), *Hope across cultures*, Cross-Cultural Advancements in Positive Psychology 14, https://doi.org/10.1007/978-3-031-24412-4_3

3.1 Introduction

The hope concept presented in the previous chapter comprises three basic elements of hope: (1) A wish or desire that is regarded as a significant and meaningful good; (2) the belief that the realization of this wish is possible (although not necessarily probable); and (3) the trust in the availability of personal, social, transcendental, or other (e.g., political, economic) resources to overcome difficulties and obstacles. The first domain of the hope concept addresses the wishes and desires along with the fundamental values of people. These can be directed to a certain state of affairs, to an event, to particular circumstances, or to specific goals related to the individual. They can also be focused on the closer social environment, on a certain institution, on society or on the entire world (e.g., the hope for a sustainable economy). The central elements here are the targets of hope based on certain values that are of particular importance and significance to individuals.

From a social-constructionist point of view, Averill and his colleagues (Averill et al., 1990; Averill & Sundararajan, 2005) considered that the nature of hope would depend on the cultural context with its particular values and norms in which the hoping person is embedded. Personal hopes are characterized by their significance and value but not by the likelihood of their achievement. The authors identified different kinds of targets people might hope for in different cultures (e.g., material goods, hedonic experiences, social relationships, and altruistic motives) and the actions performed to achieve the outcome. According to these studies, people generally hope less for materialistic and hedonic goods but more for social relationships, altruistic ends, or for an ideal self and world. However, the authors also identified differences between cultures, specifically the United States and Korea, proposed that hope is related to a cultural value structure.

Our assumption in this chapter is that what people hope for is to a certain extent related to their values and interests and also, to what they consider as desirable for a good life for themselves, their closer environment, and for society at large. Further, these values are partly influenced by cultural values. Whereas in this chapter we will focus on personal hopes in people's own life, Chap. 10 will be dedicated to hopes related to the broader environment and society. We commence with the definition, qualities, and types of basic human values and establish their conceptual connection to the phenomenon of hope. This is followed by the results of our empirical studies conducted in Switzerland, Spain, Portugal, and the Czech Republic with the aim of identifying possible universal patterns as well as cultural characteristics across countries. Our basic assumption is that the general level of hope might be influenced by the quality of basic values held by an individual and shaped by the cultural context.

3.2 Theoretical Background

3.2.1 Defining Values

Kluckhohn (1951) was one of the first authors who studied human values from a psychological perspective, conceptualizing value orientations in the context of a theory of action and performing comparative studies in several cultures. He defined values as general principles regarding what a person considers desirable and worthwhile for him−/herself and others. Values express what is important to us and guide our goals and behavior (e.g., security, autonomy, attachment, pleasure, success, etc.). Each person holds several values with varying degrees of importance. For example, a secure job can be important for one person, but unimportant for another, who wants to progress quickly in a professional career. In doing so, values drive our perception, preferences, judgements, motives and actions, and may have an effect on what people hope for and the way in which hopes tend to be fulfilled.

The original empirical studies performed by Rokeach (1973) have shaped the understanding of the nature and quality of values even more. Rokeach defined a value as an action-guiding conviction according to which a course of action (instrumental value) or a target state (terminal value) is personally or socially preferred to other courses of action or target states. Values are cross-situational higher goals that guide individuals and social groups and vary in importance. Based on his or her values, an individual chooses those attitudes, goals and behaviors that are personally and socially more desirable. Values serve as orientation in various fields of life. Rokeach assumed that people all over the world have only a few central values and that these are similar for most people but with different tones and emphases. The distinct qualities of values are a consequence of cultural influences, social institutions as well as the individual personality.

3.2.2 Basic Principles of Human Values and their Connection to Hope

Based on these classic precursors, Schwartz (1992, 1994) developed a psychological theory and a general model of universal human values. According to his theory, values emerge from three basic requirements of human beings and societies (Schwartz & Bardi, 2001):

1. Biological needs motivate people to work and satisfy their needs (e.g., self-direction values).
2. The necessity to coordinate interpersonal social interactions motivate people intrinsically to cooperation and support each other (e.g., pro-social values).
3. Social demands for group welfare and development motivate people to regulate their behavior to be socially acceptable (e.g., conformity values).

Schwartz (1994, p. 21) defined values as "desirable trans-situational goals, varying in importance, that serve as guiding principles in the life of a person or other social entity". Crucial in his definition is that values express a type of motivational goal. Understanding values as higher-level goals includes the idea that they represent the interests of an individual or group, they motivate action, they function as standards for judging desirable outcomes, and they are acquired through experience and socialization. In a broader sense, values are psychological constructs that help to understand other psychological phenomena (like anxiety and hope) based on an affective evaluation, justification, and selection of goals and actions.

Starting from the basic requirements of human social interaction and based on previous theories, Schwartz (2003, 2007, 2012) identified general principles underlying the concept of basic values. For the purpose of our study, we will draw attention to the similarities between basic values and hope:

1. Values are beliefs, which are infused with emotions. Values as well as hopes are primarily subjective feelings and not objective facts. Important values and hopes generate positive feelings such as excitement and enthusiasm (Fredrickson, 2013; Tennen et al., 2002).
2. Values refer to desirable goals and motives. The individual who values justice, fairness or kindness also hopes for the fulfilment of these values. People hope for a valuable and desirable outcome. This highlights the motivational character of values and hopes (Pettit, 2004).
3. Values transcend concrete situations. Someone for whom a certain value is especially important, hopes for it in different areas of life, e.g., within the family, at work, in society. In this sense, values and hopes can be described as abstract or general goals and wishes (Averill et al., 1990).
4. Values serve as standards or criteria. Values guide the selection of hope targets. We evaluate whether certain targets we might hope for are good or bad, desirable or undesirable and worth engaging in, in light of our esteemed values (Webb, 2013).
5. Values are hierarchically ordered by importance. Individuals and social groups develop a system of values and hopes structured according to their importance and priority (Averill & Sundararajan, 2005; Krafft & Walker, 2018b). Some values and hopes (e.g., material goods, family traditions, spirituality, etc.) can be more significant for one person and less essential for another. The hierarchical value system creates a structure of compatibility and antagonism between values (e.g., tradition vs. stimulation).
6. Relevant values guide action. Values and hopes typically foster a certain behavior (McGeer, 2008). People for whom achievement is important will work hard and engage themselves, whishing and hoping for success, often at expense of other values such as pleasure or social relationships.
7. One of the most relevant aspects that may distinguish values from hopes is that whereas hopes are consciously chosen wishes or desires, values are rarely conscious. In daily life, people generally are not aware about which values motivate their actions. Hopes, instead, are much more deliberately articulated (Pettit, 2004).

Based on these conceptual parallels between values and hopes and following Blöser and Stahl's (2017) claim that hope is related to our practical identity, we argue that human values and hope are inextricably linked together, that values influence what people may hope for and that values are meaningful sources of hope. Values and hopes both refer to desirable goals that motivate action. On the one hand, values have an effect on the importance and desirability of certain targets of hope and the actions that will be performed in order to accomplish them. For example, people who prime the value of power will hope for an influential position at work or in politics and will do everything required to triumph over other people. Due to their motivational power, values will foster particular hopes and may lead individuals to adopt a specific behavior to promote these hopes and values.

3.2.3 Ten Basic Human Values

Schwartz (1992) asked people in 20 nations about the guiding principles in their lives. Based on his general theory and as result of his empirical work, Schwartz (1994) derived four higher order value categories and ten motivationally distinct, broad, and basic value dimensions. In recent years these dimensions were refined into 19 value sub-types (Schwartz & Cieciuch, 2016). For the purpose of our study, we have chosen to work with the original ten and the four higher order values as conceptualized in the refined theory presented in Schwartz et al. (2012) and Schwartz and Cieciuch (2016). Below we describe the ten values as defined by Schwartz and his colleagues and classify them into the four higher order value dimensions:

1. *Self-transcendence*: These values are not directed to fulfill one's own particular interests but to transcend them considering the interests of others.
   (a) *Benevolence*: This value is oriented to the closer social group to which one belongs. It follows the goal of being a trustworthy and reliable member of the social group (e.g., circle of friends) and emphasizes the concern and care for the welfare of the loved ones (e.g., family). Benevolence is derived from the need for social affiliation and attachment (a sense of belonging) and promotes cooperative and supportive relationships.
   (b) *Universalism*: This value focuses on a positive relationship between oneself und the wider environment. It comprises the acceptance, tolerance, and respect of people different from oneself, it treasures equality, social justice, peace and living in harmony with all people regardless of their personal and cultural backgrounds. It also commits to the preservation of the natural environment and treasures a world of natural beauty.
2. *Openness to change*: These values are oriented to elevate one's personal level of mastery and self-competence.
   (a) *Self-direction*: The value of self-direction is derived from the need for control and mastery. It cherishes freedom, independence and autonomy to explore

and develop one's own ideas and abilities (e.g., creativity and imagination) and highlights self-determination in choosing and pursuing personal goals and actions.

(b) *Stimulation*: People with a strong interest in stimulation are continuously in search of new and exciting experiences, of adventures and challenges in life. The goal and motivation is to have a varied life full of novelty and change.

(c) *Hedonism*: The main characteristic of hedonism is the pursuit of pleasure and sensuous gratification through enjoyment and amusement. In some cases, hedonism can also be part of the higher value of self-enhancement.

3. *Conservation*: Values in the sphere of conservation emphasize the significance of social order, continuity, and coherence.

   (a) *Tradition*: This value focuses on appreciating and preserving family, cultural and religious norms, habits, and practices. Traditions symbolize the identity of a social group and the respect for its history and beliefs.

   (b) *Security*: This value can be directed to the personal and the societal sphere. At the personal level, security relates to one's health and safety in the immediate environment. At the societal level, the attention lies on harmony, safety, and stability in the broader society.

   (c) *Conformity*: This value is split into interpersonal conformity and compliance. On the one hand, conformity is about the desire not to hurt or harm other people. On the other hand, it spotlights the requirement to comply with rules, laws, and social expectations. Conformity endorses values such as obedience, self-discipline, loyalty, and politeness.

4. *Self-enhancement*: Values that foster self-enhancement are oriented to satisfy one's own individual needs and interests.

   (a) *Achievement*: Beneath this value lies the motive of performance and competence in achieving one's personal goals and being successful according to some social standards. A central motivation and goal is that of receiving social recognition. It encourages being ambitious and working hard.

   (b) *Power*: Striving for power has three components. The first domain is dominance and control over other people to compel them to act according to one's own will. The second field is having control over material and social resources. The third element refers to the inclination of preserving and cultivating one's prestige, social status, and public image (e.g., through wealth).

3.2.4 The Circular Structure of Human Values and its Effect on Hope

In addition to identifying the ten motivational value types and the four higher order value dimensions, Schwartz' theory also explains the relationships among the

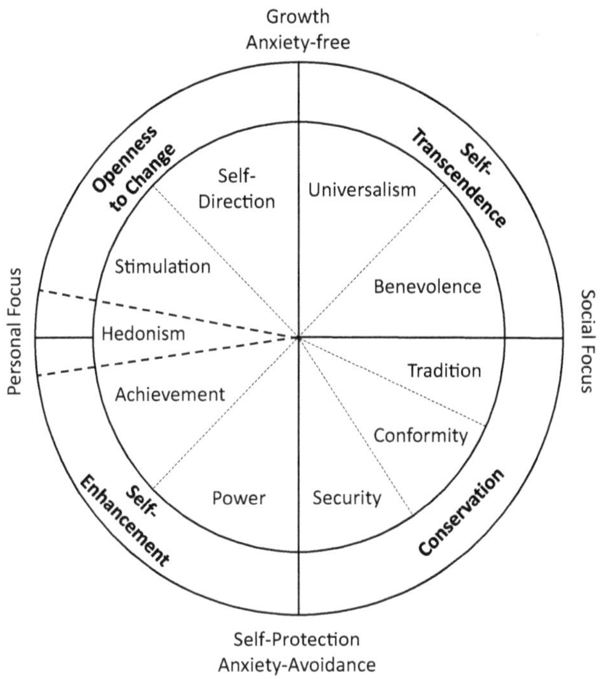

Fig. 3.1 Circular Motivational Continuum of 10 Human Values according to Schwartz (2007, 2012)

individual value orientations (Schwartz & Bilsky, 1987). In his model, values are structured in a circular psychological, motivational, and behavioral system that drives attitudes, decisions and actions. The model uses two criteria to characterize and distinguish different value types, which are significant to understand possible connections between values and hope. The ten particular values that people in almost all cultures seem to adopt can be located in a circular continuum characterized by two bipolar dimensions: personal and social focus on the one hand, and growth promotion (anxiety-free and self-expansion) and anxiety-avoidance (self-protection) on the other. The first criterion distinguishes values oriented to protect oneself against threats, to prevent possible losses and to avoid or cope with anxiety from other values that are free from anxiety, that promote new opportunities and that help people to develop and to grow (Schwartz, 2012). The second criterion distinguishes values concerning personal interests from values with a social focus. Schwartz (1992) assumes that actions oriented toward one value dimension have consequences that either contradict or coincide with actions performed arising from other value type. For example, orientation to novelty and change (stimulation values) undermines the preservation of established customs and habits (tradition values). Figure 3.1 displays the original circular model illustrating the two bipolar dimensions, the ten basic value types and the four higher order values.

The four higher order values emerge from the combination of these two criteria (Schwartz, 2003): Self-transcendence has a social focus and is anxiety-free as well as growth oriented. These values characterize people who are caring, selfless, kind, and concerned with the well-being of other people and the environment. Opposite values are those of self-enhancement, which are centered on the individual, on anxiety-avoidance and self-protection, which lead people to pursue selfish interests. Openness to change, in turn, covers values directed to fulfil individual goals but with an anxiety-free and growth-oriented attitude. These are values that drive people to be open to new challenges that want to be autonomous, and not to shy away from uncertainty. Finally, conservation values are motivated by social goals, but the underlying mood is one of anxiety-avoidance and self-protection. Individuals with these values are more concerned with security, social stability and seek to conserve the status quo.

In several philosophical and psychological writings, hope has been characterized as the opposite of anxiety, fear and despair but also as being in a dialectical relation to them (Farran et al., 1995; Govier, 2011). Following this line of thought, it could be assumed that whereas anxiety-free values will be positively related to the general feeling of hope, anxiety-avoiding values will be less connected with hope. However, in certain situations, such as an illness, hope could also be motivated from, or at least related to, anxiety and the intention to defeat it. For example, Gravlee (2020) explained that, according to Plato, desperate hope, can have a positive value when fighting for a good cause. Furthermore, aligned with theories that underline the social character of hope (Erikson, 1963; Marcel, 1951; McGeer, 2008), it can be presumed that social values will have a closer connection to hope than values focused on the individual. Based on these considerations, we assume that the values of self-transcendent and openness to change will have a strong and self-enhancement values a weak connection to hope, and that values belonging to conservation will be somewhere in between.

3.2.5 Personal and Cultural Values

Schwartz (2012) argued that values characterize cultural groups and societies, that his theory describes basic human values, which people in most cultures embrace, and that there is a universal structure of human motivations. However, he clearly distinguished between personal and cultural values (Schwartz, 2014a). The culture of a society consists of certain cultural value orientations such as egalitarianism vs. hierarchy, autonomy vs. social embeddedness and mastery vs. harmony. The culture of each society is located somewhere in between these polarities and expresses ideals of what is good and desirable, in the present and in the future. Does a society value more performance or caring, power, or social justice, traditions, or innovation? These normative standards confront people with certain expectations about how to think and behave (Schwartz, 2006, 2013).

Conceptually and methodologically, it is important to note that Schwartz (2014b, p. 6) defined societal culture "as the latent, normative value system, external to the individual, which underlies and justifies the functioning of societal institutions". This definition conceptualizes societal culture as a latent construct that cannot be observed directly but it can be inferred from prevalent social manifestations such as meaning, beliefs, symbols, and practices. Moreover, as a latent construct, societal culture is part of people's context, shaped by its material environment (e.g., its geography, natural resources, and history) and therefore external to the individual. Consequently, the normative cultural value system is not per se located in the mind of the individual, but it influences it via the organization, the practices, and policies of societal institutions (e.g., the political, legal and education systems).

From a methodological point of view, cultural values cannot be simply observed aggregating individual value scores since these are also influenced by individual characteristics. Moreover, besides the dominant or overarching cultural values, a variety of ethnic, professional, religious etc. subcultures and value systems co-exist. In each group, the meaning ascribed to a certain value can differ significantly (Steinmetz et al., 2009). For example, whereas personal achievement can be a springboard to get more power and prestige for men, for women it could be much more related to autonomy and independence (Struch et al., 2002). For young people, success might be connected to pleasure, novelty and risk taking, while for older people it might be linked to security. People belonging to a social or cultural group can internalize and share a set of values that defines the social or cultural identity of the group (Schwartz et al., 2008).

However, in any society, we encounter certain prevailing normative values that are a central element of its culture, and which influences the thoughts, goals, and behaviors of the individual through social expectations and taken-for-granted beliefs (Schwartz, 2008). In methodological terms, Schwartz argued that individuals and cultural groups differ in their responses to the values questionnaire. For this reason, he recommended making a correction for individual differences by centering the individual responses. Using centered values, the differences in the observed mean scores between samples of participants from different cultures can reflect the differences in the latent cultural values. That is, the mean scores themselves are not the cultural values but they can indicate a certain tendency when comparing them to other cultures.

3.2.6 Human Values and the Phenomenon of Hope

The interactions between basic human values, the general perception of hope and the significance of individual hopes are presuppositions that still need to be examined in more detail. The first possible connection between human values and hope is the assumption that certain values foster the overall perception of hope or, simply speaking, can increase hopefulness. Sagiv and Schwartz (2000) have already argued that particular values can promote well-being. Joshanloo and Ghaedi (2009) found that a number of values were correlated particularly with life domains promoting eudaimonic well-being.

Slezackova and colleagues (Slezackova et al., 2018) explored the role of life values in subjective well-being among Czech and Maltese university students. They found that Czech and Maltese students did not differ significantly in life satisfaction and happiness levels. However, differences were revealed in the hierarchy of their life values and their relationship to subjective well-being. This study has pointed out that cultures might differ in the importance they assign to various life values, and that cognitive and affective components of subjective well-being might be predicted by unique variables in different national samples.

Following the values-as-moderator model of Oishi et al. (1999), which postulates that the level of well-being in a country is moderated by personal values influenced by cultural characteristics, we assume that the level of hope is connected with the personal values and the targets of hope people might have. If hope, in terms of a positive future orientation, is an element of well-being (Slezackova, 2017; Slezackova & Krafft, 2017), we could expect that values may be a significant source of hope.

However, as Schwartz (2011) suggested in relation to well-being, some values can have a positive effect in promoting hope and other values can undermine it. Accordingly, this means that certain targets of hope (e.g., pro-social hopes) will have a positive effect on people's general level of hope and other types of hopes (e.g., the strive for power) may be detrimental to hope. Schwartz (2009) has already suggested that stimulation, self-direction, universalism, and benevolence are "growth" values. The more these values are attained, the more valuable and important they become. Alternately, other values such as power and security are "defensive" values. These values are only or especially important when they are lacking.

These reflections can lead to the general idea that to hope for certain things will probably affect the way we hope (Averill et al., 1990). People can hold different types of hopes such as material goods, personal achievements, hedonic pursuits, interpersonal relationships, and altruistic motives (Averill & Sundararajan, 2005), which might also have an effect on the quality of the general perception of hope. It might not be the same to hope for the achievement of a specific career goal, for a happy partnership or for more religious or spiritual experiences.

Moreover, people in different nations and cultures can coincide or differ with regard to what is most relevant to them. Hope might be related to the basic understanding of what is a good life (Krafft & Walker, 2018a). Triandis (1995), for example, distinguished between individualist and collectivist cultures based on the type of goals that people have. People in individualistic societies tend to hold and pursue more self-centered goals that reflect personal wishes, whereas people in more collectivist cultures tend to value goals related to the desires and wishes of the family and the closer social environment, including good social relationships, to be in harmony with their environment and to support others (Triandis, 1997). In the first case, the focus is on the accomplishment of one's own wishes and desires, on personal success and on novel experiences. Goals have to be achieved by one's own efforts. In the other case, people appreciate tolerance, respect, and the care for others (Eid & Diener, 2009; Park & Huebner, 2005).

3.3 The Present Study

3.3.1 Objectives

The general purpose of the current study is to explore the notion that human values are related to or influence both the general level of perceived hope as well as the formation and importance of certain individual targets of hope. Therefore, our first goal is to assess how far basic value orientations predict the level of hope in different cultures and if we could find common patterns and individual characteristics across countries. Based on previous research, we hypothesize that (1) anxiety-free values (self-transcendence and openness to change) will be positively connected to hope and that (2) anxiety-avoiding values (conservation and self-enhancement) will be only slightly, not at all or even negatively related to hope.

Before comparing mean scores of perceived hope and relate them to the ten value orientations, two prerequisites have to be tested. Firstly, we have to assess whether the items of our instrument to measure perceived hope have been interpreted similarly by the participants in each cultural sample. Secondly, we would like to assess if the ten basic values mirror the circular continuum and the two bipolar dimensions and whether some particularities emerge in the individual samples.

Our second goal is to explore the basic assumption that what people hope for can be influenced by their value orientations. While people in some cultures might be more inclined to cherish individual achievements, people in other cultures could give more importance to the quality of social relationships or to altruistic motives (Park & Huebner, 2005). Furthermore, we would like to assess which individual targets of hope have a stronger or weaker connection to the general perception of hopefulness. Our assumption here is that targets of hope oriented to foster eudaimonic well-being will be positively related to perceived hope and that material and hedonistic targets of hope will not or at least less strongly related.

3.3.2 Procedure and Participant Samples

The five samples of our study were part of the online survey of the Hope Barometer in November 2018. Participants were recruited through newspapers via online advertisement, social media, and e-mails. No incentives were offered. The inclusion criterion was a minimum age of 18. In total, 6134 people completed the questionnaire, from which 302 were excluded due to a high number of missing values, erroneous answers (e.g., always 0 or 1) and multivariate outliers.

We included five samples into the analyses with participants from German ($N = 3049$) and French speaking Switzerland ($N = 1109$), Spain ($N = 528$), Portugal ($N = 808$) and the Czech Republic ($N = 338$). Switzerland is the country with the highest GDP per capita (U$S 87,000.-) followed by the Czech Republic (U$S 42,000.-), Spain (U$S 38,000.-) and Portugal (U$S 34,000.-). In Appendix 3.1 we present the demographic structure of the five samples.

Gender distribution was quite balanced in the two Swiss samples (around 40% male and 60% female). In the other three samples, we have considerably more female than male participants. The age structure is close to that of the general population in the Swiss samples, where the national median is MED = 42.7, but below the average in Spain (MED = 43.9), Portugal (MED = 44.6), and the Czech Republic (MED = 43.3).

When looking at the structure of the education level we have to consider the diverse national education systems. Switzerland has a very popular and high quality dual vocational training system. This is the reason why almost three quarters of the participants in our samples hold a professional training diploma. In the Spanish and Portuguese samples, we find about two thirds of the participants with a tertiary or university degree. In the Czech Republic, around half of the sample has secondary education and more than 40% a university degree. In these three countries, the education level of our participants is presumably higher than the average of the population.

Regarding marital status, main activity and professional status, the structure across countries is visibly more homogeneous. Whereas in Switzerland the sample includes more people with a part-time job than in the other countries, the number of people in education or training is higher in Spain, Portugal, and the Czech Republic.

Overall, the German and French samples from Switzerland is more representative of the general population than the Spanish, Portuguese, and Czech samples, where most participants are female, younger and with a higher education level than the average of the general population. These biases must be taken into account when analyzing, comparing and interpreting the results of our study.

3.3.3 Measures

For the purpose of this study, we used instruments to measure (1) the general level hope, (2) the centrality of several targets of hope, and (3) the basic human values. The questionnaires were administered in the local language: German and French in Switzerland, Spanish in Spain, Portuguese in Portugal, and Czech in the Czech Republic.

Perceived Hope Scale

The Perceived Hope Scale (PHS) is a six-item one-dimensional self-rating instrument to measure the level of hope in a direct manner and free from any preconceptions regarding the nature and quality of hope (Krafft et al., 2017, 2021; Águeda

Marujo et al., 2021; Slezackova et al., 2020). The PHS was developed with the specific purpose to assess the level of general hope in different cultures avoiding any bias regarding potential dimensions and elements of hope. It evaluates the perceived degree of hope in one's life and specifically when facing difficult situations, the belief in the fulfillment of one's hopes and the intensity of hope vis-à-vis the feeling of anxiety, independently from possible roots and sources. The six positively worded items can be rated on a 6-point Likert scale from 0 (strongly disagree) to 5 (strongly agree). In the current study the six items achieved a high internal consistency in all samples with Cronbach alpha values between $\alpha = 0.88$ and $\alpha = 0.90$.

Hope Targets
Personal hopes are things or domains in life that are of particular important to the individual and which are considered desirable, possible, or achievable, regardless of whether their probability of occurrence is assessed as high or low. The focus is therefore on the significance of the hoped-for things in people's life, rather than on the subjectively assessed expectation of occurrence. In order to assess the centrality of several targets of hope as previously done by Staats (1989) and Erickson et al. (1975), we used a pool of 17 life domains in terms of people's personal hopes for the coming year (Krafft & Walker, 2018a, 2018b). Participants could rate their hopes on a 4-point scale from "0 = not important" to "3 = very important". The 17 areas of life cover six different categories:

1. Personal well-being (e.g., personal health, harmony)
2. Social relationships (e.g., happy marriage, family, partnership)
3. Success and material goods (e.g., more money)
4. Pleasure (e.g., more sex, romantic experiences)
5. Meaning, purpose and altruism (e.g., a meaningful task and being able to help other people)
6. Religious and spiritual experiences.

Portrait Values Questionnaire RR
The refined portrait values questionnaire (PVQ-RR) consists of 57 items assigned to 19 sub-dimensions (3 items each) of the ten values types (Schwartz et al., 2012, 2017). Every item is formulated as a short description of a person who has a high motivation regarding the value dimension addressed. The respondents are asked to indicate how much this person is like themselves on a scale ranging from 0 ("this person is not at all like me") to 5 ("this person is completely like me").

In our study, we performed all analyses using the original ten value dimensions and the four higher order value types. For our purposes and following a variant suggested by Schwartz, we calculated the overall value of the category "openness to change" using the two dimensions "self-direction" and "stimulation" and handled "hedonism" as an individual variable. The individual dimensions achieved a satisfactory to good internal consistency in all samples: Self-transcendence ($\alpha = 0.86$ to 0.88) consisting of benevolence ($\alpha = 0.78$ to 0.86) and universalism ($\alpha = 0.84$ to 0.87); openness to change ($\alpha = 0.77$ to 0.82) entailing self-direction ($\alpha = 0.78$ to 0.80) and stimulation ($\alpha = 0.71$ to 0.74); conservation ($\alpha = 0.80$ to 0.87) comprising tradition ($\alpha = 0.76$ to 0.86), security ($\alpha = 0.75$ to 0.82) and conformity ($\alpha = 0.72$ to 0.83); self-enhancement ($\alpha = 0.81$ to 0.87) involving achievement ($\alpha = 0.67$ to 0.78) and power ($\alpha = 0.79$ to 0.86) and finally hedonism ($\alpha = 0.75$ to 0.82).

3.3.4 Data Analysis

All statistical analyses were performed with IBM SPSS and AMOS version 27.0. Before commencing with the descriptive and correlational analyses, we need to demonstrate measurement invariance of the perceived hope scale across the five samples via multi-group Confirmatory Factor Analysis (MGCFA). The fit of the general model by means of maximum likelihood estimation was evaluated using the following indices: Comparative fit index (CFI) and Tucker-Lewis index (TLI) (study criterion ≥ 0.95 as ideal and ≥ 0.90 as the minimum acceptable level), root mean square error of approximation (RMSEA) (study criterion ≤ 0.08) and the standardized root mean residual SRMR (study criterion ≤ 0.08) (Hu & Bentler, 1999). The test for measurement invariance was performed in different steps, from configurational invariance (equal form), to metric invariance (equal loadings), to scalar invariance (equal intercepts), and finally to strict invariance (equal residuals). The recommended criteria to demonstrate invariance are changes in CFI and TLI between comparison and nested models of ≥ -0.010, a change in RMSEA of ≤ 0.015 and a variation in SRMR of ≤ 0.030 (for loading invariance) and ≤ 0.010 (for intercept invariance) (Chen, 2007).

One central element of Schwartz's value theory is the proposition that the single values are related to each other on a circular motivational continuum. The individual value dimensions are located on the circular continuum according to the proximity or the distance of certain motives and general life orientations they represent (e.g., anxiety avoiding vs. anxiety free and individual vs. social focus). Using multidimensional scaling (MDS) we can position the value types as points in a bi-dimensional space and evaluate if the empirical data represents the theoretical model. Following the instructions of Schwartz et al. (2012), we performed the SPSS PROXSCAL procedure for each sample independently, calculating ordinal proximity transformations between the variables in a two-dimensional space using Euclidian distances and standardizing the values with z-scores.

The main data analyses were then performed in three steps:

Step 1—Descriptive statistics and mean value comparisons: We started calculating mean values and standard deviations for perceived hope and the variables representing the ten individual and the four higher order value dimensions. We then compared the scores of the single samples via univariate analysis of variance (ANOVA). To perform mean value comparisons of the human values, Schwartz recommends making a correction for individual or cultural differences in the use of the response scale and to calculate centered value scores (Schwartz et al., 2017). For this purpose, a common mean value called MRAT was computed over all raw values. The MRAT is then subtracted from the individual raw score in order to obtain the relative importance of the individual value orientations.

Step 2—Correlation and regression analyses: Computing partial bivariate Pearson correlations we analyzed the relationships between the value dimensions and perceived hope (after controlling for demographic variables) and compared selected results between samples via correlation comparisons (Steiger, 1980). By means of multiple regression analyses, we tested the effect of the higher order value dimensions (plus hedonism) for each sample, as well as the ten individual value orientations to predict perceived hope, beyond demographic characteristics of gender, age, marital status, education, main activity, and professional status. We compared the explained variance (R^2) and the Beta coefficients to identify similarities and differences between samples.

Step 3—Targets of hope—mean values and correlations with perceived hope and human values: The last step was dedicated to assessing the centrality of several targets of hope and their connections to the basic human value dimensions. Using ANOVA, we compared the mean values of the individual samples and correlated the hope targets with the general perception of hope and with the ten value types, again controlling by demographic variables. If fundamental human values are explained in terms of trans-situational motivational goals, as suggested by Schwartz et al. (2012), we expect that individual values will substantially be correlated with specific targets of hope.

3.3.5 Results

3.3.5.1 Measurement Invariance of the PHS

The goal of this first preliminary analysis was to test measurement invariance of the perceived hope scale across the five investigated samples. Table 3.1 presents the fit indices of the multi-group CFA to assess the goodness of fit of the general sample and of the five models to test different levels of group invariance. The one-factor

Table 3.1 Multi-group CFA and analysis of group invariance

	X^2	df	CFI	TLI	RMSEA	SRMR
Total sample ($N = 5832$)	278.96	9	0.986	0.977	0.072	0.020
Country/sample invariance						
Configurational invariance (equal form)	1569.75	99	0.924	0.943	0.050	0.028
Metric invariance (equal loadings)	1604.46	104	0.923	0.944	0.050	0.027
Scalar invariance (equal intercepts)	1673.57	110	0.919	0.945	0.049	0.027
Full uniqueness (measurement residuals)	1714.61	117	0.918	0.947	0.048	0.027

Note: *CFA* Confirmatory Factor Analysis, *CFI* Comparative fit index, *TLI* Tucker-Lewis index, *RMSEA* Root mean square error of approximation, *SRMR* Standardized root mean residual

model for the total sample revealed a good model fit (CFI and TLI > 0.95, RMSEA and SRMR < 0.08). Furthermore, every single sample was tested and an acceptable to good model fit was obtained (CFI and TLI ≥ 0.94, RMSEA and SRMR ≤ 0.08). The first step of configurational invariance across the groups (equal form) also provided a good fit to the data and can therefore be used as baseline model. All further models compared to the baseline model were under the threshold values recommended by the literature (CFI and TLI > 0.01, RMSEA and SRMR < 0.015). These results indicate that the PHS reveals strong measurement invariance across the investigated cultural samples and that we can compare the individual scores. This means that perceived hope has been conceptualized in a similar form across these cultures and that correlation analyses with other constructs are possible.

3.3.5.2 Multidimensional Scaling of Basic Human Values

Regarding the basic human values, we firstly wanted to establish whether the ten categories displayed a similar pattern to Schwartz's theoretical model. The diagrams in Fig. 3.2 map the results of the multidimensional scaling analyses. In all samples the variables exhibited a good approximation to the theorized model, in which the self-transcendence categories (benevolence and universalism) are opposed to the self-enhancement variables (achievement and power) and where openness values (self-direction, stimulation and hedonism) are in contrast to the self-enhancement types (achievement and power).

Beyond these common patterns, the diagrams of the single samples exhibit some individual characteristics, worthwhile to be mentioned. In some samples (Spain, Portugal, and Czech Republic.), stimulation and hedonism were very close (distances between 0.072 and 0.177) and self-direction was in-between stimulation/hedonism and benevolence/universalism. In the Spanish group, self-direction was even adjacent to the social dimensions universalism (distance 0.254) and benevolence (0.595) and distant to the individual focused dimensions stimulation (0.895) and hedonism (0.770), which were nearer to achievement (0.452 and 0.618). This means that self-direction indicates reliance on one's own ideas and actions, not always focusing on selfish interests, but also engaging oneself for the well-being of others. Moreover, in the Portuguese sample, tradition was more distant from security and conformity than it usually is, suggesting that tradition could have a particular quality in the Portuguese society.

These results imply that our data represents Schwartz's model appropriately but that the ten basic values may be interpreted differently in various countries or cultures. Specifically, the values of self-direction and tradition seem to have additional attributes worth to be examined more in detail.

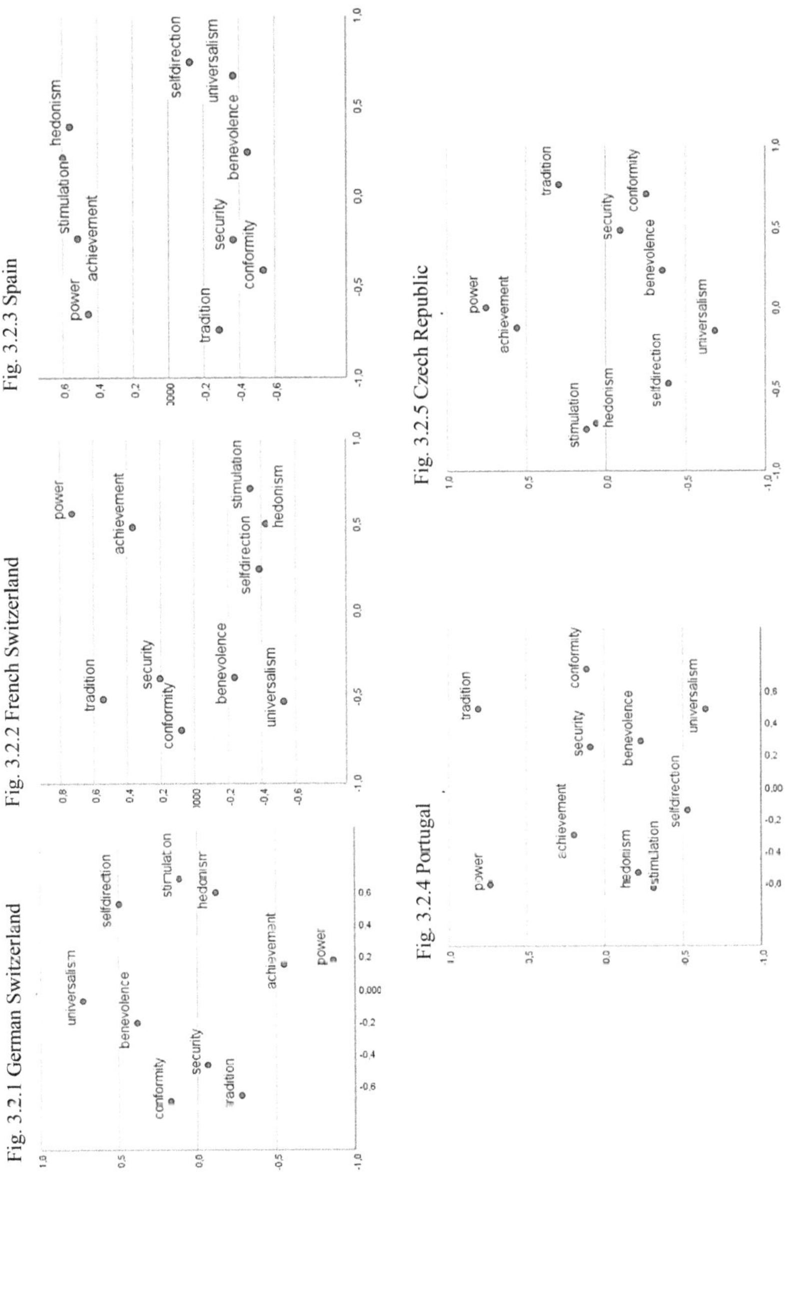

Fig. 3.2 Multivariate scaling of basic value dimensions by sample

3.3.5.3 Comparing Levels of Perceived Hope and Basic Human Values Between Samples

The next step was to compare levels of perceived hope between the samples through ANOVA and post hoc analyses. The results in Table 3.2 exhibit moderate to high levels of perceived hope, with small but significant differences between samples. Portugal and the Czech Republic display the highest levels of hope, significantly higher than the other three samples ($p < 0.01$), followed by the German Swiss and the Spanish and finally the French Swiss with the significantly lowest mean value ($p < 0.01$) Only in German Switzerland, women ($M = 3.46$; $SD = 0.95$) exhibit significant higher levels of hope than men ($M = 3.31$; $SD = 1.10$). In all other samples, the PHS scores between men and women did not differ significantly. This is important to note since in the Spanish, Portuguese, and Czech samples the number of women considerably exceeded the number of men. Furthermore, the level of hope increased with age. In all countries, older people tended to be significantly more hopeful than younger. This is also relevant to be considered, since the age structure amongst the Spanish, Portuguese and Czech participants is significantly younger than in the Swiss groups. This means that the higher levels of hope in Portugal and the Czech Republic cannot be attributed to the different gender and age structures of the samples.

Our main question was to establish to what extent differences in the general level of hope can partially be explained by the intensity of culturally colored basic human values. To compare the mean coefficients of the basic human values across cultures we used centered values as recommended by Schwartz et al. (2017). The coefficients in Table 3.2 show that across all samples the highest coefficients belonged to benevolence, universalism, self-direction, security, and hedonism and the lowest to the power dimension. In general terms, the dimension of self-transcendence was rated the highest, followed by openness to change, then by conservation and finally by self-enhancement. This pattern was similar in all samples.

Comparing the indicators of the four higher-order and the ten individual value types between samples, some noteworthy results emerged. Portugal demonstrated the second highest level of self-transcendence (after Spain), due to the pronounced level of universalism. Together with German speaking Switzerland, Portugal displayed a higher coefficient of conservation, especially due to the significantly higher level of conformity. At the same time, the Portuguese sample showed the second highest level of self-enhancement (after the Czech Republic.), due to the highest level of achievement. In comparison to the other samples, the Portuguese presented the lowest coefficient in openness to change, since both dimensions, self-direction, and stimulation, together with hedonism were the lowest.

The Czech Republic, the country with the second-highest level of hope, revealed a different pattern. First, this sample showed the highest level of self-enhancement, especially because of the highest coefficient in the power dimension. Although levels of security and conformity were the lowest of all samples, tradition was the highest (together with the German-Swiss). Furthermore, the Czechs had the second lowest scores of self-direction and hedonism after the Portuguese, but the highest level of stimulation.

Table 3.2 Mean values, standard deviations and univariate analysis of variance by sample

	Swiss German $N = 3049$		Swiss French $N = 1109$		Spain $N = 528$		Portugal $N = 808$		Czech Rep. $N = 338$		ANOVA	
	M	*SD*	*M*	*SD*	*M*	*SD*	*M*	*SD*	*M*	*SD*	*F*	sig.
Perceived Hope	3.40	1.02	2.93	1.15	3.42	0.93	3.59	0.95	3.59	0.95	63.91	<0.001
Self-transcendence	4.48	0.50	4.49	0.52	4.68	0.43	4.60	0.38	4.53	0.44	26.15	<0.001
Openness to change	4.47	0.59	4.36	0.65	4.33	0.54	4.19	0.48	4.34	0.56	41.33	<0.001
Conservation	3.90	0.59	3.80	0.59	3.72	0.58	3.88	0.47	3.71	0.59	19.25	<0.001
Self-enhancement	2.81	0.81	2.79	0.77	2.64	0.73	2.94	0.70	3.09	0.77	22.79	<0.001
Benevolence	4.96	0.54	4.86	0.61	4.90	0.49	4.83	0.42	4.83	0.52	17.43	<0.001
Universalism	4.16	0.72	4.24	0.73	4.53	0.60	4.45	0.53	4.32	0.63	53.95	<0.001
Self-direction	4.83	0.65	4.72	0.66	4.64	0.62	4.50	0.52	4.57	0.61	53.99	<0.001
Stimulation	3.76	0.92	3.65	1.07	3.71	0.98	3.57	0.90	3.88	0.93	10.08	<0.001
Hedonism	4.22	0.94	4.51	0.85	4.36	0.87	4.01	0.80	4.15	0.86	43.33	<0.001
Tradition	3.44	1.20	3.11	1.13	2.81	1.08	2.98	1.18	3.42	1.09	55.43	<0.001
Security	4.33	0.65	4.54	0.65	4.24	0.57	4.33	0.46	4.09	0.64	46.09	<0.001
Conformity	3.87	0.78	3.80	0.84	3.96	0.75	4.09	0.58	3.68	0.77	26.24	<0.001
Achievement	3.85	0.90	3.72	0.88	3.69	0.83	4.18	0.64	3.89	0.87	41.97	<0.001
Power	2.29	0.94	2.32	0.90	2.11	0.87	2.32	0.90	2.69	0.90	21.03	<0.001

The French Swiss, the group with the lowest level of perceived hope, exhibited the second lowest level of universalism and stimulation (together with Spain), the highest levels among all samples in security and hedonism and the second highest in self-direction (after the German Swiss).

People in German speaking Switzerland and in Spain displayed similar levels of perceived hope. Spain exhibited the highest scores in universalism and therefore also in self-transcendence, and it has the lowest scores in self-enhancement, in both dimensions of power and achievement (together with the French Swiss), as well as in tradition. The German Swiss presented the highest scores in benevolence, self-direction, and tradition (together with the Czechs) but the lowest in universalism. These figures bring about higher coefficients of openness to change and at the same time of conservation.

To summarize, Portugal and Spain had the highest levels of self-transcendence (especially of universalism), and both Swiss regions and the Czech Republic the lowest. The German Swiss had higher scores in openness to change and the Portuguese the lowest. Spain and the Czech, both displayed the lowest levels of conservation, however, due to different reasons: The Spanish were lower in tradition while the Czech were lower in conformity and security. Regarding self-enhancement, the Czech achieve the highest scores, especially regarding the search for power, and the Spanish the lowest.

3.3.5.4 Correlations and Regression Analyses with Perceived Hope

Partial bivariate Pearson Correlations

Before presenting the results of the hierarchical regression analyses in search of significant predictors of perceived hope, we examined the partial bivariate correlation coefficients reported in Table 3.3 (the correlation coefficients including all variables for the entire sample are presented in the Appendix 3.2). In general terms, the correlation coefficients of most dimensions of basic values with perceived hope were significant and positive, but the effect sizes were relatively small and quite similar across samples. Using the Fisher r-to-z transformations, we calculated z-values to assess the significance of the difference between two correlation coefficients from two independent samples (Eid et al., 2011).

The most striking results can be summarized as follows: Regarding the four higher order dimensions, the only significant difference is the positive correlation coefficient between self-enhancement and perceived hope in the Czech sample. This can be explained by a significant correlation coefficient of perceived hope with power and a higher correlation value with achievement. Striking is also the lower correlation score between stimulation and perceived hope in the Spanish sample. Other slightly higher correlation coefficients with perceived hope, although not achieving statistical significance, were related to the dimensions self-direction and security in the French Swiss sample. All other coefficients were similar across countries.

Table 3.3 Partial bivariate Pearson correlation coefficients of human values with perceived hope by sample

	German Swiss	French Swiss	Spain	Portugal	Czech Republic
	$N = 3049$	$N = 1109$	$N = 528$	$N = 808$	$N = 338$
Self-transcendence	0.282**	0.327**	0.243**	0.277**	0.296**
Openness to change	0.266**	0.296**	0.216**	0.247**	0.232**
Conservation	0.134**	0.197**	0.116**	0.189**	0.134*
Self-enhancement	0.059**	0.111**	0.080	−0.003	0.222**
Benevolence	0.229**	0.274**	0.223**	0.217**	0.302**
Universalism	0.252**	0.293**	0.198**	0.252**	0.223**
Self-direction	0.198**	0.247**	0.203**	0.144**	0.143**
Stimulation	0.258**	0.267**	0.143**	0.278**	0.262**
Tradition	0.130**	0.136**	0.127**	0.202**	0.225**
Security	0.125**	0.206**	0.121**	0.172**	0.163**
Conformity	0.090**	0.160**	0.072	0.083*	0.010
Achievement	0.116**	0.224**	0.095*	0.146**	0.279**
Power	0.020	0.031	0.061	−0.063	0.163**
Hedonism	0.263**	0.258**	0.211**	0.203**	0.253**

Note: **. Correlation is significant at 0.01 level; *. Correlation is significant at 0.05 level
Control variables: Gender, age, marital status, education, main activity, and professional status

Hierarchical Regression Analyses

We performed two series of hierarchical regression analyses to predict the variance of perceived hope. In the first series, we entered the demographic variables in the first step and then added the four higher order value dimensions plus hedonism in the second step (Table 3.4). In the second series of analyses, we again started with the demographic variables and included the ten individual value dimensions in the second step (Table 3.5). Initially, the higher order values presented in Table 3.4 explained between 7.4% (Spain) and 13.5% (Czech Republic) of the variance in perceived hope. When applying the ten value dimensions, the predictive effect rose to between 9.3% (Spain) and 20% (Czech Republic) (see Table 3.5). This means that basic values have a significant impact on hope but that the magnitude of the effect varies across cultures.

Considering the demographic variables, we found that these were stronger predictors of hope in Portugal. Specifically, age, marital status and professional status had significant effects on hope. Older people were much more hopeful than younger, married people and those living in a partnership more than singles, and the higher the professional position the higher the level of hope. In German Switzerland, the effects of the demographic variables were lower, but all variables had a significant effect. After the professional position, marital status and age, gender and education also significantly predicted hope. Women were slightly more hopeful than men and the higher the education the higher the level of hope. The French Swiss sample

Table 3.4 Hierarchical regression analyses with fundamental values predicting perceived hope by sample

Dependent Variable: Perceived Hope	German Swiss $N = 3049$		French Swiss $N = 1109$		Spain $N = 528$		Portugal $N = 808$		Czech Rep. $N = 338$	
	Std. β	Sig.	Std. β	Sig.	Std. β	Sig.	Std. β	Sig.	Std. β	Sig.
Step 1: Demographic variables										
Gender	0.066	<0.001	0.030	0.316	−0.055	0.188	0.024	0.443	0.066	0.215
Age	0.144	<0.001	0.073	0.049	0.129	0.070	0.145	0.007	0.059	0.428
Marital status	0.084	<0.001	0.059	0.059	0.113	0.058	0.171	<0.001	0.054	0.424
Education	0.068	<0.001	0.007	0.804	0.071	0.103	−0.005	0.873	0.069	0.186
Main activity	−0.041	0.031	0.027	0.413	0.007	0.916	0.073	0.120	<0.001	0.997
Professional status	0.118	<0.001	0.103	<0.001	0.071	0.137	0.160	<0.001	0.127	0.036
Step 2: Fundamental human values										
Self-transcendence	0.168	<0.001	0.206	<0.001	0.138	0.014	0.127	0.001	0.274	<0.001
Openness to change	0.120	<0.001	0.140	<0.001	0.078	0.155	0.140	<0.001	−0.024	0.724
Conservation	0.028	0.144	0.036	0.291	0.038	0.437	0.102	0.004	−0.050	0.438
Self-enhancement	−0.019	0.300	0.016	0.622	0.013	0.802	−0.083	0.016	0.191	0.001
Hedonism	0.172	<0.001	0.094	0.007	0.112	0.026	0.083	0.025	0.126	0.033
	Δ adj. R^2	Sig. Change	Δ adj. R^2	Sig. Change	Δ adj. R^2	Sig. Change	Δ adj. R^2	Sig. Change	Δ adj. R^2	Sig. Change
Model 1 (demographics)	0.061	<0.001	0.027	<0.001	0.075	<0.001	0.189	<0.001	0.053	0.006
Model 2 (demographics + value dimensions)	0.120	<0.001	0.132	<0.001	0.074	<0.001	0.093	<0.001	0.135	<0.001
Total adj. R^2	0.182	<0.001	0.159	<0.001	0.150	<0.001	0.282	<0.001	0.188	<0.001

Table 3.5 Hierarchical regression analyses with single value dimensions to predict perceived hope by sample

Dependent Variable: Perceived Hope	German Swiss $N = 3049$		French Swiss $N = 1109$		Spain $N = 528$		Portugal $N = 808$		Czech Rep. $N = 338$	
	Std. β	Sig.	Std. β	Sig.	Std. β	Sig.	Std. β	Sig.	Std. β	Sig.
Step 1: Demographic variables										
Gender	0.068	<0.001	0.029	0.327	−0.044	0.303	0.030	0.337	0.056	0.293
Age	0.145	<0.001	0.096	0.010	0.108	0.133	0.156	0.003	0.081	0.266
Marital status	0.084	<0.001	0.060	0.053	0.116	0.052	0.168	<0.001	0.068	0.305
Education	0.070	<0.001	−0.002	0.952	0.071	0.107	−0.001	0.966	0.032	0.544
Main activity	−0.040	0.035	0.033	0.308	−0.005	0.940	0.067	0.150	0.004	0.953
Professional status	0.112	<0.001	0.097	0.001	0.066	0.168	0.146	<0.001	0.130	0.027
Step 2: Basic human values										
Benevolence	0.071	0.001	0.095	0.011	0.121	0.020	0.042	0.280	0.195	0.004
Universalism	0.128	<0.001	0.129	<0.001	0.086	0.112	0.135	<0.001	0.172	0.009
Self-direction	0.044	0.023	0.011	0.755	0.117	0.021	0.009	0.802	−0.094	0.110
Stimulation	0.103	<0.001	0.135	<0.001	−0.016	0.764	0.161	<0.001	0.040	0.566
Tradition	0.082	<0.001	0.044	0.173	0.136	0.010	0.186	<0.001	0.217	0.001
Security	−0.022	0.342	0.010	0.792	−0.052	0.368	0.021	0.614	−0.046	0.513
Conformity	−0.017	0.422	0.004	0.917	−0.045	0.406	−0.077	0.036	−0.212	0.001
Achievement	0.019	0.399	0.137	<0.001	−0.043	0.468	0.062	0.152	0.197	0.005
Power	−0.043	0.043	−0.099	0.004	0.035	0.525	−0.129	<0.001	−0.003	0.960
Hedonism	0.159	<0.001	0.079	0.025	0.131	0.014	0.040	0.313	0.102	0.110
Model summary	Δ adj. R^2	Sig. Change	Δ adj. R^2	Sig. Change	Δ adj. R^2	Sig. Change	Δ adj. R^2	Sig. Change	Δ adj. R^2	Sig. Change
Model 1 (demographics)	0.061	<0.001	0.027	<0.001	0.075	<0.001	0.189	<0.001	0.053	0.006
Model 2 (demographics + value dimensions)	0.127	<0.001	0.149	<0.001	0.093	<0.001	0.131	<0.001	0.200	<0.001
Total adj. R^2	0.188	<0.001	0.177	<0.001	0.168	<0.001	0.320	<0.001	0.253	<0.001

displayed a much lower effect of demographics on hope, similar to the results of the Czech sample, where only professional status had a positive impact.

Observing the results in Table 3.4, it is evident that self-transcendence, hedonism, and openness to change were significant predictors of hope in almost all samples, and that conservation and self-enhancement only had small effects on hope in one or two cases. The Swiss samples and Spain showed similar results. In French speaking Switzerland, self-transcendence clearly had the strongest effect on hope. However, people in Switzerland also presented the lowest mean values in self-transcendence (Table 3.2).

The results for Portugal and the Czech Republic, the two countries with the highest mean levels of hope, were remarkably different. In the Portuguese sample, conservation emerged as a positive and self-enhancement as a negative predictor of hope. A more detailed analysis in Table 3.5 reveals the relevance of tradition and the negative impact of power seeking. Furthermore, stimulation (belonging to openness) and universalism (as part of self-transcendence) appear to be significant. A different picture emerged for Czech sample. Here self-transcendence and self-enhancement had a significant impact on hope (Table 4). Whereas conformity had a negative effect, benevolence, universalism, tradition, and achievement stood out as having a positive impact on hope (Table 3.5).

The detailed results in Table 3.5 show that security, conformity, and power had no or sometimes even a negative impact on hope, which indicate that these values are oriented to self-protection and are anxiety-based, as suggested by Schwartz and Cieciuch (2016). Alternately, tradition, displayed a positive effect on hope in four samples and achievement also showed a positive impact in French Switzerland and the Czech Republic. Moreover, stimulation seemed to have a stronger impact on hope than self-direction (except in Spain), aligned with its growth orientation and anxiety-free quality proposed by Schwartz. Hedonism was positively related to hope in Switzerland and Spain but not in Portugal and the Czech Republic.

Overall, our results suggest that self-transcendent values of benevolence and universalism were almost always positively related to hope, reinforcing, and expanding their anxiety-free character. Openness to change was also related to hope in most cases, with exception of the Czech Republic. Stimulation and hedonism (the willingness to experience new challenges and to enjoy life) seemed to be more significant to hope than self-direction (freedom to think, act and unfold one's ideas and abilities). Conservation and self-enhancement values were hardly and sometimes even negatively related to hope, as power orientation and conformity showed. However, the value of tradition (culture, family, and religion) and in some cases also achievement (personal success and competence) did not only seem to be anxiety-avoiding, but also hope enhancing, as results from the Czech Republic and in Portugal (for tradition) demonstrate.

3.3.5.5 Targets of Hope

In the conceptual section of this chapter, we explained that national circumstances, cultural conditions, and values have an impact on what people might hope for. One of the cultural factors that may influence the targets of hope is the degree of individualism/collectivism and long-term/short-term orientation. While individualistic cultures tend to emphasize individual achievement orientation (e.g., agency, autonomy, and personal independence), collectivistic cultures emphasize relationship orientation, i.e., interdependence, relational goals, social support, and relational harmony (Uchida & Ogihara, 2012). Long-term vs. short-term orientation associates the connection of the past with current and future actions. A higher degree of long-term orientation indicates that society views adaptation and pragmatic problem-solving as a necessity. On the other hand, in societies with a lower degree in this index (short-term) traditions are kept and honored, while steadfastness is valued (Hofstede, 2001). The comparison of these two cultural dimensions between Czech Republic, Portugal, Spain, and Switzerland shows that Czech Republic and Switzerland score significantly higher in individualism and long-term orientation than Portugal and Spain. Portugal shows the lowest levels in both dimensions compared to the other three countries (Hofstede-Insights, 2022). However, the comparisons should be interpreted with caution, since data came from different and non-representative samples. In the final step of our study, we therefore compared and analyzed the targets of hope of the investigated samples and correlated these targets with perceived hope and the dimensions of basic values.

Comparison of Mean Values

Based on the mean scores of the 17 targets of hope and the ANOVA effects in Table 3.6, we firstly describe the main similarities and the more striking particularities of the specific countries.

In all five samples, the main targets of hope were good health, a happy partnership, family or marriage and harmony in life (with only small differences between the countries). This was followed by personal independence, good and trusting relationships, and having a meaningful task in life. In all countries, these targets of hope, which represent dimensions of eudaimonic well-being, were considerably more important than materialistic and hedonic goals such as more sex and more money.

Significant differences appeared between the somewhat "younger" and "poorer" national samples (Spain, Portugal, and the Czech Republic) and Switzerland. Whereas in Switzerland it was much more cherished to be engaged in a meaningful task than being successful at the workplace or university, the younger sample in Spain, Portugal and the Czech Republic considered having success in their activities as more important than having a meaningful task. Moreover, having a secure job was more important for people in Portugal and Spain, and of less value in Switzerland

Table 3.6 Targets of hope—mean values, standard deviations and univariate analysis of variance by sample

	German Swiss $N = 3049$		French Swiss $N = 1109$		Spain $N = 528$		Portugal $N = 808$		Czech Rep. $N = 338$		ANOVA	
	M	*SD*	*M*	*SD*	*M*	*SD*	*M*	*SD*	*M*	*SD*	*F*	Sig.
Good health	2.77	0.54	2.67	0.63	2.82	0.49	2.85	0.40	2.60	0.72	21.74	<0.001
Happy partnership, family, marriage	2.67	0.67	2.70	0.63	2.62	0.70	2.71	0.61	2.74	0.62	2.62	0.033
Harmony in life	2.53	0.70	2.61	0.62	2.54	0.64	2.68	0.54	2.49	0.76	10.07	<0.001
Good and trusting relationships with other people	2.47	0.72	2.36	0.74	2.57	0.60	2.62	0.60	2.37	0.73	38.02	<0.001
Personal independence and self-determination	2.50	0.71	2.26	0.79	2.37	0.77	2.45	0.73	2.23	0.77	12.64	<0.001
Being engaged in meaningful and satisfying tasks	2.33	0.75	2.21	0.75	2.33	0.71	2.59	0.60	2.13	0.76	39.96	<0.001
More fun with friends	2.09	0.85	2.19	0.78	2.20	0.75	2.16	0.79	2.00	0.89	6.33	<0.001
A secure job	2.07	1.04	2.13	0.96	2.29	0.89	2.35	0.76	1.68	1.08	34.26	<0.001
Order in my life	2.24	0.81	1.57	0.98	2.29	0.74	2.30	0.78	1.85	0.90	158.82	<0.001
More time to relax	2.04	0.91	2.01	0.88	2.12	0.81	2.17	0.78	1.91	0.88	7.36	<0.001
Helping other people	1.92	0.95	2.08	0.87	2.33	0.66	2.50	0.65	2.12	0.79	116.37	<0.001
Success at the workplace, at school/university etc.	1.89	0.97	2.03	0.91	2.35	0.72	2.56	0.65	2.17	0.88	118.22	<0.001
More free time	1.86	0.89	1.94	0.87	2.18	0.79	2.18	0.77	1.98	0.91	21.84	<0.001
More safety in your personal environment	1.87	1.00	1.84	0.98	2.10	0.84	2.18	0.79	1.83	1.09	21.76	<0.001
More sex and romantic experiences	1.76	0.99	1.70	1.04	1.90	0.93	1.90	0.93	2.02	0.96	11.64	<0.001
More money	1.55	0.97	1.78	0.89	1.63	0.84	2.03	0.77	1.51	0.88	51.66	<0.001
More religious and spiritual experiences	0.76	1.00	0.65	0.92	0.82	0.95	1.36	1.10	1.09	1.09	74.70	<0.001

and the least in the Czech Republic. Another remarkable difference between the countries relates to the desire to help other people. In almost all age categories, Portuguese participants showed a significant higher wish to be able to help other people, followed by the Spanish and Czech and finally the Swiss samples.

Comparison of Correlation Coefficients Between Hope Targets and Perceived Hope

Earlier, in the conceptual section of this chapter, we proposed that the everyday perception of hope may be associated with the different targets people might hope for and that this could differ between cultures. In Table 3.7 we present the partial correlation coefficients between the 17 hope targets and the general perception of hope in the five national samples (after controlling for demographic variables). Our findings revealed that certain hopes and desires are closer linked to the general level of perceived hope in most samples and that some cultural differences exist. Across all samples, perceived hope correlated the strongest with the following targets of hope: to help other people, having good and trusting relationships with other people, being engaged in a meaningful task, a happy partnership, family, or marriage and more religious and spiritual experiences. On the other hand, hoping for more money and for a secure job were either not, only slightly or even negatively related to hope. In general terms, the hedonic and materialistic items (e.g., money, success, fun with friends, sex and romantic experiences, time to relax) seemed to be less associated with perceived hope than the social and eudaimonic items (e.g., helping other people, a meaningful task, good relationships to other people).

Besides these general patterns, some minor but noteworthy differences between samples emerged. Portugal displayed the highest correlation coefficients for helping other people, having a meaningful task, religious experiences, and good relationships with other people, and the lowest for success. The Spanish sample exhibited a stronger correlation with success and a happy partnership, family and marriage and the weakest for helping other people. The German Swiss sample showed the lowest coefficients with success and a secure job and a negative correlation between perceived hope and hoping for more money. The Czech sample presented a slightly higher correlation coefficient with good health and the lowest with more free time, more fun with friends and a happy partnership or family. The French Swiss showed a stronger association between hope and harmony in life.

To summarize, the Portuguese seemed to relate hope with altruistic, social, and religious wishes and the Spanish with family and performance. For the German Swiss the materialistic and safety targets are the least associated with hope and the Czech participants linked hope to less hedonic experiences.

Table 3.7 Partial bivariate Pearson correlation coefficients of targets of hope with perceived hope by sample

	German Swiss $N = 3049$	French Swiss $N = 1109$	Spain $N = 528$	Portugal $N = 808$	Czech Rep. $N = 338$
Success at the workplace, at school etc.	0.058**	0.102**	0.184**	0.065	0.139*
Happy partnership, family, marriage	0.185**	0.193**	0.265**	0.206**	0.135*
More free time	0.081**	0.106**	0.120**	0.139**	0.057
More sex and romantic experiences	0.054**	0.095**	0.133**	0.133**	0.206**
More religious and spiritual experiences	0.183**	0.188**	0.175**	0.262**	0.259**
More money	−0.092**	−0.042	−0.001	−0.013	0.052
More fun with friends	0.104**	0.114**	0.142**	0.134**	0.062
More safety in your personal environment	−0.007	0.032	0.061	0.130**	0.108*
Good health	0.169**	0.151**	0.154**	0.150**	0.235**
A secure job	0.010	0.068*	0.080	0.028	0.012
Good and trusting relationships with other people	0.225**	0.242**	0.201**	0.258**	0.193**
Being engaged in meaningful and satisfying tasks	0.198**	0.170**	0.226**	0.277**	0.180**
Order in my life	0.063**	0.143**	0.115**	0.069*	0.088
Personal independence and self-determination	0.115**	0.123**	0.140**	0.091*	0.135*
More time to relax	0.074**	0.036	0.062	0.123**	0.116*
Harmony in life	0.141**	0.237**	0.163**	0.155**	0.201**
Helping other people	0.260**	0.251**	0.134**	0.290**	0.209**

Note: **. Correlation is significant at 0.01 level. *. Correlation is significant at 0.05 level
Control variables: Gender, age, marital status, education, main activity, and professional status

Comparison of Correlation Coefficients between Hope Targets and Basic Values

We found it interesting to examine the correlations between the targets of hope and the single value dimensions, after controlling for demographic variables. The question was: What do people holding certain human values focus their hopes on? The tables in Appendix 3.3 exhibit the correlation coefficients in the five samples and reflect common patterns and national particularities. Firstly, most of the coefficients were significant, but only a few achieved a moderate effect of $r = 0.20$ and higher, on which we will focus our attention.

Some noteworthy findings were common to all samples. Starting with the values of self-transcendence, people higher in benevolence and universalism wished to help other people, to be engaged in a meaningful task, to have good and trusting relationships with other people and enjoy a harmonious life. Moreover, benevolence and universalism were not related to the desire to possess or earn more money. On the other hand, to hope for more money was above all, significantly related to self-enhancement values of achievement and power. Another general finding was the positive relationship between the values of self-direction and stimulation with the desire of more personal independence and self-determination, which can be interpreted as the wish to escape or be liberated (at least in part) from daily external demands and pressures. Hedonism seemed to exhibit some universal patterns too, since it was related to the wish of having fun with friends, with romantic experiences, more free time, and time to relax, and with good relationships with other people in all samples. The values of conservation displayed varied results. All three values, tradition, security, and conformity were generally related to the desire of order in one's life. People for whom security is especially important, also seem to hope for a secure job, for good health, for harmony in life, and for more safety in their personal environment. Tradition was frequently related to the wish for more religious and spiritual experiences, and conformity to some extent with the inclination to help other people. Finally, the achievement value clearly correlated with the desire to be successful at the workplace, university or in other activities. This effect was particularly strong in the Czech Republic.

In addition to these more or less universal features, some remarkable particularities can be highlighted. For example, whereas in Spain and Portugal hedonism (meaning the value of enjoying life and having a good time), had a moderate correlation with the desire for more money, in Switzerland this was much less the case. The wish for success at the workplace and other activities may be the consequence of or be nourished by different underlying values. In German speaking Switzerland and prominently in the Czech Republic, for example, the desire for success is related to the values of achievement and power. In French speaking Switzerland, Spain, and Portugal instead, the motives seem to be slightly different since success is more connected to achievement and security. Furthermore, in Portugal (and to a lesser extent also in Spain) hoping for success seemed to be related to self-direction, stimulation, and hedonism, which in Switzerland and the Czech Republic was barely the case.

The wish for a happy family, partnership or marriage was generally and almost exclusively linked to the value of benevolence. However, in French Switzerland and in the Czech Republic it was also a matter of security. On the other hand, whereas wishing to have more sex and romantic experiences was clearly related to the value of hedonism, in the Czech Republic, in particular, it was also about the search for stimulation, achievement and exerting power. Hoping for good and trustworthy relationships with other people, besides being connected to benevolence, universalism, and hedonism, was also a matter of security in Portugal and of conformity in French Switzerland. More personal independence and self-determination was not only about self-direction and stimulation, but in Spain, Portugal, and the Czech Republic it was also related to universalism and security.

These findings suggest that some universal features regarding what most people in different cultures hope exist, and that these targets of hope are related to some universal values, particularly the values of self-transcendence. Furthermore, our results indicate that personal hopes of all types are indeed related to different basic values, but that people from with diverse cultural backgrounds seem to develop personal hopes endorsed by similar as well as by specific motives.

In the next section, we connect the vast and differentiated empirical findings of our study and discuss them in the light of our research interest and the theoretical background presented at the beginning of the chapter.

3.3.6 General Findings and Discussion

3.3.6.1 Common Patterns across Cultures

The purpose of the current study was to explore the relation of human values with the general level of perceived hope as well as with individual targets of hope among samples from five countries. We first tested group invariance with five language versions of the Perceived Hope Scale (Krafft et al., 2017, 2021; Águeda Marujo et al., 2021; Slezackova et al., 2020) across the investigated samples and found that the general perception of hope was understood similarly in two Swiss regions, Spain, Portugal, and the Czech Republic. We then tested the location of the ten basic human values in a bi-dimensional space, achieving similar pictures to the circular continuum proposed by Schwartz (2012), but with some cultural particularities in the location of the single value types. Specifically, self-direction stood closer to universalism and benevolence in Spain, Portugal, and the Czech Republic, indicating a certain social orientation besides its individual focus. Tradition seemed to have a particular meaning for the Portuguese participants, which has to be investigated more in detail.

Before discussing cultural differences, we first would like to highlight results that seem to be common to all samples and represent possible universal characteristics. Despite huge differences in national GDP per capita, participants in all samples displayed similar moderate to high levels of perceived hope above the center of the scale. Regarding the human values, in all countries the highest scores were obtained for self-transcendence values. This underlines the importance of the family and of cooperative and supportive social relationships as well as an attitude of respect, tolerance, and harmony with the wider social and natural environment. The values of self-direction and hedonism, representing openness to change, personal mastery and pleasurable experiences, were the second most important values after self-transcendence. At the next level of importance were security and conformity values, which promote safe and harmonious social relations. Tradition and stimulation, instead, were something lower and ranked clearly after achievement values, which promote engagement and individual performance. At the end of the list, we found power values, which tend to promote hierarchical structures and could be detrimental for cooperative social relationships. In line with previous research findings (Schwartz, 2012; Fischer & Schwartz, 2011), our results suggest that there are some widely recognized universal value priorities, beyond individual and cultural influences.

These findings are supported by the importance people in different countries ascribed to certain targets of hope. In all samples, people hoped above all for good health, a happy family, marriage or partnership, a harmonious life, good and trusting relationships with other people, personal independence and being engaged in meaningful and fulfilling tasks. These targets of hope represent life domains that foster eudaimonic well-being (Ryff, 1995; Ryan & Deci, 2001; Seligman, 2004). Likewise, in all countries the hope for more money, more sex, and romantic experiences as well as for religious and spiritual experiences were located at the bottom of the list (see also Krafft & Walker, 2018b). Beyond these common patterns, our results indicate that in some countries people hoped for success at the workplace or at university and a secure job, reinforcing the positive role of achievement and the desire for security in people's life.

In the next step, we assessed the role of value types as predictors of perceived hope. We expected that self-transcendence and openness to change, which have been conceptualized as anxiety-free and growth-oriented values, would have a positive impact on hope and that the values of conservation and self-enhancement, which are anxiety-based, would be less or not at all related with hope. Our results confirmed that values of self-transcendence and openness to change are indeed positively connected to hope and that security, conformity and power are barely related to hope. However, our findings also indicated that tradition and achievement can also count as significant predictors of hope, suggesting that these values are not only anxiety-based but could also be hope enhancing.

Again, these findings are reinforced and broadened by the correlation coefficients between perceived hope and selected targets of hope. Prosocial and religious (transcendence) targets of hope, such as the wish to help other people, to enjoy good social relationships, to perform a meaningful task, to have a happy family, marriage, or partnership and to face religious experiences, demonstrated the strongest correlations with hope, while materialistic and security-oriented hopes (e.g., more money and a secure job) displayed the weakest correlation. These results are in line with previous studies of Averill and his colleagues (Averill et al., 1990; Averill & Sundararajan, 2005).

Finally, we investigated which targets of hope might express which types of basic human value orientations. People high in benevolence and universalism hoped the most for altruistic and prosocial life domains such as helping other people, having a meaningful task, good social relationships, and harmony in life. A hedonistic orientation was expressed by maintaining hopes such as having fun with friends, enjoying romantic experiences, having more free time and time to relax as well as holding good social relationships. Security values were related to the desire for a secure job, good health and a harmonious life, more safety in the personal environment and order in one's life. Tradition had a close connection to the wish for religious experiences, while conformity was related to the desire to help other people and achievement was expressed by the wish to be successful at work, at school, university etc. Moreover, the results of our study revealed that certain targets of hope were grounded in more than one value dimension, as proposed by Schwartz, (2012). For example, the desire to help other people was connected to benevolence, universalism, and conformity. The wish to maintain good social relationships was linked to benevolence, universalism, hedonism, and conformity. Those who longed for a harmonious life cherished values of self-transcendence and security.

To summarize, the level of perceived hope is not linked to the economic wealth of a country. People in poorer countries can display similar or even higher levels of hope than people in a rich country. Our findings highlight moreover the importance of the basic values of self-transcendence (caring for the wellbeing of others) and of openness to change (self-mastery, looking for new challenges and novel experiences) as favorable sources of hope. Furthermore, our study indicates that tradition, religious experiences, and achievement are not only anxiety-based but could also act as hope-related values. In general terms, the wish for domains that nurture eudaimonic well-being are positively related to hope, demonstrating that the more people wish for eudaimonic life targets, the more they hope. This is apparently not the case for materialistic targets of hope.

3.3.6.2 Individual Characteristics of Single Cultures

Beyond the common patterns found across all samples, our results revealed noteworthy distinctive characteristics in the specific samples. First, Portuguese and Czech participants showed the highest levels of hope and the French Swiss the lowest, signaling that the perception of hope is barely dependent on the wealth of a nation.

Portugal displayed high levels of universalism, conformity and achievement. Besides self-transcendence, openness to change and hedonism, the conservative value of tradition had a significant impact on hope, highlighting the importance of family, cultural and religious habits and norms as possible sources of hope. This may also reflect notably higher levels of collectivism and short-term orientation compared to the levels of these cultural dimensions in the other three countries (Hofstede-Insights, 2022). Due to their unsteady economic and social situation, Portuguese people also ascribed importance to success (in terms of achievement and security) and to a secure job but additionally to the possibility to help other people. Furthermore, to maintain good social relationships with other people is not only a matter of benevolence and universalism but also of security. The desire to be successful in life seemed motivated by achievement and security, but also by self-direction, stimulation and hedonism. However, for the Portuguese, the desire to help other people, to be engaged in a meaningful task and to enjoy religious and spiritual experiences were more strongly related to the general perception of hope than in other countries.

In the Spanish sample, people exhibited higher scores in universalism than the Swiss and the Czech and the lowest scores in self-enhancement (achievement and power) but also in tradition. Whereas universalism and stimulation do not predict hope at all, hedonism, tradition, benevolence and self-direction do. Similar to Portugal, Spanish participants wished for a secure job and success at the workplace/university, but with the difference, that they do not value helping other people that much, which also yielded the lowest correlation with hope compared to all other samples. This seems to be in contradiction with the higher scores of universalism and would need to be explored more in detail in future studies.

For the Czechs, the underlying patterns and dynamics are slightly different. In comparison to the other countries, participants of the Czech sample were higher in tradition, stimulation and power and lower in security, conformity and hedonism. Besides benevolence and universalism, people higher in tradition and in achievement exhibited higher levels of hope. On the contrary, conformity had a significant negative effect on hope. Moreover, the wish for more free time and more fun with friends (the hedonic orientation) had no effect on hope. Interestingly, the pleasure related to romantic experiences was also a matter of achievement and power. This means that for Czech people (at least in our sample), achievement and to some extent power, had a stronger significance and effect on hope than pleasure, leisure and social conformity, which can be also explained by higher levels of individualism, which emphasizes individual achievement orientation.

The Swiss population, the country with the highest GDP per capita in our study, exhibited a somewhat differentiated picture with aspects distinguishing the two major language regions. While the German Swiss were higher in benevolence, self-direction, and tradition but the lowest in universalism, the French Swiss, who are the participants in our study with the lowest level of perceived hope, were higher in security, hedonism and self-direction but lower in universalism, stimulation and achievement. However, in the French sample, stimulation and achievement significantly predicted hope and self-direction not at all. Interestingly, hedonism (enjoying life) had a stronger effect on hope for the German Swiss and achievement for the French. Especially in the German part of Switzerland, success, a secure job and more money were of minor importance to hope, whereas performing a meaningful task was much more relevant.

To summarize, the level of hope can be similar or even higher in some poorer countries than in a rich country. Moreover, within a rich country, two regions with different cultural backgrounds may show significant differences in the level of hopefulness. These differences can be the consequence of several reasons. Beyond the values of self-transcendence and openness to change, Portuguese participants obtain hope from traditional family and cultural habits and norms, from the wish to help other people but do also yearn for success and achievement. In Spain, people experience similar conditions than in Portugal, but exhibit lower levels of hope, probably because the prosocial and altruistic motives are less pronounced. Central values in the Czech sample, the country with the highest level of hope together with Portugal, are the seemingly contradictory values of benevolence, tradition and achievement, which are the most salient predictors of hope. In Switzerland, the German and the French population present some common patterns but also striking differences. A meaningful task has a higher value than a secure job or success and self-transcendence values have a similar effect on hope in both regions. Tradition is more important and relevant for hope in the German part and achievement for the French speaking population.

3.4 Limitations

The current study has a number of limitations that must be addressed. The design of the study is cross-sectional, thus we are not able to infer causalities between variables. If self-transcendent values foster hope or if the consequence of being hopeful is to care for the well-being of others, this should be investigated in future cross-sectional studies. Another limitation is the different sample sizes and the lacking of national representativeness of our samples. The Swiss samples reflected the demographic structure of the population much better than the Spanish, the Portuguese and the Czech groups. In the latter countries, the participants were younger and had a better education than the average of the population. Furthermore, most participants were recruited via online platforms. Population groups, especially older people and persons living in rural areas with little online skills or access, were underrepresented. However, the main finding obtained from our results are independent from demographic differences or represent at least the characteristics of a sub-group of the general population.

3.5 Conclusions

We started this chapter with the conceptualization of hope as a wish or desire for a valuable good whose realization is regarded as possible but not necessarily as probable and with the assumption that personal values and cultural characteristics could have an effect on the general levels of hope as well as on the significance of particular targets of hope. Our findings support the notion that certain human values can positively influence both the general level of perceived hope as well as the formation and meaning of certain individual targets of hope. Specifically, anxiety-free and growth-oriented values (self-transcendence and openness to change) revealed positive effects on hope and were significantly related to the most important hope targets. Moreover, values and hope targets with a social and transcendent focus such as tradition and spirituality usually exhibit a stronger connection to hope than values and hopes with an individual and materialistic focus, with exception of the positive effect of personal achievement. On the one hand, our study suggests that many presumably universal features of the general perception of hope, of the most relevant hope targets of the population and of their connection to basic human values exist. On the other hand, it discloses some significant and several subtle cultural particularities, worth to be investigated more in detail in future psychological empirical studies.

Appendix 3.1: Demographic Structure of the Samples

	German Swiss	French Swiss	Spain	Portugal	Czech Rep.
	N/n	*N/n*	*N/n*	*N/n*	*N/n*
	%	%	%	%	%
Total	3049	1109	528	808	338
Age (M)	43.71	44.16	37.79	37.49	30.92
Age (SD)	15.92	14.15	14.78	15.53	11.90
Gender					
Male	1255	472	134	153	117
	41.2%	42.6%	25.4%	18.9%	34.6%
Female	1794	637	394	655	221
	58.8%	57.4%	74.6%	81.1%	65.4%
Marital status					
Still living with my parents	234	69	139	222	56
	7.7%	6.2%	26.3%	27.5%	16.6%
Single, unmarried	526	160	76	149	62
	17.3%	14.4%	14.4%	18.4%	18.3%
Living in a partnership with separate households	263	93	20	25	42
	8.6%	8.4%	3.8%	3.1%	12.4%
Living together in a partnership	592	226	69	99	75
	19.4%	20.4%	13.1%	12.3%	22.2%
Married	1111	395	186	236	86
	36.4%	35.6%	35.2%	29.2%	25.4%
Divorced/separated	267	143	34	68	13
	8.8%	12.9%	6.4%	8.4%	3.8%
Widowed	56	23	4	9	4
	1.8%	2.1%	0.8%	1.1%	1.2%
Education					
Did not finish school	9	5	1	0	0
	0.3%	0.5%	0.2%	0.0%	0.0%
Primary school	105	71	12	1	9
	3.4%	6.4%	2.3%	0.1%	2.7%
Secondary school	255	68	87	227	157
	8.4%	6.1%	16.5%	28.1%	46.4%
Professional training/diploma	2050	687	68	6	28
	67.2%	61.9%	12.9%	0.7%	8.3%
Tertiary education/university	630	278	360	574	144
	20.7%	25.1%	68.2%	71.0%	42.6%
Main activity					
In education or training	202	68	159	283	131
	6.6%	6.1%	30.1%	35.0%	38.8%
Household/raising children	123	56	18	6	15

(continued)

	German Swiss	French Swiss	Spain	Portugal	Czech Rep.
	4.0%	5.0%	3.4%	0.7%	4.4%
Part-time job	617	230	46	70	19
	20.2%	20.7%	8.7%	8.7%	5.6%
Fulltime job	1580	562	269	404	162
	51.8%	50.7%	50.9%	50.0%	47.9%
Unemployed	109	62	17	17	5
	3.6%	5.6%	3.2%	2.1%	1.5%
Retired	418	131	19	28	6
	13.7%	11.8%	3.6%	3.5%	1.8%
Professional status					
No position in an organization	407	208	95	173	71
	13.3%	18.8%	18.0%	21.4%	21.0%
In education/training	170	69	106	140	58
	5.6%	6.2%	20.1%	17.3%	17.2%
Employee	1248	519	181	313	146
	40.9%	46.8%	34.3%	38.7%	43.2%
Junior/middle management	729	143	65	79	31
	23.9%	12.9%	12.3%	9.8%	9.2%
Senior management/board of directors	147	70	42	29	7
	4.8%	6.3%	8.0%	3.6%	2.1%
Entrepreneur/business owner	348	100	39	74	25
	11.4%	9.0%	7.4%	9.2%	7.4%
Religion					
Catholic	770	330	277	405	91
	25.3%	29.8%	52.5%	50.1%	26.9%
Protestant	822	203	4	21	9
	27.0%	18.3%	0.8%	2.6%	2.7%
Another Christian church	141	24	1	7	4
	4.6%	2.2%	0.2%	0.9%	1.2%
Muslim	43	13	2	2	1
	1.4%	1.2%	0.4%	0.2%	0.3%
Jewish	6	3	0	0	0
	0.2%	0.3%	0.0%	0.0%	0.0%
Hindu	4	0	0	1	0
	0.1%	0.0%	0.0%	0.1%	0.0%
Buddhist	22	6	1	6	1
	0.7%	0.5%	0.2%	0.7%	0.3%
I am a spiritual person outside the traditional world religions.	204	130	55	160	109
	6.7%	11.7%	10.4%	19.8%	32.2%
Without religion or confession	989	382	164	174	103
	32.4%	34.4%	31.1%	21.5%	30.5%
Something different	48	18	24	32	20
	1.6%	1.6%	4.5%	4.0%	5.9%

Appendix 3.2: Partial Bivariate Pearson Correlation Coefficients for the Total Sample ($N = 5832$)

	1	2	3	4	5	6	7	8	9	10	11	12	13	14
1. Perceived Hope	1.000													
2. Self-transcendence	0.297**	1.000												
3. Openness to change	0.268**	0.422**	1.000											
4. Conservation	0.158**	0.403**	0.146**	1.000										
5. Self-enhancement	0.082**	0.022	0.283**	0.287**	1.000									
6. Benevolence	0.259**	0.751**	0.354**	0.455**	0.125**	1.000								
7. Universalism	0.256**	0.931**	0.373**	0.291**	−0.040**	0.457**	1.000							
8. Self-direction	0.203**	0.375**	0.885**	0.161**	0.193**	0.342**	0.316**	1.000						
9. Stimulation	0.257**	0.332**	0.790**	0.073**	0.300**	0.242**	0.313**	0.415**	1.000					
10. Hedonism	0.230**	0.331**	0.428**	0.169**	0.215**	0.336**	0.260**	0.278**	0.471**	1.000				
11. Tradition	0.165**	0.187**	0.098**	0.741**	0.265**	0.293**	0.089**	0.077**	0.090**	0.097**	1.000			
12. Security	0.122**	0.354**	0.220**	0.740**	0.327**	0.420**	0.244**	0.258**	0.092**	0.277**	0.426**	1.000		
13. Conformity	0.107**	0.422**	0.059**	0.850**	0.162**	0.403**	0.345**	0.088**	0.001	0.099**	0.379**	0.512**	1.000	
14. Achievement	0.156**	0.193**	0.380**	0.346**	0.793**	0.273**	0.109**	0.305**	0.342**	0.269**	0.259**	0.385**	0.240**	1.000
15. Power	0.030*	−0.070**	0.189**	0.212**	0.949**	0.030*	−0.110**	0.105**	0.231**	0.154**	0.226**	0.245**	0.097**	0.562**

Note: **. Correlation is significant at 0.01 level; *. Correlation is significant at 0.05 level;
Control variables: Country, gender, age, marital status, education, main activity and professional status

Appendix 3.3: Partial Bivariate Pearson Correlation Coefficients Between Targets of Hope and Basic Value Dimensions

Appendix 3.3.1: German Switzerland

	Benevolence	Universalism	Self-direction	Stimulation	Hedonism	Tradition	Security	Conformity	Achievement	Power
Success at the workplace, at school etc.	0.089**	0.039*	0.063**	0.142**	0.112**	0.095**	0.141**	0.103**	0.387**	0.210**
Happy partnership, family, marriage	0.268**	0.143**	0.034	0.087**	0.194**	0.135**	0.174**	0.143**	0.120**	0.009
More free time	0.103**	0.090**	0.063**	0.106**	0.260**	0.045**	0.154**	0.077**	0.076**	0.032
More sex and romantic experiences	0.134**	0.082**	0.029	0.170**	0.254**	0.063**	0.107**	0.076**	0.150**	0.106**
More religious and spiritual experiences	0.093**	0.189**	0.029	0.079**	−0.038*	0.249**	0.051**	0.059**	0.011	0.004
More money	0.025	−0.062**	0.063**	0.096**	0.112**	0.129**	0.179**	0.066**	0.300**	0.343**
More fun with friends	0.250**	0.145**	0.106**	0.228**	0.424**	0.121**	0.141**	0.105**	0.139**	0.047**
More safety in your personal environment	0.200**	0.082**	0.051**	0.035*	0.154**	0.244**	0.404**	0.254**	0.171**	0.110**
Good health	0.182**	0.128**	0.096**	0.072**	0.178**	0.123**	0.311**	0.144**	0.112**	0.023
A secure job	0.153**	0.067**	0.016	0.002	0.082**	0.159**	0.308**	0.200**	0.195**	0.102**
Good and trusting relationships with other people	0.366**	0.296**	0.111**	0.153**	0.231**	0.138**	0.163**	0.188**	0.111**	−0.012
Being engaged in meaningful tasks	0.194**	0.258**	0.171**	0.166**	0.094**	0.131**	0.139**	0.151**	0.168**	0.030
Order in my life	0.223**	0.095**	0.089**	0.021	0.083**	0.264**	0.365**	0.287**	0.225**	0.117**
Personal independence and self-determination	0.125**	0.124**	0.353**	0.205**	0.137**	0.055**	0.166**	0.040*	0.147**	0.070**
More time to relax	0.135**	0.143**	0.103**	0.104**	0.238**	0.121**	0.229**	0.142**	0.107**	0.060**
Harmony in life	0.272**	0.214**	0.124**	0.089**	0.230**	0.155**	0.268**	0.226**	0.103**	−0.009
Helping other people	0.395**	0.490**	0.059**	0.160**	0.149**	0.173**	0.162**	0.277**	0.074**	−0.052**

Note: **. Correlation is significant at 0.01 level; *. Correlation is significant at 0.05 level
Control variables: Gender, age, marital status, education, main activity, and professional status

Appendix 3.3.2: French Switzerland

	Benevolence	Universalism	Self-direction	Stimulation	Hedonism	Tradition	Security	Conformity	Achievement	Power
Success at the workplace, at school etc.	0.082**	0.029	0.103**	0.097**	0.107**	0.075**	0.208**	0.074*	0.269**	0.186**
Happy partnership, family, marriage	0.369**	0.176**	0.155**	0.064*	0.224**	0.150**	0.249**	0.159**	0.126**	−0.007
More free time	0.106**	0.105**	0.090**	0.070*	0.282**	0.062*	0.112**	0.042	0.042	0.048
More sex and romantic experiences	0.059*	0.010	0.033	0.184**	0.262**	0.004	0.024	−0.047	0.128**	0.136**
More religious and spiritual experiences	0.130**	0.228**	0.045	0.090**	0.025	0.229**	0.087**	0.110**	0.084**	0.090**
More money	0.007	−0.039	0.017	0.045	0.093**	0.058*	0.155**	0.045	0.211**	0.329**
More fun with friends	0.302**	0.181**	0.133**	0.152**	0.303**	0.087**	0.144**	0.090**	0.100**	0.053
More safety in your personal environment	0.125**	0.058*	0.030	0.019	0.145**	0.216**	0.345**	0.172**	0.159**	0.112**
Good health	0.199**	0.116**	0.055	0.061*	0.146**	0.138**	0.346**	0.182**	0.140**	0.094**
A secure job	0.137**	0.098**	0.063*	0.014	0.124**	0.107**	0.319**	0.196**	0.170**	0.162**
Good and trusting relationships with other people	0.348**	0.310**	0.105**	0.106**	0.232**	0.098**	0.169**	0.254**	0.147**	0.002
Being engaged in meaningful tasks	0.254**	0.272**	0.178**	0.171**	0.156**	0.052	0.145**	0.162**	0.188**	0.057
Order in my life	0.175**	0.063*	0.021	−0.047	0.056	0.287**	0.338**	0.319**	0.191**	0.177**
Personal independence and self-determination	0.117**	0.152**	0.324**	0.239**	0.239**	0.039	0.131**	0.028	0.119**	0.050
More time to relax	0.094**	0.097**	0.093**	0.026	0.218**	0.108**	0.144**	0.103**	0.054	0.120**
Harmony in life	0.251**	0.212**	0.183**	0.053	0.251**	0.124**	0.248**	0.212**	0.135**	0.051
Helping other people	0.392**	0.508**	0.113**	0.154**	0.142**	0.139**	0.122**	0.251**	0.055	−0.059*

Note: **. Correlation is significant at 0.01 level; *. Correlation is significant at 0.05 level
Control variables: Gender, age, marital status, education, main activity, and professional status

Appendix 3.3.3: Spain

	Benevolence	Universalism	Self-direction	Stimulation	Hedonism	Tradition	Security	Conformity	Achievement	Power
Success at the workplace, at school etc.	0.215**	0.153**	0.182**	0.169**	0.156**	0.080	0.201**	0.124**	0.276**	0.059
Happy partnership, family, marriage	0.218**	0.099*	0.045	0.001	0.147**	0.061	0.103*	0.090*	0.021	−0.059
More free time	0.180**	0.195**	0.118**	0.136**	0.223**	0.055	0.125**	0.089*	0.012	0.082
More sex and romantic experiences	0.109*	0.074	0.086	0.196**	0.340**	0.044	0.072	0.014	0.056	0.126**
More religious and spiritual experiences	0.076	0.166**	0.133**	0.105*	0.055	0.301**	0.148**	0.081	0.138**	0.142**
More money	0.087*	0.015	0.076	0.262**	0.196**	0.107*	0.185**	0.030	0.260**	0.377**
More fun with friends	0.250**	0.184**	0.121**	0.218**	0.438**	0.077	0.097*	0.048	0.096*	0.086*
More safety in your personal environment	0.200**	0.064	0.020	0.038	0.169**	0.160**	0.310**	0.153**	0.095*	0.133**
Good health	0.154**	0.054	0.014	0.045	0.203**	0.114**	0.217**	0.160**	0.009	0.060
A secure job	0.187**	0.130**	0.067	0.077	0.093*	0.137**	0.294**	0.262**	0.100*	0.103*
Good and trusting relationships with other people	0.224**	0.266**	0.224**	0.189**	0.238**	0.069	0.172**	0.093*	0.067	0.004
Being engaged in meaningful tasks	0.230**	0.375**	0.229**	0.220**	0.138**	0.130**	0.236**	0.151**	0.148**	0.058
Order in my life	0.183**	0.138**	0.061	0.028	0.050	0.213**	0.341**	0.317**	0.094*	0.055
Personal independence and self-determination	0.262**	0.248**	0.335**	0.238**	0.183**	0.060	0.269**	0.127**	0.159**	0.063
More time to relax	0.114**	0.217**	0.112*	0.134**	0.256**	0.107*	0.252**	0.143**	0.100*	0.124**
Harmony in life	0.231**	0.189**	0.194**	0.099*	0.199**	0.206**	0.311**	0.200**	0.114**	0.057
Helping other people	0.353**	0.461**	0.216**	0.164**	0.180**	0.066	0.233**	0.175**	0.030	−0.069

Note: **. Correlation is significant at 0.01 level; *. Correlation is significant at 0.05 level
Control variables: Gender, age, marital status, education, main activity, and professional status

Appendix 3.3.4: Portugal

	Benevolence	Universalism	Self-direction	Stimulation	Hedonism	Tradition	Security	Conformity	Achievement	Power
Success at the workplace, at school etc.	0.176**	0.049	0.227**	0.197**	0.241**	0.049	0.247**	0.148**	0.371**	0.193**
Happy partnership, family, marriage	0.236**	0.1[illegible]5**	0.032	0.051	0.105**	0.106**	0.124**	0.073*	0.113**	0.000
More free time	0.136**	0.161**	0.072*	0.117**	0.258**	0.044	0.180**	0.119**	0.085*	−0.021
More sex and romantic experiences	0.156**	0.066	0.108**	0.229**	0.342**	0.051	0.181**	0.046	0.151**	0.136**
More religious and spiritual experiences	0.028	0.178**	−0.113**	0.034	−0.018	0.211**	−0.003	0.087*	−0.065	−0.079*
More money	0.059	−0.047	0.146**	0.144**	0.202**	0.055	0.187**	0.053	0.310**	0.334**
More fun with friends	0.245**	0.176**	0.131**	0.263**	0.473**	0.001	0.188**	0.143**	0.182**	0.026
More safety in your personal environment	0.176**	0.174**	0.159**	0.162**	0.215**	0.078*	0.335**	0.165**	0.178**	0.039
Good health	0.232**	0.150**	0.180**	0.111**	0.213**	0.039	0.319**	0.178**	0.165**	0.011
A secure job	0.158**	0.065	0.140**	0.048	0.138**	0.093**	0.323**	0.192**	0.199**	0.114**
Good and trusting relationships with other people	0.358**	0.318**	0.146**	0.133**	0.214**	−0.008	0.247**	0.124**	0.136**	−0.084*
Being engaged in meaningful tasks	0.269**	0.282**	0.204**	0.208**	0.178**	0.029	0.198**	0.078*	0.231**	−0.036
Order in my life	0.169**	0.142**	0.146**	0.122**	0.170**	0.090*	0.260**	0.189**	0.146**	0.087*
Personal independence and self-determination	0.170**	0.209**	0.293**	0.206**	0.210**	0.044	0.247**	0.110**	0.207**	0.092**
More time to relax	0.181**	0.213**	0.167**	0.160**	0.298**	0.038	0.256**	0.147**	0.153**	0.003
Harmony in life	0.268**	0.217**	0.150**	0.084*	0.170**	0.066	0.285**	0.180**	0.181**	0.041
Helping other people	0.316**	0.443**	0.097**	0.161**	0.131**	0.155**	0.161**	0.202**	0.093**	−0.142**

Note: **. Correlation is significant at 0.01 level; *. Correlation is significant at 0.05 level
Control variables: Gender, age, marital status, education, main activity, and professional status

Appendix 3.3.5: Czech Republic

	Benevolence	Universalism	Self-direction	Stimulation	Hedonism	Tradition	Security	Conformity	Achievement	Power
Success at the workplace, at school etc.	0.135*	0.071	0.096	0.174**	0.131*	0.076	0.153**	0.034	0.463**	0.321**
Happy partnership, family, marriage	0.231**	0.111*	0.107	0.042	0.091	0.182**	0.241**	0.178**	0.167**	0.083
More free time	0.081	0.093	0.103	0.212**	0.272**	0.026	0.110*	0.067	0.069	0.052
More sex and romantic experiences	0.145**	0.104	0.070	0.267**	0.335**	0.075	0.176**	0.069	0.257**	0.213**
More religious and spiritual experiences	0.007	0.286**	0.059	0.202**	−0.064	0.184**	0.037	0.023	0.065	0.004
More money	0.059	−0.084	0.010	0.076	0.157**	0.080	0.209**	0.121*	0.231**	0.406**
More fun with friends	0.146**	0.153**	0.069	0.226**	0.394**	0.079	0.091	0.138*	0.123*	0.097
More safety in your personal environment	0.243**	0.026	−0.012	0.017	0.214**	0.218**	0.391**	0.251**	0.096	0.184**
Good health	0.252**	0.178**	0.060	0.052	0.185**	0.090	0.394**	0.149**	0.224**	0.124*
A secure job	0.118*	0.021	−0.055	−0.005	0.139*	0.268**	0.239**	0.169**	0.097	0.207**
Good and trusting relation-ships with other people	0.283**	0.256**	0.108*	0.198**	0.213**	0.040	0.089	0.025	0.070	−0.003
Being engaged in meaningful tasks	0.151**	0.263**	0.220**	0.224**	0.068	0.106	0.111*	0.049	0.187**	0.124*
Order in my life	0.210**	0.121*	0.009	−0.018	−0.088	0.329**	0.279**	0.325**	0.178**	0.140*
Personal independence and self-determination	0.104	0.254**	0.330**	0.231**	0.135*	−0.010	0.194**	−0.045	0.173**	0.069
More time to relax	0.153**	0.139*	0.104	0.185**	0.207**	0.097	0.269**	0.131*	0.097	0.132*
Harmony in life	0.232**	0.226**	0.096	0.032	0.087	0.097	0.218**	0.170**	0.070	−0.044
Helping other people	0.289**	0.400**	0.090	0.165**	0.181**	0.179**	0.190**	0.182**	0.105	−0.006

Note: **. Correlation is significant at 0.01 level; *. Correlation is significant at 0.05 level
Control variables: Gender, age, marital status, education, main activity, and professional status

References

Águeda Marujo, H., Velez, M. J., Gonçalves, S. P., Neto, L. M., Krafft, A. M., & Casais, M. (2021). The value of hope: Validation of the perceived hope scale in the Portuguese population. *Current Psychology*, 1–9. https://doi.org/10.1007/s12144-021-02115-6.

Averill, J. R., Catlin, G., & Chon, K. K. (1990). *Rules of hope: Recent research in psychology*. Springer.

Averill, J. R., & Sundararajan, L. (2005). Hope as rhetoric: Cultural narratives of wishing and coping. In J. Eliott (Ed.), *Interdisciplinary perspectives on hope* (pp. 133–165). Nova Science.

Blöser, C., & Stahl, T. (2017). Fundamental Hope and practical identity. *Philosophical Papers, 46*(3), 345–371. https://doi.org/10.1080/05568641.2017.1400918

Chen, F. F. (2007). Sensitivity of goodness of fit indexes to lack of measurement invariance. *Structural Equation Modeling: A Multidisciplinary Journal, 14*(3), 464–504. https://doi.org/10.1080/10705510701301834

Eid, M., & Diener, E. (2009). Norms for experiencing emotions in different cultures: Inter-and intranational differences. In E. Diener (Ed.), *Culture and well-being* (pp. 169–202). Springer. https://doi.org/10.1007/978-90-481-2352-0_9

Eid, M., Gollwitzer, M., & Schmitt, M. (2011). *Statistik und Forschungsmethoden Lehrbuch*. Beltz.

Erickson, R. C., Post, R. D., & Paige, A. B. (1975). Hope as a psychiatric variable. *Journal of Clinical Psychology, 31*(2), 324–330. https://doi.org/10.1002/1097-4679(197504)31:2<324::AID-JCLP2270310236>3.0.CO;2-Q

Erikson, E. (1963). *Childhood and society* (2d ed., rev. and enl.). W.W. Norton & Co.

Farran, C. J., Herth, K. A., & Popovich, J. M. (1995). *Hope and hopelessness: Critical clinical constructs*. Sage Publications, Inc.

Fischer, R., & Schwartz, S. (2011). Whence differences in value priorities? Individual, cultural, or artifactual sources. *Journal of Cross-Cultural Psychology, 42*(7), 1127–1144. https://doi.org/10.1177/0022022110381429

Fredrickson, B. L. (2013). Positive emotions broaden and build. *Advances in Experimental Social Psychology, 47*(1), 1–53. https://doi.org/10.1016/B978-0-12-407236-7.00001-2

Govier, T. (2011). Hope and its opposites. *Journal of Social Philosophy, 42*(3), 239–253.

Gravlee, G. S. (2020). Hope in ancient Greek philosophy. In S. van den Heuvel (Ed.), *Historical and multidisciplinary perspectives on Hope* (pp. 3–23). Springer. https://doi.org/10.1007/978-3-030-46489-9_1

Hofstede, G. (2001). *Culture's consequences: Comparing values, behaviors, institutions, and organizations across nations* (2nd ed.). Sage Publications.

Hofstede-Insights. (2022, March 8). *Compare countries on Hofstede's cultural dimensions*. Retrieved March 8, from https://www.hofstede-insights.com/product/compare-countries/

Hu, L. T., & Bentler, P. M. (1999). Cutoff criteria for fit indexes in covariance structure analysis: Conventional criteria versus new alternatives. *Structural Equation Modeling: A Multidisciplinary Journal, 6*(1), 1–55. https://doi.org/10.1080/10705519909540118

Joshanloo, M., & Ghaedi, G. (2009). Value priorities as predictors of hedonic and eudaimonic aspects of Well-being. *Personality and Individual Differences, 47*(4), 294–298. https://doi.org/10.1016/j.paid.2009.03.016

Kluckhohn, C. (1951). Values and value orientations in the theory of action: An explanation in definition and classification. In T. Parsons & E. Shills (Eds.), *Toward a general theory of action* (pp. 388–433). Harvard University Press. https://doi.org/10.4159/harvard.9780674863507.c8

Krafft, A. M., Guse, T., & Maree, D. (2021). Distinguishing perceived Hope and dispositional optimism: Theoretical foundations and empirical findings beyond future expectancies and cognition. *Journal of Well-Being Assessment, 4*, 217–243. https://doi.org/10.1007/s41543-020-00030-4

Krafft, A. M., Martin-Krumm, C., & Fenouillet, F. (2017, April 1). Adaptation, further elaboration, and validation of a scale to measure hope as perceived by people. *Assessment*. https://doi.org/10.1177/1073191117700724.

Krafft, A. M., & Walker, A. M. (2018a). Exploring the concept and experience of Hope –theoretical and methodological foundations. In A. M. Krafft, P. Perrig-Chiello, & A. M. Walker (Eds.), *Hope for a good life: Results of the Hope barometer international research program* (pp. 3–19). Springer Int. https://doi.org/10.1007/978-3-319-78470-0_1

Krafft, A. M., & Walker, A. M. (2018b). Exploring the concept and experience of Hope – Empirical findings and the virtuous circle of Hope. In A. M. Krafft, P. Perrig-Chiello, & A. M. Walker (Eds.), *Hope for a good life: Results of the Hope barometer international research program* (pp. 21–60). Springer Int. https://doi.org/10.1007/978-3-319-78470-0_2

Marcel, G. (1951). *Homo Viator. Introduction to a Metaphysic of Hope*. Harper.

McGeer, V. (2008). Trust, hope and empowerment. *Australasian Journal of Philosophy, 86*(2), 237–254. https://doi.org/10.1080/00048400801886413

Oishi, S., Diener, E., Suh, E., & Lucas, R. E. (1999). Value as a moderator in subjective Well-being. *Journal of Personality, 67*(1), 157–184. https://doi.org/10.1111/1467-6494.00051

Park, N., & Huebner, E. S. (2005). A cross-cultural study of the levels and correlates of life satisfaction among adolescents. *Journal of Cross-Cultural Psychology, 36*(4), 444–456. https://doi.org/10.1177/0022022105275961

Pettit, P. (2004). Hope and its place in mind. *The Annals of the American Academy of Political and Social Science, 592*(1), 152–165. https://doi.org/10.1177/0002716203261798

Rokeach, M. (1973). *The nature of human values*. Free Press.

Ryan, R. M., & Deci, E. L. (2001). On happiness and human potentials: A review of research on hedonic and eudaimonic Well-being. *Annual Review of Psychology, 52*(1), 141–166. https://doi.org/10.1146/annurev.psych.52.1.141

Ryff, C. D. (1995). Psychological Well-being in adult life. *Current Directions in Psychological Science, 4*(4), 99–104. https://doi.org/10.1111/1467-8721.ep10772395

Sagiv, L., & Schwartz, S. H. (2000). Value priorities and subjective Well-being: Direct relations and congruity effects. *European Journal of Social Psychology, 30*(2), 177–198. https://doi.org/10.1002/(SICI)1099-0992(200003/04)30:2<177::AID-EJSP982>3.0.CO;2-Z

Schwartz, S. H. (1992). Universals in the content and structure of values: Theoretical advances and empirical tests in 20 countries. In *Advances in experimental social psychology* (Vol. 25, pp. 1–65). Academic Press. https://doi.org/10.1016/S0065-2601(08)60281-6.

Schwartz, S. H. (1994). Are there universal aspects in the structure and contents of human values? *Journal of Social Issues, 50*(4), 19–45. https://doi.org/10.1111/j.1540-4560.1994.tb01196.x

Schwartz, S. H. (2003). A proposal for measuring value orientations across nations. *Questionnaire Package of the European Social Survey, 2003*, 259–290.

Schwartz, S. H. (2006). A theory of cultural value orientations: Explication and applications. *Comparative Sociology, 5*(2), 137–182.

Schwartz, S. H. (2007). Value orientations: Measurement, antecedents and consequences across nations. In *Measuring attitudes cross-nationally: Lessons from the European social survey* (pp. 161–193). Sage

Schwartz, S. H. (2008). *Cultural value orientations: Nature and implications of national differences*. Publishing house of SU HSE.

Schwartz, S. H. (2009). Basic values: How they motivate and inhibit prosocial behavior. In M. Mikulincer & P. Shaver (Eds.), *Prosocial motives, emotions, and behavior: The better angels of our nature* (pp. 221–241). American Psychological Association Pres. https://doi.org/10.1037/12061-012

Schwartz, S. H. (2011). Studying values: Personal adventure, future directions. *Journal of Cross-Cultural Psychology, 42*(2), 307–319. https://doi.org/10.1177/0022022110396925

Schwartz, S. H. (2012). An overview of the Schwartz theory of basic values. *Online readings in Psychology and Culture, 2*(1), 1–20. https://doi.org/10.9707/2307-0919.1116

Schwartz, S. H. (2013). Culture matters: National value cultures, sources, and consequences. In understanding culture (pp. 137-160). Psychology Press. In C.-Y. Chiu, Y. Y. Hong, S. Shavitt, & R. S. Wyer Jr. (Eds.), *Understanding culture: Theory, research and application* (pp. 127–150). Psychology Press.

Schwartz, S. H. (2014a). Societal value culture: Latent and dynamic. *Journal of Cross-Cultural Psychology, 45*(1), 42–46. https://doi.org/10.1177/0022022113513404
Schwartz, S. H. (2014b). Rethinking the concept and measurement of societal culture in light of empirical findings. *Journal of Cross-Cultural Psychology, 45*(1), 5–13. https://doi.org/10.1177/0022022113490830
Schwartz, S. H., & Bardi, A. (2001). Value hierarchies across cultures: Taking a similarities perspective. *Journal of Cross-Cultural Psychology, 32*(3), 268–290. https://doi.org/10.1177/0022022101032003002
Schwartz, S. H., & Bilsky, W. (1987). Toward a universal psychological structure of human values. *Journal of Personality and Social Psychology, 53*(3), 550–562.
Schwartz, S. H., & Cieciuch, J. (2016). Implications of definitions of value. The ITC International Handbook of Testing and Assessment, 106–119. Oxford University Press
Schwartz, S. H., Cieciuch, J., Vecchione, M., Davidov, E., Fischer, R., Beierlein, C., Ramons, A., Verkasalo, M., Lönnkvist, J.-E., Demirutku, K., Dirilen-Gumus, O., & Konty, M. (2012). Refining the theory of basic individual values. *Journal of Personality and Social Psychology, 103*(4), 663. https://doi.org/10.1037/a0029393
Schwartz, S. H., Cieciuch, J., Vecchione, M., Torres, C., Dirilen-Gumus, O., & Butenko, T. (2017). Value tradeoffs propel and inhibit behavior: Validating the 19 refined values in four countries. *European Journal of Social Psychology, 47*(3), 241–258. https://doi.org/10.1002/ejsp.2228
Schwartz, S. J., Zamboanga, B. L., & Weisskirch, R. S. (2008). Broadening the study of the self: Integrating the study of personal identity and cultural identity. *Social and Personality Psychology Compass, 2*(2), 635–651. https://doi.org/10.1111/j.1751-9004.2008.00077.x
Seligman, M. E. (2004). *Authentic happiness: Using the new positive psychology to realize your potential for lasting fulfillment*. Simon & Schuster.
Slezackova, A. (2017). *Hope and Well-being: Psychosocial correlates and benefits*. Centre for Resilience and Socio-Emotional Health, L'Univesità ta' Malta.
Slezackova, A., Cefai, C., Cejkova, E., & Gassman, S. (2018). The role of life values in subjective Well-being among Czech and Maltese university students. *Horizons of Psychology/Psihološka obzorja, 27*, 35–47. https://doi.org/10.20419/2018.27.483
Slezackova, A., & Krafft, A. (2017). Hope: A driving force of optimal human development. In J. Mohan & M. Sehgal (Eds.), *Idea of excellence: Multiple perspectives* (pp. 1–12). Panjab University. ISBN 81-85322-59-7.
Slezackova, A., Prošek, T., Malatincová, T., & Krafft, A. M. (2020). Psychometrické vlastnosti české verze Škály prožívané naděje: faktorová struktura a vnitřní konzistence [Psychometric characteristics of the Czech version of The Perceived Hope Scale: Factor structure and internal consistency]. *Československá psychologie/Czechoslovak Psychology, 64*(3), 288–305.
Staats, S. (1989). Hope: A comparison of two self-report measures for adults. *Journal of Personality Assessment, 53*(2), 366–375. https://doi.org/10.1207/s15327752jpa5302_13
Steiger, J. H. (1980). Tests for comparing elements of a correlation matrix. *Psychological Bulletin, 87*(2), 245–251. https://doi.org/10.1037/0033-2909.87.2.245
Steinmetz, H., Schmidt, P., Tina-Booh, A., Wieczorek, S., & Schwartz, S. H. (2009). Testing measurement invariance using multigroup CFA: Differences between educational groups in human values measurement. *Quality & Quantity, 43*(4), 599. https://doi.org/10.1007/s11135-007-9143-x
Struch, N., Schwartz, S. H., & Van Der Kloot, W. A. (2002). Meanings of basic values for women and men: A cross-cultural analysis. *Personality and Social Psychology Bulletin, 28*(1), 16–28. https://doi.org/10.1177/0146167202281002
Tennen, H., Affleck, G., & Tennen, R. (2002). Clipped feathers: The theory and measurement of hope. *Psychological Inquiry, 13*(4), 311–317.

Triandis, H. C. (1995). *Individualism and collectivism*. Westview Press.

Triandis, H. C. (1997). Cross-cultural perspectives on personality. In R. Hogan, J. Johnson, & S. Briggs (Eds.), *Handbook of personality psychology* (pp. 439–464). Academic Press.

Uchida, Y., & Ogihara, Y. (2012). Personal or interpersonal construal of happiness: A cultural psychological perspective. *International Journal of Wellbeing, 2*, 354–369.

Webb, D. (2013). Pedagogies of hope. *Studies in Philosophy and Education, 32*(4), 397–414. https://doi.org/10.1007/s11217-012-9336-1

Andreas Krafft holds a doctoral degree in Management Sciences at the University of St. Gallen (Switzerland) with special focus on Organizational Psychology, Culture and Development. He has academic specializations in Social Psychology of Organizations, Work and Health Psychology as well as Positive Psychology from the University of Zürich. Andreas is associate researcher for Futures Studies and lecturer at the Institute of Systemic Management and Public Governance at the University of St. Gallen. Furthermore, he teaches at the University of Zürich in the field of Work and Health, at the Master of Applied Positive Psychology at the University of Lisbon, Portugal, as well as at the Master of Futures Studies from the Free University Berlin. He is co-president of swissfuture, the Swiss Society for Futures Studies, member of the executive board of SWIPPA (the Swiss Positive Psychology Association) and of the DACH-PP (German speaking Association of Positive Psychology). Since many years he leads the International Research Network of the Hope Barometer.

Alena Slezackova, Ph.D., is an Associate Professor of Psychology and a Vice Head of the Dept. of Psychology and Psychosomatics, Faculty of Medicine, Masaryk University, in Brno, Czech Republic. Her scientific interests include mainly hope, mental health, and well-being. She also has a special interest in the research and practice of mindfulness. Alena is a founder and director of the Czech Positive Psychology Centre (CPPC), a member of the Advisory Council of the International Positive Psychology Association (IPPA), and a member of the Executive Board of the European Network for Positive Psychology (ENPP). She has been a member of several international research projects, and she serves on the editorial boards of five academic psychological journals. Alena is the author of the first comprehensive monograph on positive psychology in the Czech language and dozens of scientific publications in positive psychology and health psychology.

Helena Águeda Marujo has a PhD in Psychology. She is Associate Professor at the Instituto Superior de Ciências Sociais e Politicas of the University of Lisbon, where she holds the positions of Executive Coordinator of master's and PhDs programs in Development Human Resources Policies; of Scientific Coordinator of the Postgraduate Degree in Applied Positive Psychology; of researcher at the Centre for Administration and Public Policy (CAPP); and of member of the Ethics Committee. She is the Coordinator of the UNESCO Chair in Education for Global Peace Sustainability at the University of Lisbon. Helena is a member of the Advisory Board of the International Positive Psychology Association and of the Board of Directors of the European Positive Psychology Network.

Valle Flores-Lucas is Associate Professor at Valladolid University, in the psychology department. She led the Postgraduate course on Positive Psychology and Humour sense at Valladolid University. Her research work has been centred on two main research lines: developmental language and communication disorders. In the last years, she started another research line in the field of Positive Psychology mainly in the study of hope and its relations with other positive strengths and its applications on education. She is member of the Spanish Positive Psychology Society.

Chapter 4
Long-term Future Expectations and Collective Hope

Andreas M. Krafft, JohnBosco Chika Chukwuorji, Rajneesh Choubisa, Stella Conte, Valle Flores-Lucas, Tharina Guse, Elżbieta Kasprzak, Helena Agueda Marujo, Chitra S. Nair, Dorit Redlich-Amirav, Mark Sinclair, Alena Slezackova, Patryk Stecz, Olga Varsos, and Eduardo Wills Herrera

Abstract The purpose of this chapter is to extend and explore the definition of collective hope as the shared desire for a better future not only for oneself, but for the

---

A. M. Krafft (✉)
Institute of Systemic Management and Public Governance, University of St. Gallen, St. Gallen, Switzerland
e-mail: andreas.krafft@unisg.ch

J. C. Chukwuorji
Department of Psychology, University of Nigeria, Nigeria, Nsukka

R. Choubisa
Department of Humanities and Social Sciences, Birla Institute of Technology and Science, (BITS), Pilani, India

S. Conte
Department of Psychology, University of Cagliari, Cagliari, Italy

V. Flores-Lucas
Department of Psychology, University of Valladolid, Valladolid, Spain

T. Guse
Department of Psychology, University of Pretoria, Pretoria, South Africa

E. Kasprzak
Department of Work and Organisational Psychology, Institute of Psychology, Kazimierz Wielki University of Bydgoszcz, Bydgoszcz, Poland

H. A. Marujo
Instituto Superior de Ciências Sociais e Politicas, University of Lisbon, Lisbon, Portugal

C. S. Nair
K. N. M. Government Arts and Science College Kanjiramkulam, University of Kerala, Kanjiramkulam, India

D. Redlich-Amirav
Sackler Faculty of Medicine, Tel Aviv University, Tel Aviv-Yafo, Israel

M. Sinclair
Mentor Education, Windsor, VIC, Australia

A. M. Krafft et al. (eds.), *Hope across cultures*, Cross-Cultural Advancements in Positive Psychology 14, https://doi.org/10.1007/978-3-031-24412-4_4

entire social community, the belief that a better future for all is possible but not necessarily guaranteed or even likely, and the trust in the human capacity to cooperate and support each other towards the realization of a better world despite current struggles and challenges. Conceptually we chose an interdisciplinary approach, integrating insights from Positive Psychology, Futures Studies, and Pragmatic Hope Philosophy. After introducing the concept of collective hope we present the nature and role of images of the future in terms of probable, possible and desired future trends and scenarios. Based on data collected with the Hope Barometer across 12 countries in November 2019 (N = 10,665), we evaluated people's long-term future expectations regarding the general quality of life, social trends and expected as well as wished-for future scenarios. We then related these expectations to perceived hope and social well-being. Our results suggest that long-term social expectations are significantly more pessimistic in European than in non-European countries and that personal hope levels are significantly higher in countries outside Europe. Moreover, an overwhelming majority of participants in this study preferred a social-sustainable over an individualist-competitive future scenario. Whereas future prospects had a significant effect on hope and (social) well-being, desirable images of the future hardly displayed an effect. Our findings highlight the importance of encouraging people to develop new positive pictures of the future which could foster hope, belief, and trust in a flourishing and sustainable world and to get engaged in its realization.

4.1 Introduction

Until now, research fields in psychology dedicated to future and prospective thinking (Oettingen, 2012; Baumeister et al., 2018; Seligman et al., 2016), positive and negative future expectations (Scheier & Carver, 1987; Seligman, 1990) and hope (Snyder, 1994; Scioli et al., 2011) have primarily been focused on personal goals. In this chapter, we will go beyond personal hopes of the individual and address collective social expectations and hopes in a global context. Our focus of analysis will be the wider societal future trends and scenarios as perceived by people in

A. Slezackova
Department of Medical Psychology and Psychosomatics, Faculty of Medicine, Masaryk University, Brno, Czech Republic

P. Stecz
Department of Clinical Psychology and Psychopathology, Institute of Psychology, University of Łódź, Łódź, Poland

O. Varsos
Centre for Positive Change, Melbourne, Australia

E. W. Herrera
Interdisciplinary Center for Development Studies (CIDER), School of Management, University of Los Andes, Bogotá, Cundinamarca, Colombia

different countries and their impact on perceived hope (Krafft et al., 2019) as well as on personal and social well-being (Keyes, 2014). For this purpose, we followed an interdisciplinary approach, integrating Positive Psychology, the humanistic discipline of Futures Studies and the philosophy of collective hope as theoretical foundations guiding our empirical research. Accordingly, the current chapter broadens the scope of analysis as recommended by authors like Lomas et al. (2021), Wissing (2018, 2022), and Marujo and Neto (2014), incorporating an interdisciplinary perspective, highlighting the importance of social processes, and taking into account the cultural context shaping hope and well-being.

4.2 Theoretical Background

4.2.1 Collective Hope

Conceptually, we define hope as a wish or desire, whose fulfilment is believed to be possible (although not necessarily probable), as well as the trust in the availability of personal, social, or other resources for realizing this wish. Collective hope represents a particular form of hope, namely shared desires for a better world (Braithwaite, 2004; Kleist & Jansen, 2016; McGeer, 2004; Shade, 2019; Stahl, 2019; Stitzlein, 2019). This kind of social hope refers to common wishes and beliefs that people share with others for the realization of certain values and dreams of a community (Blöser & Stahl, 2019). Collective hope connects people to other people, with whom they build a community with common interests and goals (Stahl, 2019). From this larger social perspective, collective hope is therefore the wish or desire for a better future, the belief in the possibility (although not likelihood) that a better future for a community of people might be possible, and the trust in some collective resources to positively deal with current problems and challenges (such as environmental degradation).

Therefore, collective hope begins with shared visions for a better future of society (Braithwaite, 2004; Rorty, 2002). Instead of focusing only on individual goals, people engage in a larger community to pursue overarching social, environmental and economic goals. At the core of collective hope is an interest in shaping the world in a positive way so that all members of a community can live better.

According to Rorty (1998), the value of collective hope lies not just in the hope of a better future, but also in the belief that people can shape a better future together through collective goals and efforts. This basic belief can also be formulated as: We can take the current problems of humanity in our hands and change something together. Social oriented hope is filled with a belief in future possibilities and a trust in the powers of collective determination and action. An essential question, therefore, is: What kind of common wishes and desires people do hold for the future and what do they believe in? In order to change things together, a community needs specific ideals. According to Rorty (1999), we must dream the future. Positive pictures of the future aim to mobilize a greater number of people to realize them.

The belief in the possibilities of the dreamed vision lies not in the evidence, but in the inspirational quality of the vision itself. Common visions offer people an image of an ideal future to work for (Gutiérrez, 2001). These ideals serve to broaden individual perspectives and widen personal horizons. The more conscious these ideals are, the more they can motivate individuals to act and work together.

4.2.2 Futures Studies and Images of the Future

The discipline that deals with prospective thinking by systematically exploring and creating alternative images of the future of society is called Futures Studies. The main purpose of Futures Studies, as Bell (1996, 2009) defines it, is to maintain or improve the welfare of humankind and the life-sustaining capacities of the Earth itself. Whereas Positive Psychology is primarily concerned with the good life and the flourishing of the individual, families and institutions, the scope of Futures Studies is about the nature of the good society and the flourishing of the entire world including the natural environment as well as the well-being of future generations (Bell, 1997, 2004). Both Positive Psychology and Futures Studies aim to contribute to human betterment and to make the world a better place in which to live. Taking the societal perspective, Futures Studies deals with long-term trends and scenarios, with overarching goals and values, and studies the images of the future held by diverse groups of people.

4.2.3 Images and Scenarios of the Future

Researchers in the field of Futures Studies do not predict the future but try to uncover how people think about the future (Bell, 1997). The pictures that people consciously or unconsciously maintain about the future affect their decisions, choices, and actions in the present (Hicks, 2003). On a broader scale, collective images of the future are influenced by psychological and cultural factors and can determine social progress or stagnation (Holden, 2002). Therefore, the main focus is to create and evaluate alternative images of the future, including peoples' general expectations, hopes and fears (Dator, 1996). These general hopes and worries regarding a good or a threatening future can influence the way people engage themselves at both the personal and the societal level.

One essential instrument to study people's images of the future is the development and evaluation of different future scenarios (Hicks, 2003). Basically, future scenarios are like cognitive maps, short portraits, or stories about the future, in which different trends are taken into account. The purpose of scenarios is to guide people's attention and imagination by highlighting the consequences of different trends and to anticipate a range of possible future developments. Therefore, the word "futures" is used in plural because there is not only one future but many possible futures.

Usually, people are focused on the immediate future, engrossed in their daily challenges but they are not used to think about long-term trends and prospects. The task of researchers in Futures Studies is to encourage and guide people to become aware of their long-term expectations, to open up the horizon for imagining new future opportunities and to identify and become conscious about desirable futures, both for themselves and the world (Bell, 2003; Eckersley, 2002; Hicks, 2003). This means that researchers must challenge prevalent ways of thinking and daily habits, consider, and evaluate new possibilities and alternatives, and analyze values, norms, goals, attitudes, and preferences of the population (Bell, 2004). In sum, Futures Studies aims to explore probable (what is likely to be), possible (what can or could be) and preferable (what ought to be) images of the future as seen by different people.

4.2.3.1 Probable Futures

Probable futures are defined by people's beliefs and subjective estimation concerning the future they expect to be most likely. For a systematic investigation of the probable, people are assisted to consider past, present, and future trends and developments. One frequently asked question is what the most probable future would be if things continue to unfold the way they have done until now. What would the most probable future be, if we continue to behave as we usually do (Bell, 2003)?

4.2.3.2 Possible Futures

Guiding people to imaging possible futures seeks to draw their attention to alternative scenarios and to new future opportunities. The fundamental purpose here is to encourage individuals to think about what could be if things change, or if they took an alternative route, and to believe that a different future is possible. Basically, considering possible futures fosters new perspectives, increase future options, and broaden possible choices. Often, people are encouraged to think about completely unconventional and creative scenarios. It involves constructing a variety of clear and powerful, both positive and negative images of the future (Bell, 1996).

4.2.3.3 Desirable Futures

After contemplating the many possible future scenarios, and considering that some futures are better than others, the core question that remains is: which of these scenarios are the most and the less desired by people? This comprises an assessment of the value judgements, the general goals, preferences, and the priorities of different groups of individuals. Central to this question is what people consider to be the characteristics of a good society (Bell, 2004). In order to know what is the desirable, people are asked which futures they want to achieve and which futures they want to avoid (Hicks, 2003).

The contemplation of probable, possible and desirable future scenarios creates positive and negative images of the future, which in extreme cases tell stories of ideal and feared futures in the form of utopias and dystopias. Four typical scenarios usually evolve (Hicks, 2003):

1. More of the same: Basically, everything will remain the same or continue to unfold as it always did.
2. Technological development: New technologies will solve current problems and enable continued progress.
3. Catastrophe: Current developments will lead to multiple economic, environmental, and social crises.
4. Sustainable development: New forms of production, consumption, and behavior are evidence of a change in consciousness and will give rise to new kinds of social norms and structures.

4.2.4 Global Futures, Hopes and Fears and their Impact on Well-being

In many empirical studies, researchers discovered a huge discrepancy between what people expect will happen in the future and what they would wish to happen (Eckersley et al., 2007; Inayatullah, 2000, 2002). People's expectations regarding global future trends and scenarios are often in sharp contradiction to what they hope for the world (Hicks, 1996). Furthermore, another paradox is the dissonance found between people's optimistic view of their personal life and the pessimistic assessment of social and global futures (Rubin, 2002; Toffler, 1974). Particularly young people are hopeful with regard to their future job opportunities, their families, and their expected living conditions. In contrast, the images of the future of society and the world are influenced by the global problems such as environmental crises, population growth, economic turmoil and health issues. The negative view of the global future can be an effect of people's perception of growing complexity, uncertainty, and loss of personal control (Brunstad, 2002).

Psychologically speaking, the inner tension and lack of coherence existing between probable, possible, and desirable futures can be a source of mistrust, anger, anxiety, and apathy (Eckersley et al., 2007; Grund & Brock, 2019; Hickman, 2020; Searle & Gow, 2010). Based on a sense of powerlessness of being unable to change anything beyond one's own life, people focus on what they can influence, that is, short sighted but attainable personal goals. However, these are often deprived of a deeper meaning and purpose, which in turn increases the negative view toward the larger society and the disengagement from global issues (Eckersley et al., 2007).

In recent years, researchers started to emphasize that personal well-being is not only determined by pleasurable experiences and satisfaction with personal domains in life, such as the family, work, closer friends and so on, but that social issues and developments and the perception of the future of the world may also have a significant impact on well-being (Eckersley et al., 2007; Keyes, 2014). Researchers in the field of Positive Psychology have already revealed that psychological well-being is closely related to a greater meaning and purpose in life and the attachment to something larger than the self (Delle Fave & Soosai-Nathan, 2014; Delle Fave et al., 2011, 2013, 2016; Ryff, 1989; Ryff & Keyes, 1995). However, the connection between global threats and personal well-being is something that still has to be investigated more in detail.

In short, Eckersley (1999, p. 88) noticed that a "failure to provide a broad cultural framework of hope, meaning and purpose in young people's lives could be weakening their resilience, making them more vulnerable to these problems". Likewise, Hicks (2012, p. 7) argued that "clarifying hopes for the future can enhance motivation in the present and thus positive action for change." Researchers in the field of Futures Studies clearly distinguished between optimism/pessimism on the one hand, and hopefulness/hopelessness on the other (Slaughter, 2002; Nordensvard, 2014). Optimistic (unrealistic) visions based on the belief that at the end, everything will be fine, could be detrimental if they fail encouraging people to action. What is needed is an active hope that motivates people to commit themselves to overcome the problems and difficulties the world is facing. Moreover, people with pessimistic images of the future can remain hopeful if the negative expectations do not lead to helplessness (Grund & Brock, 2019; Nordensvard, 2014). The combination of negative future scenarios with images of preferred futures can motivate people to become engaged in addressing contemporary problems, and therefore preventing the negative expectations from becoming a reality. This could foster the achievement of the desired future conditions (Eckersley et al., 2007).

4.2.5 *Personal and Social Well-being*

In order to examine the relationship between global expectations for the future and well-being, it is necessary to briefly present different concepts of well-being. Researchers in Positive Psychology have identified two types of well-being (Delle Fave, 2020; Delle Fave et al., 2011; Ryan & Deci, 2001): Hedonic well-being is basically related to positive experiences and emotions and comprises feeling good and being satisfied with one's life (Diener, 2000). Eudaimonic well-being, on the other hand, is a more complex psychological construct and addresses the way people relate to and function in the world (Ryff, 1989; Ryff & Keyes, 1995; Ryff & Singer, 2008).

In his model of complete mental health, Keyes (2002, 2014) has differentiated two domains of eudaimonic well-being: The psychological and the social sphere. Psychological well-being is about personal growth and optimal development as an individual. It comprises experiencing purpose and meaning in life, maintaining good personal relations with other people, feeling competent in relation to one's tasks and having an overall good view of oneself (e.g., being a good, loveable, responsible, and engaged person) (Ryff, 1989). Social well-being, on the other hand, refers to the relationship of the individual to the wider community and society. A positive relationship between the individual and the social environment is typically characterized by shared social goals and values (Massimini & Delle Fave, 2000), by meaningful and accepted social norms and structures, by a sense of belonging and feeling part of society, by mutual appreciation, respect, and recognition with other people, by having something to contribute to the community, and by experiencing a positive development of society and the world at large.

According to Keyes and Haidt (2010), a person can flourish when he or she achieves a harmonious balance between feeling good, functioning well as an individual and interacting positively with others as member of a community embedded in elevating social structures. However, Keyes (2014) recognized that especially the relationship between the individual and society and its contribution to well-being still requires more investigation. Delle Fave and her colleagues (Delle Fave et al., 2011) noticed that social issues seem to be less relevant for individual well-being, which could have detrimental effects for collective welfare.

In this sense, Frank Polak, one of the fathers of humanistic Futures Studies, formulated a provocative thesis: "The rise and fall of images of the future precedes or accompanies the rise and fall of cultures. As long as a society's image of the future is positive and flourishing, the flower of culture is in full bloom. Once the image begins to decay and lose its vitality, however, the culture cannot long survive." (Polak, 1961/1973, p. 19). For Polak, images of the future are like a mirror of the respective zeitgeist. In his eyes, the degree of optimism or pessimism is a measure of the health and well-being of the population. The lack of positive images of the future is therefore an obstacle to social progress, especially because it can turn the future into a projection field of fears instead of hopes.

4.3 The Present Study

4.3.1 Aim and Objectives

The aim of our study was to investigate the long-term expectations concerning the future quality of life, both in general and in several life and social domains, as well as the outlooks regarding probable and desirable long-term future scenarios (in 20 years' time) across 12 countries and relate these images of the future to people's perceived personal hope and well-being.

Based on measures developed by Eckersley (1999), our first objective was to identify similarities and differences across countries in how people perceive future prospects regarding the general quality of life as well as particular social domains in their country, such as family life, mental health of the population, the natural environment etc.

The second objective was to evaluate expected and desirable social scenarios across countries. Firstly, we analyzed the subjective likelihood people ascribe to two possible scenarios portraying a flourishing and a declining future full of crises. Afterwards, we assessed the desirability of two other scenarios describing a (modern) competitive and individualistic society, on the one hand, and a (post-modern) sustainable and communal society, on the other (Eckersley, 1999; Eckersley et al., 2007).

Our third objective was to assess the relationship of future expectations and scenarios with the general level of perceived hope as well as with hedonic, psychological, and social well-being. Specifically, we wanted to establish the association of future expectations and future scenarios on perceived hope and social well-being.

We assumed that the expectation of negative future trends and scenarios will have a significant negative association with hope and well-being and that positive scenarios will display a positive relationship. Moreover, desired scenarios could have a positive connection with hope and well-being.

4.3.2 *Procedure and National Samples*

Data was collected as part of the Hope Barometer in November 2019 (a few months before the outbreak of the COVID19-pandemic) through announcements in online newspapers, social media, and e-mails. No incentives were offered. We selected 12 countries displaying a robust database of at least 200 participants. People younger than 18 were excluded from the analysis. A total of 10,759 people completed the questionnaire, from which 94 were removed due to a high number of missing values and obvious erroneous answers (e.g., always 0 or 1).

Participants were from Australia ($N = 474$), Colombia ($N = 311$), the Czech Republic ($N = 469$), India ($N = 1092$), Israel ($N = 884$), Italy ($N = 272$), Nigeria ($N = 665$), Poland ($N = 481$), Portugal ($N = 507$), South Africa ($N = 574$), Spain ($N = 529$) and Switzerland ($N = 3935$). The questionnaire was administered in English (Australia, Northern and Southern India, Nigeria, and South Africa), Spanish (Colombia and Spain), Czech (Czech Republic), Hebrew (Israel), Italian (Italy and Switzerland), Polish (Poland), Portuguese (Portugal), Malayalam (Southern India) as well as French and German (Switzerland).

The demographic structure of the samples is exhibited in Appendix 4.1. Gender distribution was quite balanced in Australia, Colombia, India, South Africa, and Switzerland. In the Czech Republic, Israel, Italy, Poland, Portugal and Spain, more women than men (about 70/30) and in Nigeria more men than women took part in the survey. The mean age ranged between the youngest people participating in Colombia (M = 26.29, SD = 8.63) and the oldest in Australia (M = 47.53, SD = 13.05) and Switzerland (M = 46.82, SD = 15.67).

4.3.3 Measures

Long-Term Future Expectations and Scenarios

Long-term future expectations and scenarios were measured implementing questionnaires developed by the Australian futurologist Richard Eckersley (Eckersley, 1999; Eckersley et al., 2007). Participants were initially asked to imagine their country in twenty years' time (around 2040) and to rate on a five-point Likert-scale (from 1 to 5) if the general quality of life would be better, the same or worse than it is today. Afterwards, they could assess their long-term expectations in eleven social domains (e.g., public health, family life, employment, natural environment, etc.). Participants were not asked to assess their own life but the general outlooks in their country. The Cronbach alpha coefficients of the twelve items exhibit good scores in all samples between $\alpha = 0.89$ and $\alpha = 0.97$.

The next step was to assess the likelihood of two scenarios in 2040. The first scenario describes a world in which a larger population, environmental destruction, new diseases, and ethnic and regional conflicts would drive the world into times of crises. In the second scenario the world would continue a path of economic and technological development, enabling humanity to overcome the obstacles it faces and to enter a new age of sustainability, peace, and prosperity. The two scenarios could be rated on a six-point scale from 1 (very unlikely) to 6 (very likely).

To assess the desirability of future states in 2040, two additional scenarios were provided. The first scenario portrayed a fast-paced, internationally competitive society, with the emphasis on the individual, wealth generation, and technological advancements. The second scenario represented a greener, more harmonious society, where the emphasis is on cooperation, community and family, more equal distribution of wealth, and greater economic self-sufficiency. Both scenarios were rated on a six-point scale from 1 (highly undesired) to 6 (highly desired).

Perceived Hope

To assess the general level of personal hope we employed the Perceived Hope Scale (PHS) (Krafft et al., 2019, 2021; Marujo et al., 2021; Slezackova et al., 2020). The PHS consists of six items to measure the level of hope as perceived by people in a direct manner and free from any preconceptions regarding the nature and quality of hope. The PHS is especially suitable to assess the level of general hope in different cultures since it avoids any bias regarding potential sources, roots, dimensions, and elements of hope. The items of the PHS evaluate the degree of hope in general ("I feel hopeful"), in one's life ("I am hopeful with regard to my life") and in difficult situations, the belief in the possibility of fulfilment of one's hopes and the intensity of general hope vis-à-vis the feeling of anxiety ("In my life hope outweighs anxiety"). The six positively worded items were rated on a 6-point Likert scale from 0 (strongly disagree) to 5 (strongly agree). In the current study the six items achieved a high internal consistency in all samples with Cronbach alpha values between $\alpha = 0.79$ and $\alpha = 0.90$.

Hedonic, Psychological, and Social Well-being

For a differentiated evaluation of hedonic, eudaimonic and especially social well-being, we reverted to Keyes' (2002; Keyes et al., 2008) Mental Health Continuum (MHC-SF). The MHC-SF comprises 14 positively worded items, with three items representing hedonic well-being (happy, interested in life, and satisfied), six items evaluating psychological well-being (functioning well in one's personal life) and five items describing social well-being (the relationship between oneself and the larger community/society). Participants were asked to rate how often in the past month they felt in a specific manner. Items are rated on a six-point scale from 1 (never) to 6 (every day). Reliability coefficients were good in all samples, achieving levels between $\alpha = 0.78$ and $\alpha = 0.92$ for hedonic well-being, between $\alpha = 0.80$ and $\alpha = 0.89$ for psychological well-being, and between $\alpha = 0.80$ and $\alpha = 0.88$ for social well-being.

4.3.4 Data Analysis

We started our analysis by calculating mean values and standard deviations of the long-term future expectations, presenting the rank order among countries, and comparing the results via univariate analysis of variance (ANOVA). Afterwards we computed the ascribed likelihood to the crisis and the flourishing scenarios for each country, compared both mean values and assessed if the differences were significant (ANOVA). In order to evaluate the gap between both scenarios, we devised two groups of participants for every country: The first group contains people that have judged the crisis scenario 1 to be more likely than the flourishing scenario 2 and the second group those who considered the flourishing scenario 2 to be more likely than the crisis scenario 1. We then calculated the proportion of people belonging to each group and the mean values of both scenarios and compared them with and between the groups (scenario 1 vs. scenario 2 within groups and scenarios 1 and 2 vs. scenarios 1 and 2 across groups).

A similar procedure was performed with both scenarios judged as more or less desirable (the individualistic-competitive and the social-sustainable). After calculating mean values and standard deviations and comparing mean values of both scenarios via ANOVA, we created two groups of participants for each national sample and compared their individual scores within and between groups. Group 1 comprised people who assessed the individualistic-competitive scenario 1 to be more desirable than the social-sustainable scenario 2. Group 2 consisted of participants believing that the social-sustainable scenario 2 would be more desirable than the individual-competitive scenario 1.

The final step assessed the mean levels of perceived hope as well as hedonic, psychological, and social well-being across countries. Before starting with the analyses, we tested group invariance for the PHS across the 12 countries via multi-group confirmatory factor analysis (MGCFA). We applied the nested model procedure to examine configurational, metric, scalar, and full invariance by means of

Maximum Likelihood estimation. The goodness of the models was assessed with the Comparative fit index (CFI) and Tucker-Lewis index (TLI) (study criterion ≥ 0.95 as ideal and ≥ 0.90 as the acceptable level), the root mean square error of approximation (RMSEA) (study criterion ≤ 0.08) and the standardized root mean residual SRMR (study criterion ≤ 0.08) (Hu & Bentler, 1999). The recommended criteria to demonstrate invariance are changes in CFI and TLI between comparison and nested models of $\geq -.010$, a change in RMSEA of ≤ 0.015 and a variation in SRMR of ≤ 0.030 (for loading invariance) and ≤ 0.010 (for intercept invariance) (Chen, 2007).

Performing ANOVA, we compared the mean values of hope and well-being of the different groups of participants, those believing in the likelihood of the crisis or the flourishing scenario, as well as of both groups supporting the individual-competitive or the social-sustainable scenario more. Afterwards, we computed partial bivariate correlations between expectations and scenarios with perceived hope and the well-being indicators (controlling for demographic variables). Finally, we performed a series of hierarchical regression analyses for every country to predict perceived hope, on the one hand, and social well-being, on the other. As predictor variables we employed the composite score of future social expectations in the first analyses, both "likely" scenarios (crisis and flourishing) in the second series of analyses, and both desirable scenarios (individual-competitive and social-sustainable) in the third wave of analyses (after demographic variables).

4.3.5 *Results*

4.3.5.1 Future Expectations

Participants were asked to think about their country in twenty years' time, around 2040, and to consider whether they believe that the overall quality of life will be better than it is now, about the same, or worse than it is now. Afterwards we invited the participants to assess different life domains, and indicate whether they expect these to get better, remain the same, or get worse until 2040.

Results in Fig. 4.1 and Table 4.1 point out that Nigeria, Colombia, and Portugal were the countries with the most optimistic expectations regarding future quality of life, and likewise in almost all individual life domains. The most negative countries with regards to the future development of the quality of life were Switzerland, Spain, South Africa, and Italy (all samples $F = 110.89$, $\eta2 = 0.107$, $p < 0.001$). Looking at the single life domains, the countries with the most negative outlooks were Switzerland, India, and South Africa.

In most countries, the life domains with the most positive prospects were physical health, employment opportunities, the fight against racism and the general economy. India was the exception, with a negative outlook on the domain of physical health, the Czech Republic concerning the negative prospects about future employment opportunities, Poland on the subject of rising racism and Spain about the adverse development of the general economy. The greatest concerns in almost all countries

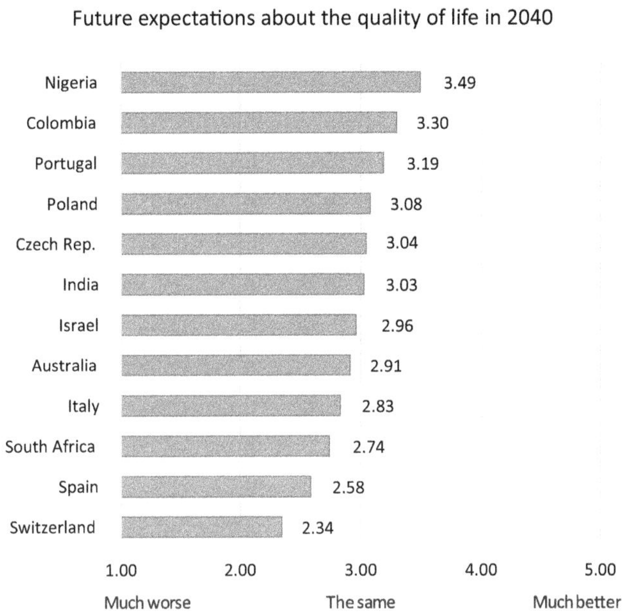

Fig. 4.1 Mean values of quality of life 2040 across countries

were related to the increasing gap between the rich and the poor, the deterioration of the natural environment, of family life and of the mental health of the population.

4.3.5.2 Expected Future Scenarios

In the next step, we presented two scenarios describing different possible futures: a crisis and a flourishing image of 2040. We asked the participants to assess how likely or unlikely these scenarios are, in their opinion.

In Table 4.2 we present the mean values and standard deviations of the ascribed likelihood to the respective scenarios in each country. Figure 4.2 reveals that for participants in most countries the crisis scenario (1) was considered more likely than the flourishing scenario (2), with exception of Nigeria and Israel where both scenarios exhibit a similar likelihood. Differences between the country samples regarding the likelihood of the crisis scenario are rather low but significant (all samples $F = 20.13$, $\eta 2 = 0.021$, $p < 0.001$). Whereas people in South Africa, Italy, Switzerland, Poland, and Spain were the most pessimistic about a future full of crises, people in Australia, Colombia, Czechia, and Israel were a little bit less concerned. Likewise, participants in Switzerland, Poland, Spain, Czechia, Portugal, and South Africa showed the lowest endorsement of a flourishing scenario. On the other hand, people in Nigeria, Israel and Colombia were the most positive about a flourishing future (scenario 2). Here the differences between the countries were slightly more pronounced (all samples $F = 91.04$, $\eta 2 = 0.090$, $p < 0.001$).

Table 4.1 Mean values and standard deviations of future expectations across countries

	Australia		Colombia		Czech Rep.		India		Israel		Italy		Nigeria		Poland		Portugal		South Africa		Spain		Switzerland	
	M	SD	M	SD	M	SD	M	SD	M	SD	M	SD	M	SD	M	SD	M	SD	M	SD	M	SD	M	SD
Quality of life 2040	2.91	1.17	3.30	1.11	3.04	0.95	3.03	1.29	2.96	1.16	2.83	1.11	3.49	1.26	3.08	1.16	3.19	1.04	2.74	1.36	2.58	0.99	2.34	0.95
The country's economy	2.99	1.01	3.57	1.00	3.00	0.86	2.91	1.33	3.07	1.05	2.84	1.08	3.39	1.32	3.00	1.13	3.27	1.12	2.88	1.21	2.88	1.18	2.60	0.91
Employment prospects	2.76	1.02	3.31	1.08	2.99	0.87	2.76	1.30	2.93	1.01	2.89	1.11	3.23	1.32	3.13	1.03	3.26	1.16	2.48	1.35	2.92	1.20	2.32	0.95
Gap between rich and poor	2.47	1.06	3.03	1.10	2.42	0.88	2.49	1.76	2.48	1.04	2.39	1.03	3.01	1.34	2.62	1.00	3.05	1.16	2.48	1.27	2.60	1.21	1.87	0.95
Family life	2.96	0.93	3.39	1.04	2.83	0.82	2.69	1.18	2.98	0.89	3.01	0.93	3.55	1.12	2.86	0.95	3.35	0.98	3.05	1.14	3.14	1.00	2.70	0.83
Our natural environment	2.50	1.19	2.92	1.31	2.61	1.05	2.34	1.25	2.75	1.17	2.79	1.18	3.47	1.14	2.48	1.18	3.10	1.29	2.56	1.26	2.48	1.30	2.53	1.08
The physical health of the population	2.93	1.10	3.36	0.99	2.96	0.93	2.68	1.22	3.40	1.00	2.99	1.08	3.37	1.19	2.80	1.13	3.39	1.10	2.66	1.26	3.16	1.09	2.75	0.99
The mental health of the population	2.50	1.14	3.01	1.13	2.53	0.92	2.63	1.17	2.91	1.02	2.51	1.08	3.28	1.27	2.40	1.12	3.10	1.24	2.56	1.24	2.71	1.19	2.21	0.90
Substance abuse	2.51	1.05	2.89	1.06	2.69	0.78	2.37	1.17	2.85	0.94	2.58	0.98	2.91	1.30	2.56	0.96	3.08	1.05	2.38	1.20	2.74	1.12	2.48	0.93
Crime and violence	2.62	1.05	3.49	0.95	2.91	0.81	2.44	1.18	2.92	0.99	2.79	0.99	3.17	1.25	2.87	0.97	3.16	1.09	2.40	1.32	3.00	1.14	2.28	0.96
Racism	3.19	1.03	3.96	0.90	3.03	0.92	2.57	1.25	2.96	1.12	2.81	1.13	3.29	1.22	3.00	1.10	3.50	1.00	2.97	1.25	3.15	1.16	2.54	1.03
Justice and equality	2.86	1.00	3.31	1.00	2.91	0.83	2.58	1.24	2.85	1.03	2.79	1.00	3.09	1.34	2.74	1.01	3.35	1.12	2.65	1.28	3.12	1.14	2.65	1.02

Table 4.2 Mean values, standard deviations and mean value comparisons of the likelihood of scenarios across countries and between different groups of participants

Country	Crisis scenario 1		Flourishing scenario 2		Differences in mean values between scenarios		Group 1: Crisis scenario 1 more likely than flourishing scenario 2				Group 2: Flourishing scenario 2 more likely than crisis scenario 1			
	M	SD	M	SD	t	Sig	n	%	M_{CS1}*	M_{FS2}*	n	%	M_{CS1}*	M_{FS2}*
Australia	3.91	1.31	3.54	1.30	3.579	<0.001	313	66.0%	4.58	3.02	161	34.0%	2.59	4.56
Colombia	3.95	1.16	3.71	1.17	2.200	0.029	205	65.9%	4.55	3.25	106	34.1%	2.80	4.61
Czech Rep.	3.95	1.08	3.37	0.98	6.941	<0.001	320	68.2%	4.49	2.94	149	31.8%	2.80	4.30
India	4.04	1.15	3.64	1.12	6.893	<0.001	764	70.0%	4.57	3.23	328	30.0%	2.82	4.62
Israel	3.96	1.20	3.93	1.40	0.387	0.699	532	60.2%	4.58	3.34	352	39.8%	3.01	4.83
Italy	4.37	1.35	3.60	1.29	5.864	<0.001	194	71.3%	4.89	3.08	78	28.7%	3.08	4.87
Nigeria	4.08	1.15	4.00	1.33	1.114	0.266	446	67.1%	4.67	3.61	219	32.9%	2.86	4.79
Poland	4.35	1.12	3.23	1.25	11.465	<0.001	376	78.2%	4.77	2.80	105	21.8%	2.86	4.75
Portugal	4.07	1.27	3.51	1.44	6.220	<0.001	349	68.8%	4.58	2.98	158	31.2%	2.96	4.68
South Africa	4.41	1.26	3.52	1.41	9.918	<0.001	441	76.8%	4.84	3.13	133	23.2%	2.99	4.83
Spain	4.22	1.23	3.24	1.26	11.474	<0.001	414	78.3%	4.61	2.89	115	21.7%	2.81	4.52
Switzerland	4.36	1.33	2.90	1.36	43.336	<0.001	3250	82.6%	4.70	2.57	685	17.4%	2.74	4.45

Note: *All differences in mean values within and between groups are significant at $p < 0.01$

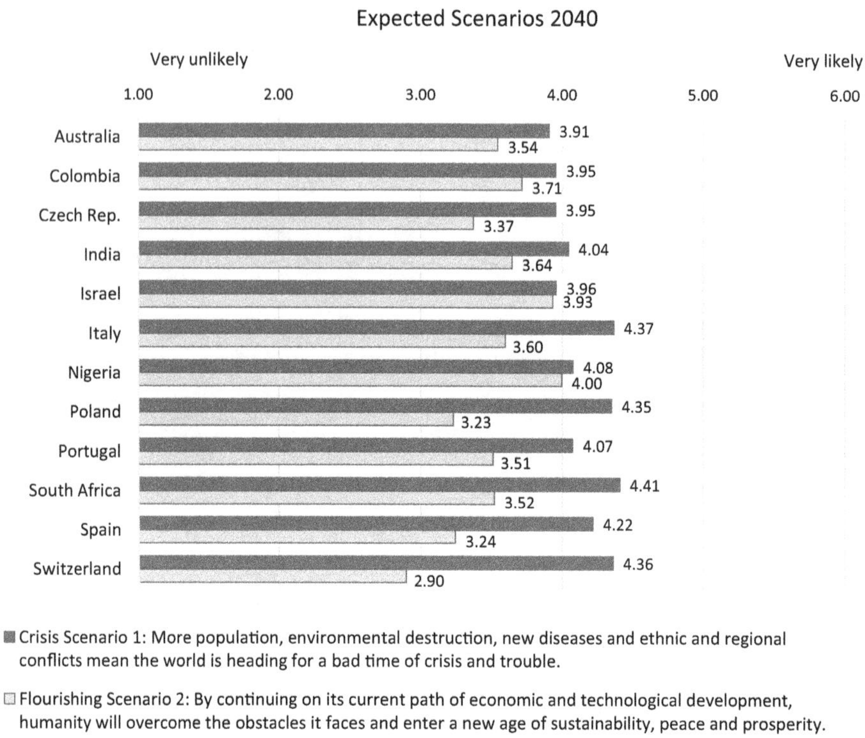

Fig. 4.2 Mean values of expected scenarios 2040 by country

In order to assess how many people were positive and how many negative about the future, we divided the samples into two groups: those who considered the crisis scenario more likely than the flourishing scenario (group 1) and those who deemed the flourishing scenario more likely than the crisis scenario (group 2). Table 4.2 displays the distribution of both groups along with the mean values of scenario 1 and 2 for each group. Between 60.2% of the participants in Israel and 82.6% in Switzerland judged the crisis scenario to be more likely than the flourishing scenario. In Switzerland, Poland, Spain and South Africa, people were especially concerned about the future prospects of their countries, since between 76.8% and 82.6% of the participants considered the crisis scenario more likely than the flourishing scenario. Remarkably, in all countries the mean values of scenario 1 and 2 (MCS1 and MFS2) differ significantly from each other, both within the single groups as well as between the two groups (MCS1 and MFS2 for group 1 vs. group 2) ($p < 0.001$). Further, the samples from Switzerland, Poland, Spain, and South Africa presented the largest gap between both scenarios.

4.3.5.3 Desirable Future Scenarios

After assessing the likelihood of the crisis and flourishing scenarios, we portrayed two new scenarios describing possible futures in 2040: the first, describing an individualist and competitive (modern) society and the second, other describing a sustainable and social oriented (post-modern) future. We asked the participants to judge how desirable or undesirable these scenarios were to them.

Similar to the previous analysis, we divided the national samples into two groups. Group 1 consisted of participants that supported the individualist-competitive scenario more than the social-sustainable scenario. Group 2 included people that esteemed the social-sustainable scenario as more desirable than the individualist-competitive scenario. Comparing mean values of both scenarios among the national samples as well as within the two groups (MIC1 and MSS2) and between groups (MIC1 and MSS2 of group 1 vs. MIC1 and MSS2 of group 2) provided significant differences in all countries ($p < 0.001$).

The results in Fig. 4.3 and Table 4.3 reveal that participants in all countries preferred the social-sustainable scenario 2 more than the individualistic-competitive

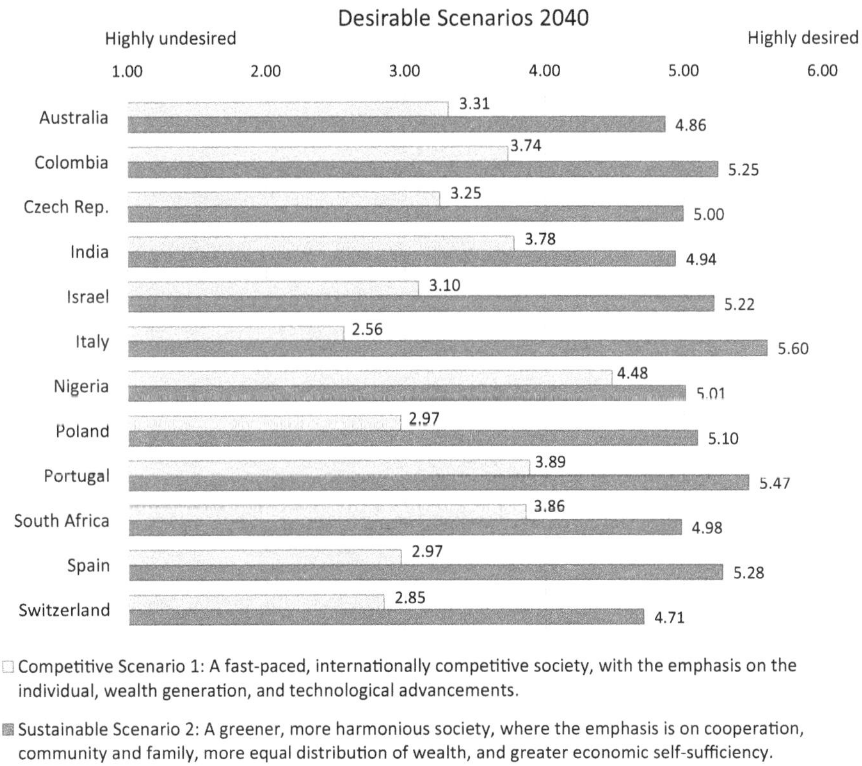

Fig. 4.3 Mean values of desirable scenarios 2040 by country

Table 4.3 Mean values, standard deviations, and mean value comparisons of the desirability of scenarios across countries and between different groups of participants

Country	Competitive Scenario 1		Sustainable Scenario 2		Differences in mean values between scenarios		Group 1: Competitive scenario 1 more desirable than sustainable scenario 2				Group 2: Sustainable scenario 2 more desirable than competitive scenario 1			
	M	SD	M	SD	t	Sig.	n	%	M_{IC1} *	M_{SS2} *	n	%	M_{IC1} *	M_{SS2} *
Australia	3.31	1.41	4.86	1.26	−15.779	<0.001	51	10.8%	5.16	2.88	423	89.2%	3.09	5.10
Colombia	3.74	1.35	5.25	0.97	−14.961	<0.001	36	11.6%	4.86	3.56	275	88.4%	3.59	5.47
Czech Rep.	3.25	1.18	5.00	1.00	−21.304	<0.001	38	8.1%	4.95	3.13	431	91.9%	3.10	5.16
India	3.78	1.36	4.94	0.96	−21.327	<0.001	127	11.6%	4.90	3.15	965	88.4%	3.63	5.18
Israel	3.10	1.52	5.22	0.82	−33.719	<0.001	61	6.9%	4.97	3.11	823	93.1%	2.96	5.37
Italy	2.56	1.26	5.60	1.14	−26.396	<0.001	10	3.7%	4.70	3.00	262	96.3%	2.48	5.70
Nigeria	4.48	1.49	5.01	1.15	−9.789	<0.001	88	13.2%	5.13	3.65	577	86.8%	4.38	5.22
Poland	2.97	1.57	5.10	0.93	−20.968	<0.001	51	10.6%	5.16	2.96	430	89.4%	2.71	5.35
Portugal	3.89	1.44	5.47	1.28	−19.242	<0.001	35	6.9%	5.29	3.71	472	93.1%	3.78	5.60
South Africa	3.86	1.45	4.98	1.26	−13.828	<0.001	92	14.3%	4.84	3.04	492	85.7%	3.70	5.30
Spain	2.97	1.36	5.28	1.40	−27.401	<0.001	31	5.9%	5.00	3.03	498	94.1%	2.84	5.42
Switzerland	2.85	1.38	4.71	1.22	−52.479	<0.001	485	12.3%	4.42	2.29	3450	87.7%	2.63	5.05

Note: * All differences in mean values within and between groups are significant at $p < 0.01$

scenario (between 85.7% in South Africa and 94.1% in Spain). Participants in Nigeria, South Africa and Portugal exhibited the highest scores in support of an individual-competitive future, and those in Poland, Spain, Switzerland, and Italy the lowest. The differences between the countries were the most pronounced (all samples $F = 128.02$, $\eta 2 = 0.122$, $p < 0.001$). Moreover, participants in Italy, Portugal, and Spain displayed the strongest support for the social-sustainable future, however, the differences between countries were significant but rather small (all samples $F = 39.44$, $\eta 2 = 0.041$, $p < 0.001$). In Nigeria, South Africa and India, the gap between the desirability of both scenarios was the lowest, suggesting that the individualistic-competitive scenario is to a certain extent also a worthwhile development. The largest gap between both scenarios was perceived in Italy, Spain, Poland, and Israel, followed by Switzerland and the Czech Republic (all samples $F = 55.85$, $\eta 2 = 0.057$, $p < 0.001$). These results suggest that people in poorer and economically less developed countries may desire to catch up with the wealthier and more competitive countries in the West, but in a social and sustainable way.

Finally, we calculated the difference between the desired social-sustainable and the expected flourishing scenario and found that the gap was significantly wider in the European countries. Specifically, it was more pronounced in Spain ($M = 2.04$), Italy ($M = 2.00$), Portugal ($M = 1.96$) and Poland ($M = 1.87$) than in the non-European countries, where it was the smallest in Nigeria ($M = 1.02$), Israel ($M = 1.29$), India ($M = 1.30$) and Australia ($M = 1.32$) (all samples $F = 26.84$, $\eta 2 = 0.028$, $p < 0.001$).

4.3.5.4 Group Invariance of the Perceived Hope Scale (PHS)

In order to be able to compare mean values of perceived hope across countries and correlate these values with the future expectations and scenarios, we first tested the measurement invariance of the PHS. Table 4.4 presents the fit indices of the MGCFA to assess the goodness of fit for the general sample and of the five models to test different levels of group invariance. The one-factor model for the total sample

Table 4.4 Multi-group CFA and analysis of group invariance for the PHS

	X^2	df	CFI	TLI	RMSEA	SRMR
Total sample (N = 10,193)	471.80	9	0.985	0.976	0.071	0.020
Country/sample invariance						
Configurational Invariance (equal form)	4746.93	288	0.854	0.909	0.039	0.055
Metric Invariance (equal loadings)	4774.00	293	0.854	0.910	0.039	0.055
Scalar Invariance (equal intercepts)	4881.22	299	0.851	0.910	0.039	0.055
Structural co-variances	4899.70	300	0.850	0.910	0.039	0.056
Full uniqueness (measurement residuals)	4908.80	306	0.850	0.912	0.038	0.056

Note: *CFA* Confirmatory Factor Analysis, *CFI* Comparative fit index, *TLI* Tucker-Lewis index, *RMSEA* Root mean square error of approximation, *SRMR* Standardized root mean residual

revealed a good model fit (CFI and TLI > 0.95, RMSEA and SRMR < 0.08). The first step of configurational invariance across the groups (equal form) provides a good fit to the data for the TLI, RMSEA and SRMR but not for the CFI. According to Marsh (1994) and Marsh et al. (1996) the difference between the TLI and the CFI is that the TLI also penalizes model complexity (thereby appropriately rewarding model parsimony). This property of the TLI has been noted as particularly useful in tests across multiple groups (Vandenberg & Lance, 2000). We therefore focused our assessment on the TLI, the RMSEA and the SRMR. All models compared to the baseline model were under the threshold values recommended by the literature (TLI > .01, RMSEA and SRMR < 0.015) with exception of the TLI = 0.003 in the full uniqueness model. These results suggest (with caution due to the CFI results) that the PHS exposes a strong invariance across the samples of the investigated countries and that we could continue to compare individual scores. This would indicate that perceived hope has been conceptualized in a similar form across countries and that correlation analyses with other constructs are possible.

4.3.5.5 Perceived Hope and Well-being

In all samples, participants report moderate to high levels (above the center of the scale) of perceived hope, relatively high levels of hedonic and psychological well-being, but only moderate levels (around the center of the scale) of social well-being (Table 4.5). Comparing scores between country samples, the first remarkable finding is that the non-European countries displayed significant higher levels of hope than the European countries. Whereas Nigeria, Australia and India, followed by South Africa, Israel and Colombia, showed the highest levels of perceived hope, Switzerland, Poland and Spain, followed by the Czech Republic, Italy and Portugal presented the lowest (all samples $F = 70.12$, $\eta 2 = 0.071$, $p < 0.001$). Moreover, participants in Nigeria, Australia and Colombia reported the highest levels of hedonic, psychological, and social well-being. Poland, Italy, and Israel exhibited the lowest levels of hedonic well-being (all samples $F = 20.76$, $\eta 2 = 0.022$, $p < 0.001$). Furthermore, people in Poland, Czechia and India exhibit the lowest levels in psychological well-being (all samples $F = 30.76$, $\eta 2 = 0.032$, $p < 0.001$) and people in Italy, Switzerland, and Poland the lowest in social well-being (all samples $F = 79.07$, $\eta 2 = 0.079$, $p < 0.001$).

Further, we compared mean values of perceived hope and well-being indicators between the two groups of participants that expected either the crisis scenario (group 1) or the flourishing scenario (group 2) to be more likely (see Table 4.5). With exception of India and Nigeria, people who expected the flourishing scenario to be more probable than the crisis scenario displayed significantly higher levels of perceived hope. Given that most people judged the crisis scenario to be more likely than the flourishing scenario (see Table 4.2), the consequence is that most people belong to those displaying weaker levels of hope. Similar results emerge when comparing mean values of hedonic, psychological, and social well-being. Those who expected the crisis scenario more likely to become true, expressed lower levels

Table 4.5 Mean values and mean value comparisons between groups of "likely" scenarios of perceived hope and well-being

Country	Perceived Hope				Hedonic well-being				Psychological well-being				Social well-being			
	M	M_{GE1}	M_{GE2}	Sig.	M	M_{GE1}	M_{GE2}	Sig.	M	M_{GE1}	M_{GE2}	Sig.	M	M_{GE1}	M_{GE2}	Sig.
Australia	3.71	3.63	3.86	0.007	4.76	4.67	4.93	0.013	4.73	4.64	4.90	0.007	3.85	3.66	4.20	<0.001
Colombia	3.55	3.46	3.72	0.008	4.72	4.60	4.96	0.002	4.62	4.55	4.74	0.092	3.87	3.75	4.11	0.010
Czech Rep.	3.41	3.28	3.69	<0.001	4.46	4.31	4.76	<0.001	4.09	3.92	4.45	<0.001	3.10	2.88	3.59	<0.001
India	3.69	3.68	3.71	0.616	4.43	4.44	4.42	0.846	4.33	4.29	4.40	0.130	3.81	3.69	4.08	<0.001
Israel	3.60	3.39	3.92	<0.001	4.36	4.17	4.64	<0.001	4.45	4.31	4.67	<0.001	3.38	3.08	3.82	<0.001
Italy	3.43	3.27	3.82	<0.001	4.34	4.21	4.66	0.002	4.58	4.44	4.92	<0.001	2.90	2.67	3.46	<0.001
Nigeria	4.21	4.20	4.24	0.404	4.79	4.74	4.90	0.034	4.90	4.86	4.99	0.073	3.86	3.79	4.00	0.025
Poland	3.26	3.15	3.63	<0.001	3.98	3.88	4.33	0.001	4.04	3.94	4.42	<0.001	3.03	2.85	3.67	<0.001
Portugal	3.50	3.36	3.81	<0.001	4.64	4.54	4.86	0.001	4.54	4.46	4.72	0.007	3.51	3.30	3.96	<0.001
South Africa	3.65	3.58	3.89	0.002	4.46	4.41	4.64	0.031	4.54	4.47	4.78	0.003	3.66	3.52	4.11	<0.001
Spain	3.28	3.18	3.63	<0.001	4.58	4.50	4.90	<0.001	4.41	4.33	4.71	<0.001	3.48	3.31	4.08	<0.001
Switzerland	3.24	3.15	3.67	<0.001	4.43	4.36	4.79	<0.001	4.36	4.29	4.69	<0.001	2.99	2.84	3.69	<0.001

Note: M_{GE1} Mean values for group 1, which expected the crisis scenario 1 to be more likely than the flourishing scenario 2, M_{GE2} Mean values for group 2, which expected the flourishing scenario 2 to be more likely than the crisis scenario 1 of hedonic well-being (except in India), psychological well-being (not significant in Colombia, India, and Nigeria), and particularly of social well-being.

A similar analysis is presented in Table 4.6, comparing mean values between the groups of participants preferring an individual-competitive future (group 1) and those favoring a social-sustainable future (group 2). With only few exceptions, there seems to be no differences between both groups in hedonic, psychological, and social well-being. Only in India and South Africa, people who preferred a social-sustainable future were higher in psychological well-being than those who preferred an individualist-competitive scenario in the first place. With regards to perceived hope, only in Czechia, India, Nigeria, and South Africa people who preferred a social and sustainable future exhibited higher levels of hope than those favoring the individual-competitive scenario.

4.3.5.6 Partial Bivariate Correlations and Hierarchical Regression Analyses

We report the partial bivariate correlation coefficients for every single country between future expectations and scenarios, on the one hand, and perceived hope and hedonic, psychological, and social well-being, on the other, in Appendix 4.2.1–4.2.12. First, the overall findings indicate that most of the future oriented variables correlated positively and significantly with the hope and well-being indicators, but with notable differences between countries. The correlations of the expected crisis scenario displayed significant negative coefficients with hope and well-being, while the flourishing scenario showed positive effects in most countries. Furthermore, the correlation coefficients between both "desirable" scenarios and hope and well-being are either very low or not significant at all. For a better comparison of the effects between countries, we performed a series of hierarchical regression analyses with perceived hope and social well-being as dependent variables.

Predictors of Perceived Hope

In the first series of analyses to predict perceived hope, we entered the demographic variables in step 1 and alternatively in separate analyses the composite score of future expectations 2040 (Table 4.7), the two "expected" scenarios (crisis and flourishing) (Table 4.8), and both "desirable" future scenarios (individualist-competitive and social-sustainable) (Table 4.9) in step 2.

Results in Table 4.7 indicate that long-term future expectations had a significant and moderate positive predictive effect on perceived hope in all countries. The explained variance of hope was the highest in Israel, South Africa, Poland, Spain, and Italy and the lowest in India, the Czech Republic, Nigeria, and Portugal. Essentially, the more pessimistic the long-term future expectations, the weaker the perceived personal hope of the country sample.

Table 4.6 Mean values and mean value comparisons between groups of "desirable" scenarios of perceived hope and well-being

Country	Perceived Hope				Hedonic well-being				Psychological well-being				Social well-being			
	M	M_{GD1}	M_{GD2}	Sig.	M	M_{GD1}	M_{GD2}	Sig.	M	M_{GD1}	M_{GD2}	Sig.	M	M_{GD1}	M_{GD2}	Sig.
Australia	3.71	3.79	3.70	0.490	4.76	4.92	4.74	0.268	4.73	4.87	4.71	0.300	3.85	3.75	3.86	0.583
Colombia	3.55	3.58	3.54	0.791	4.72	4.80	4.72	0.637	4.62	4.81	4.59	0.209	3.87	3.97	3.86	0.594
Czech Rep.	3.41	3.11	3.44	0.044	4.46	4.34	4.47	0.505	4.09	4.05	4.09	0.799	3.10	3.05	3.11	0.750
India	3.69	3.47	3.72	0.002	4.43	4.46	4.43	0.813	4.33	3.99	4.37	<0.001	3.81	3.67	3.83	0.191
Israel	3.60	3.52	3.61	0.457	4.36	4.33	4.36	0.853	4.45	4.48	4.45	0.854	3.38	3.34	3.38	0.783
Italy	3.43	3.38	3.43	0.894	4.34	4.20	4.34	0.677	4.58	4.68	4.57	0.721	2.90	3.04	2.89	0.681
Nigeria	4.21	4.04	4.24	0.004	4.79	4.63	4.82	0.065	4.90	4.90	4.90	0.980	3.86	3.81	3.87	0.655
Poland	3.26	3.12	3.27	0.288	3.98	3.97	3.98	0.970	4.04	3.95	4.05	0.566	3.03	2.86	3.05	0.300
Portugal	3.50	3.48	3.50	.918	4.64	4.59	4.64	0.785	4.54	4.45	4.55	0.579	3.51	3.70	3.49	0.315
South Africa	3.65	3.52	3.67	0.181	4.46	4.33	4.48	0.236	4.54	4.30	4.58	0.033	3.66	3.69	3.65	0.812
Spain	3.28	3.15	3.29	0.419	4.58	4.28	4.60	0.089	4.41	4.26	4.42	0.378	3.48	3.26	3.49	0.312
Switzerland	3.24	3.24	3.24	0.974	4.43	4.56	4.42	0.015	4.36	4.47	4.34	0.018	2.99	3.06	2.97	0.152

Note: M_{GD1} Mean values for group 1, which considered the individualistic scenario 1 to be more desirable than the social-sustainable scenario 2, M_{GE2} Mean values for group 2, which considered the social-sustainable scenario 2 to be more desirable than the individualistic scenario 1

Table 4.7 Hierarchical Regression Analyses for perceived hope with future expectations 2040 by country

	Australia		Colombia		Czech Rep.		India		Israel		Italy	
	Std. β	Sig.	Std. β	Sig.	Std. β	Sig.	Std. β	Sig.	Std. β	Sig.	Std. β	Sig.
Step 1: Demographic variables												
Gender	−0.039	0.390	0.018	0.746	0.109	0.016	0.111	<0.001	0.074	0.019	0.083	0.164
Age	0.056	0.274	0.262	0.001	0.186	0.037	0.120	0.032	0.028	0.485	0.068	0.399
Family Status	0.115	0.017	0.021	0.768	0.103	0.131	0.022	0.668	0.112	0.002	−0.026	0.707
Education	0.075	0.091	0.012	0.837	−0.011	0.817	0.092	0.003	0.057	0.087	−0.008	0.894
Main activity	0.014	0.760	−0.125	0.128	−0.051	0.559	−0.048	0.252	0.038	0.299	−0.060	0.433
Professional Status	0.080	0.077	0.117	0.100	0.079	0.133	0.144	<0.001	0.091	0.007	0.138	0.028
Step 2: Future Expectations												
Future expectations 2040	0.276	<0.001	0.286	<0.001	0.207	<0.001	0.122	<0.001	0.386	<0.001	0.307	<0.001
	Adj. R^2	Sig.	Adj. R^2	Sig.	Adj. R^2	Sig.	Adj. R^2	Sig.	Adj. R^2	Sig.	Adj. R^2	Sig.
Model 1: Step 1	0.040	<0.001	0.034	0.011	0.056	<0.001	0.062	<0.001	0.045	<0.001	0.015	0.123
Model 2: Step 1 and 2	0.111	<0.001	0.111	<0.001	0.096	<0.001	0.076	<0.001	0.191	<0.001	0.105	<0.001
Change in R^2 Model 2	0.072		0.077		0.040		0.014		0.146		0.090	

	Nigeria		Poland		Portugal		South Africa		Spain		Switzerland	
	Std. β	Sig.	Std. β	Sig.	Std. β	Sig.	Std. β	*Sig.*	Std. β	Sig.	Std. β	Sig.
Step 1: Demographic variables												
Gender	0.011	0.774	0.121	0.007	−0.032	0.407	−0.012	0.775	0.046	0.273	0.092	<0.001
Age	0.065	0.210	0.111	0.051	0.194	0.003	−0.003	0.947	0.134	0.070	0.160	<0.001
Family Status	0.053	0.283	0.149	0.005	0.165	0.005	0.174	<0.001	−0.090	0.175	0.041	0.015
Education	0.023	0.550	−0.091	0.065	0.004	0.919	−0.031	0.447	0.024	0.566	0.109	<0.001
Main activity	−0.073	0.071	−0.047	0.445	0.133	0.026	−0.040	0.363	0.141	0.049	0.005	0.788
Professional Status	0.043	0.288	0.103	0.032	0.055	0.228	0.038	0.345	0.135	0.004	0.122	<0.001
Step 2: Future Expectations												
Future expectations 2040	0.211	<0.001	0.349	<0.001	0.226	<0.001	0.369	<0.001	0.325	<0.001	0.293	<0.001
	Adj. R^2	Sig.	Adj. R^2	Sig.	Adj. R^2	Sig.	Adj. R^2	Sig.	Adj. R^2	Sig.	Adj. R^2	Sig.
Model 1: Step 1	0.008	0.078	0.053	<0.001	0.204	<0.001	0.014	0.031	0.042	<0.001	0.072	<0.001
Model 2: Step 1 and 2	0.050	<0.001	0.168	<0.001	0.253	<0.001	0.143	<0.001	0.144	<0.001	0.155	<0.001
Change in R^2 Model 2	0.042		0.115		0.049		0.129		0.102		0.083	

Table 4.8 Hierarchical Regression Analyses for perceived hope with expected scenarios 2040 by country

	Australia		Colombia		Czech Rep.		India		Israel		Italy	
	Std. β	Sig.	Std. β	Sig.	Std. β	Sig.	Std. β	Sig.	Std. β	Sig.	Std. β	Sig.
Step 1: Demographic variables												
Gender	−0.034	0.464	0.038	0.484	0.103	0.023	0.104	0.001	0.069	0.033	0.059	0.326
Age	0.003	0.952	0.240	0.003	0.157	0.080	0.131	0.020	0.003	0.933	0.068	0.399
Family Status	0.120	0.015	−0.004	0.959	0.100	0.146	0.017	0.752	0.089	0.017	−0.005	0.945
Education	0.101	0.026	0.010	0.865	−0.006	0.902	0.096	0.002	0.053	0.115	−0.005	0.936
Main activity	0.036	0.447	−0.081	0.322	−0.065	0.458	−0.059	0.163	0.023	0.531	−0.062	0.419
Professional Status	0.072	0.123	0.114	0.107	0.095	0.072	0.157	<0.001	0.102	0.003	0.115	0.068
Step 2: Expected future scenarios												
Crisis scenario 1	−0.023	0.641	−0.037	0.516	−0.111	0.039	−0.014	0.627	−0.112	0.001	−0.119	0.063
Flourishing scenario 2	0.174	0.001	0.292	<0.001	0.063	0.242	0.039	0.191	0.290	<0.001	0.248	<0.001
	Adj. R^2	Sig.	Adj. R^2	Sig.	Adj. R^2	Sig.	Adj. R^2	Sig.	Adj. R^2	Sig.	Adj. R^2	Sig.
Model 1: Step 1	0.040	<0.001	0.034	0.011	0.056	<0.001	0.062	<0.001	0.045	<0.001	0.015	0.123
Model 2: Step 1 and 2	0.069	<0.001	0.122	<0.001	0.076	0.003	0.062	0.372	0.167	<0.001	0.103	<0.001
Change in R^2 Model 2	0.030		0.088		0.020		<0.001		0.122		0.088	

	Nigeria		Poland		Portugal		South Africa		Spain		Switzerland	
	Std. β	Sig.	Std. β	Sig.	Std. β	Sig.	Std. β	*Sig.*	Std. β	Sig.	Std. β	Sig.
Step 1: Demographic variables												
Gender	0.045	0.252	0.089	0.052	−0.008	0.831	−0.012	0.775	0.061	0.150	0.087	<0.001
Age	0.064	0.221	0.092	0.112	0.177	0.006	−0.029	0.576	0.063	0.403	0.147	<0.001
Family Status	0.044	0.376	0.168	0.002	0.147	0.012	0.151	0.003	−0.090	0.180	0.030	0.082
Education	0.028	0.480	−0.104	0.040	0.006	0.894	0.010	0.804	0.046	0.276	0.132	<0.001
Main activity	−0.091	0.025	−0.075	0.242	0.131	0.028	0.002	0.956	0.172	0.018	−0.007	0.684
Professional Status	0.047	0.251	0.110	0.026	0.051	0.258	0.063	0.121	0.100	0.036	0.114	<0.001
Step 2: Expected future scenarios												
Crisis scenario 1	0.064	0.094	−0.118	0.019	−0.040	0.371	−0.039	0.346	0.007	0.885	−0.103	<0.001
Flourishing scenaric 2	0.155	<0.001	0.200	<0.001	0.205	<0.001	0.305	<0.001	0.289	<0.001	0.190	<0.001
	Adj. R^2	Sig.	Adj. R^2	Sig.	Adj. R^2	Sig.	Adj. R^2	Sig.	Adj. R^2	Sig.	Adj. R^2	Sig.
Model 1: Step 1	0.008	0.078	0.053	<0.001	0.204	<0.001	0.014	0.031	0.042	<0.001	0.072	<0.001
Model 2: Step 1 anc 2	0.033	<0.001	0.126	<0.001	0.251	<0.001	0.111	<0.001	0.119	<0.001	0.135	<0.001
Change in R^2 Model 2	0.025		0.073		0.047		0.097		0.078		0.063	

Table 4.9 Hierarchical Regression Analyses for perceived hope with desirable scenarios 2040 by country

Perceived Hope	Australia		Colombia		Czech Rep.		India		Israel		Italy	
	Std. β	Sig.	Std. β	Sig.	Std. β	Sig.	Std. β	Sig.	Std. β	Sig.	Std. β	Sig.
Step 1: Demographic variables												
Gender	−0.033	0.489	0.026	0.652	0.081	0.077	0.105	0.001	0.082	0.020	0.098	0.117
Age	0.027	0.611	0.244	0.004	0.140	0.121	0.118	0.035	−0.012	0.785	0.088	0.297
Family Status	0.114	0.021	−0.006	0.936	0.112	0.107	0.010	0.850	0.111	0.005	−0.036	0.627
Education	0.097	0.033	−0.014	0.820	−0.023	0.640	0.092	0.002	0.035	0.331	0.031	0.628
Main activity	0.027	0.567	−0.083	0.329	−0.040	0.654	−0.054	0.202	0.018	0.658	−0.037	0.648
Professional Status	0.086	0.064	0.095	0.196	0.088	0.100	0.157	<0.001	0.115	0.002	0.160	0.015
Step 2: Desirable Future Scenarios												
Competitive Scenario 1	0.170	<0.001	0.130	0.025	−0.007	0.880	0.004	0.899	−0.040	0.247	0.063	0.324
Sustainable Scenario 2	0.082	0.082	0.088	0.122	0.101	0.033	0.133	<0.001	0.040	0.254	0.042	0.509
	Adj. R^2	Sig.	Adj. R^2	Sig.	Adj. R^2	Sig.	Adj. R^2	Sig.	Adj. R^2	Sig.	Adj. R^2	Sig.
Model 1: Step 1	0.040	<0.001	0.034	0.011	0.056	<0.001	0.062	<0.001	0.045	<0.001	0.015	0.123
Model 2: Step 1 and 2	0.062	0.001	0.048	0.036	0.063	0.072	0.078	<0.001	0.047	0.168	0.012	0.563
Change in R^2 Model 2	0.023		0.015		0.007		0.016		0.002		−0.003	

Table 4.10 Hierarchical Regression Analyses for social well-being with future expectations 2040 by country

	Australia		Colombia		Czech Rep.		India		Israel		Italy	
	Std. β	Sig.	Std. β	Sig.	Std. β	Sig.	Std. β	Sig.	Std. β ta	Sig.	Std. β	Sig.
Step 1: Demographic variables												
Gender	−0.085	0.007	−0.080	0.053	−0.058	0.083	−0.112	<0.001	0.074	0.003	0.017	0.716
Age	0.046	0.193	0.031	0.619	0.160	0.017	0.041	0.327	0.019	0.534	0.075	0.249
Family Status	0.002	0.943	−0.056	0.311	−0.136	0.008	0.142	<0.001	−0.037	0.194	−0.017	0.760
Education	0.020	0.512	0.071	0.119	−0.037	0.313	0.074	0.002	0.037	0.161	−0.009	0.842
Main activity	−0.068	0.030	0.039	0.536	−0.005	0.935	−0.007	0.830	0.027	0.359	0.008	0.900
Professional Status	−0.004	0.896	0.017	0.757	0.071	0.069	−0.107	<0.001	−0.012	0.654	0.067	0.185
Step 2: Hedonic and psychological well-being												
Hedonic wellbeing	0.075	0.128	0.064	0.340	−0.026	0.603	0.071	0.024	0.095	0.010	0.136	0.040
Psychological wellbeing	0.600	<0.001	0.605	<0.001	0.667	<0.001	0.540	<0.001	0.463	<0.001	0.465	<0.001
Step 3: Future Expectations												
Future expectations 2040	0.256	<0.001	0.112	0.012	0.148	<0.001	0.171	<0.001	0.316	<0.001	0.197	<0.001
	Adj. R^2	Sig.	Adj. R^2	Sig.	Adj. R^2	Sig.	Adj. R^2	Sig.	Adj. R^2	Sig.	Adj. R^2	Sig.
Model 1: Step 1	0.019	0.021	0.010	0.179	0.036	0.001	0.095	<0.001	0.028	<0.001	0.038	0.012
Model 2: Step 1 and 2	0.525	<0.001	0.482	<0.001	0.475	<0.001	0.454	<0.001	0.417	<0.001	0.400	<0.001
Model 3: Step 1, 2 and 3	0.583	<0.001	0.491	0.012	0.495	<0.001	0.481	<0.001	0.504	<0.001	0.434	<0.001
Change in R^2 Model 3	0.059		0.009		0.020		0.027		0.087		0.034	

(continued)

Table 4.10 (continued)

	Australia		Colombia		Czech Rep.		India		Israel		Italy	
	Std. β	Sig.	Std. β	Sig.	Std. β	Sig.	Std. β	Sig.	Std. β ta	Sig.	Std. β	Sig.
	Nigeria		Poland		Portugal		South Africa		Spain		Switzerland	
	Std. β	Sig.	Std. β	Sig.	Std. β	Sig.	Std. β	*Sig.*	Std. β	Sig.	Std. β	Sig.
Step 1: Demographic variables												
Gender	−0.112	0.001	−0.032	0.352	−0.083	0.010	0.993	0.019	−0.026	0.421	0.023	0.062
Age	0.019	0.663	0.139	0.001	0.078	0.137	0.603	0.169	0.129	0.023	0.086	<0.001
Family Status	−0.024	0.555	−0.073	0.071	−0.019	0.701	0.005	0.950	−0.035	0.490	−0.006	0.629
Education	−0.055	0.091	−0.019	0.612	0.030	0.382	0.655	0.873	0.017	0.593	0.052	<0.001
Main activity	−0.043	0.207	0.023	0.619	0.029	0.556	0.626	0.165	−0.121	0.027	−0.008	0.593
Professional Status	−0.003	0.927	−0.011	0.757	−0.002	0.948	0.113	0.212	0.059	0.107	0.014	0.262
Step 2: Hedonic and psychological well-being												
Hedonic wellbeing	0.208	<0.001	0.119	0.024	0.154	0.001	0.182	<0.001	0.119	0.030	0.095	<0.001
Psychological wellbeing	0.360	<0.001	0.524	<0.001	0.510	<0.001	0.473	<0.001	0.522	<0.001	0.469	<0.001
Step 3: Future Expectations												
Future expectations 2040	0.175	<0.001	0.205	<0.001	0.156	<0.001	0.195	<0.001	0.201	<0.001	0.276	<0.001
	Adj. R^2	Sig.	Adj. R^2	Sig.	Adj. R^2	Sig.	Adj. R^2	Sig.	Adj. R^2	Sig.	Adj. R^2	Sig.
Model 1: Step 1	0.024	0.001	0.041	<0.001	0.076	<0.001	0.032	<0.001	−0.001	0.494	0.062	<0.001
Model 2: Step 1 and 2	0.319	<0.001	0.486	<0.001	0.478	<0.001	0.486	<0.001	0.461	<0.001	0.411	<0.001
Model 3: Step 1, 2 and 3	0.347	<0.001	0.521	<0.001	0.500	<0.001	0.518	<0.001	0.496	<0.001	0.480	<0.001
Change in R^2 Model 3	0.028		0.035		0.022		0.032		0.035		0.069	

Table 4.11 Hierarchical Regression Analyses for social well-being with expected future scenarios 2040 by country

	Australia		Colombia		Czech Rep.		India		Israel		Italy	
	Std. β	Sig.	Std. β	Sig.	Std. β	Sig.	Std. β	Sig.	Std. β	Sig.	Std. β	Sig.
Step 1: Demographic variables												
Gender	−0.080	0.014	−0.071	0.084	−0.056	0.091	−0.121	<0.001	0.066	0.012	0.007	0.877
Age	−0.003	0.939	0.024	0.700	0.150	0.023	0.047	0.267	−0.001	0.980	0.080	0.217
Family Status	0.001	0.975	−0.064	0.237	−0.143	0.005	0.136	0.001	−0.053	0.077	−0.007	0.902
Education	0.040	0.204	0.072	0.113	−0.025	0.480	0.078	0.001	0.022	0.409	−0.007	0.885
Main activity	−0.051	0.113	0.056	0.360	−0.021	0.749	−0.014	0.652	0.013	0.669	0.008	0.899
Professional Status	−0.019	0.552	0.020	0.703	0.094	0.017	−0.094	<0.001	−0.007	0.801	0.054	0.286
Step 2: Hedonic and psychological well-being												
Hedonic wellbeing	0.067	0.189	0.047	0.482	−0.029	0.550	0.088	0.006	0.126	0.001	0.164	0.013
Psychological wellbeing	0.640	<0.001	0.606	<0.001	0.654	<0.001	0.543	<0.001	0.483	<0.001	0.429	<0.001
Step 3: Expected future scenarios												
Crisis Scenario 1	−0.074	0.032	−0.044	0.312	−0.063	0.111	−0.125	<0.001	−0.142	<0.001	−0.086	0.096
Flourishing Scenario 2	0.141	<0.001	0.133	0.005	0.143	<0.001	0.092	<0.001	0.128	<0.001	0.145	0.007
	Adj. R^2	Sig.	Adj. R^2	Sig.	Adj. R^2	Sig.	Adj. R^2	Sig.	Adj. R^2	Sig.	Adj. R^2	Sig.
Model 1: Step 1	0.019	0.021	0.010	0.179	0.036	0.001	0.095	<0.001	0.028	<0.001	0.038	0.012
Model 2: Step 1 and 2	0.525	<0.001	0.482	<0.001	0.475	<0.001	0.454	<0.001	0.417	<0.001	0.400	<0.001
Model 3: Step 1, 2 and 3	0.556	<0.001	0.500	0.002	0.505	<0.001	0.477	<0.001	0.464	<0.001	0.429	0.001
Change in R^2 Model 3	0.031		0.018		0.030		0.023		0.047		0.029	

(continued)

Table 4.11 (continued)

	Nigeria		Poland		Portugal		South Africa		Spain		Switzerland	
	Std. β	Sig.	Std. β	Sig.	Std. β	Sig.	Std. β	Sig.	Std. β	Sig.	Std. β	Sig.
Step 1: Demographic variables												
Gender	−0.090	0.006	−0.042	0.206	−0.062	0.046	−0.070	019	−0.016	0.616	0.015	0.215
Age	0.013	0.770	0.137	0.001	0.068	0.189	−0.067	0.081	0.084	0.143	0.068	<0.001
Family Status	−0.030	0.468	−0.075	0.062	−0.035	0.468	−0.013	0.725	−0.037	0.464	−0.018	0.172
Education	−0.050	0.126	−0.025	0.492	0.025	0.464	0.009	0.756	0.031	0.335	0.069	<0.001
Main activity	−0.057	0.097	0.007	0.885	0.033	0.494	−0.020	0.540	−0.101	0.067	−0.017	0.230
Professional Status	0.004	0.914	−0.006	0.863	−0.009	0.813	0.046	0.124	0.035	0.329	0.004	0.750
Step 2: Hedonic and psychological well-being												
Hedonic wellbeing	0.221	<0.001	0.124	0.017	0.167	<0.001	0.209	<0.001	0.153	0.005	0.104	<0.001
Psychological wellbeing	0.365	<0.001	0.516	<0.001	0.498	<0.001	0.464	<0.001	0.497	<0.001	0.487	<0.001
Step 3: Expected future scenarios												
Crisis Scenario 1	−0.062	0.056	−0.114	0.002	−0.071	0.046	−0.082	0.007	0.001	0.985	−0.127	<0.001
Flourishing Scenario 2	0.088	0.007	0.165	<0.001	0.160	<0.001	0.145	<0.001	0.193	<0.001	0.159	<0.001
	Adj. R^2	Sig.	Adj. R^2	Sig.	Adj. R^2	Sig.	Adj. R^2	Sig.	Adj. R^2	Sig.	Adj. R^2	Sig.
Model 1: Step 1	0.024	0.001	0.041	<0.001	0.076	<0.001	0.032	<0.001	−0.001	0.494	0.062	<0.001
Model 2: Step 1 and 2	0.319	<0.001	0.486	<0.001	0.478	<0.001	0.486	<0.001	0.461	<0.001	0.411	<0.001
Model 3: Step 1, 2 and 3	0.329	0.004	0.538	<0.001	0.516	<0.001	0.517	<0.001	0.493	<0.001	0.468	<0.001
Change in R^2 Model 3	0.009		0.051		0.038		0.031		0.032		0.057	

Finally, the results in Table 4.12 indicate that there were almost no or very little associations between the desired scenarios and social well-being. The individualistic-competitive scenario displayed a small positive association with social well-being, primarily in South Africa, Switzerland, and Colombia. In most countries the social-sustainable scenario showed no relation to social well-being, with exception of South Africa and Italy, where a slight negative relationship emerged. This implies that the social-sustainable scenario, which has been considered as highly desirable by a large majority in all countries, does not foster a sense of social well-being. The mood seems to be even direr in South Africa and Italy because the more people wished for a social-sustainable future, the lower their social well-being seemed to be.

4.4 Discussion

The aim of our study was to investigate the long-term expectations concerning the future quality of life, both in general and in several life and social domains, as well as the outlooks regarding probable and desirable long-term future scenarios (in 20 years' time) across 12 countries and relate these images of the future to people's perceived personal hope and hedonic, psychological, and particularly social well-being. We defined the broader concept of collective hope as a wish or desire for a better common future, the belief that the realization of a better future for all is possible (although not necessarily probable) and the trust in the availability of personal, social, and other resources to deal with current challenges and to overcome obstacles and setbacks. Our study was therefore focused on what people believe will happen in the future, what they long for and the relationship thereof to hope and well-being.

Many authors from the field of Futures Studies have already argued that people's images of the future could have a substantial effect on the evolution and the well-being of society (Boulding, 1994; Dator, 1996; Hicks, 1996; Polak, 1961/1973). Hopes and fears of the population often influence their decisions and actions in the present. Whereas fears might prevent people from following daring new paths, hope can encourage them to take necessary actions for a positive transformation (Hicks, 2012). The results from our study support previous research in showing that many people, especially in western countries, have a very clear picture about their desirable future, but at the same time have lost their belief and hope in a flourishing global future (Brunstad, 2002; Gidley & Hampson, 2005). In their eyes, technological and economic development will not solve the burning problems humanity is currently facing and would have to deal with in the future.

In previous studies, researchers revealed that future expectations of the population (especially of young people) regarding the general quality of life and specific social domains are overall pessimistic (Eckersley, 1999; Hicks, 2003; Stewart, 2002). In our study across 12 countries a more differentiated picture emerged. Our results demonstrated that people in certain (poorer) countries like Nigeria, Colombia and Portugal held prevalently optimistic outlooks regarding future quality of life in

Table 4.12 Hierarchical Regression Analyses for social well-being with desired future scenarios 2040 by country

	Australia		Colombia		Czech Rep.		India		Israel		Italy	
	Std. β	Sig.	Std. β	Sig.	Std. β	Sig.	Std. β	Sig.	Std. β	Sig.	Std. β	Sig.
Step 1: Demographic variables												
Gender	−0.099	0.004	−0.057	0.167	−0.070	0.043	−0.132	<0.001	0.084	0.002	0.027	0.577
Age	0.001	0.981	0.030	0.623	0.134	0.049	0.069	0.111	−0.002	0.945	0.084	0.209
Family Status	0.007	0.837	−0.072	0.187	−0.131	0.013	0.122	0.002	−0.052	0.100	−0.032	0.581
Education	0.037	0.251	0.077	0.089	−0.038	0.309	0.079	0.001	0.014	0.623	−0.007	0.886
Main activity	−0.056	0.092	0.073	0.235	−0.009	0.897	−0.030	0.349	0.008	0.796	0.039	0.537
Professional Status	−0.006	0.853	−0.003	0.960	0.077	0.057	−0.084	0.001	−0.001	0.975	0.072	0.163
Step 2: Hedonic and psychological well-being												
Hedonic wellbeing	0.098	0.062	0.058	0.380	−0.017	0.741	0.065	0.043	0.165	<0.001	0.164	0.015
Psychological wellbeing	0.638	<0.001	0.626	<0.001	0.685	<0.001	0.574	<0.001	0.504	<0.001	0.488	<0.001
Step 3: Desired future scenarios												
Individualistic Scenario 1	0.073	0.033	0.147	0.001	0.011	0.768	0.061	0.007	0.036	0.191	0.001	0.991
Sustainable Scenario 2	0.057	0.089	−0.050	0.225	−0.006	0.870	−0.014	0.542	0.018	0.507	−0.096	0.053
	Adj. R^2	Sig.	Adj. R^2	Sig.	Adj. R^2	Sig.	Adj. R^2	Sig.	Adj. R^2	Sig.	Adj. R^2	Sig.
Model 1: Step 1	0.019	0.021	0.010	0.179	0.036	0.001	0.095	<0.001	0.028	<0.001	0.038	0.012
Model 2: Step 1 and 2	0.525	0.000	0.482	0.000	0.475	0.000	0.454	0.000	0.417	0.000	0.400	0.000
Model 3: Step 1, 2 and 3	0.528	0.052	0.503	0.001	0.473	0.923	0.456	0.024	0.417	0.402	0.405	0.132
Change in R^2 Model 3	0.004		0.021		−0.002		0.003		0.000		0.005	

Social Well-being	Nigeria		Poland		Portugal		South Africa		Spain		Switzerland	
	Std. β	Sig.	Std. β	Sig.	Std. β	Sig.	Std. β	Sig.	Std. β	Sig.	Std. β	Sig.
Step 1: Demographic variables												
Gender	−0.094	0.005	−0.076	0.033	−0.063	0.059	−0.044	0.154	−0.032	0.343	0.037	0.004
Age	−0.002	0.967	0.110	0.014	0.078	0.149	−0.072	0.069	0.127	0.031	0.071	<0.001
Family Status	−0.032	0.444	−0.053	0.203	−0.018	0.718	−0.010	791	−0.043	0.417	−0.023	0.101
Education	−0.055	0.097	−0.030	0.444	0.037	0.296	0.031	0.322	0.026	0.442	0.080	<0.001
Main activity	−0.064	0.062	0.008	0.864	0.006	0.898	−0.038	0.255	−0.136	0.017	−0.027	0.066
Professional Status	0.006	0.856	−0.018	0.640	0.007	0.849	0.043	0.160	0.032	0.397	0.007	0.560
Step 2: Hedonic and psychological well-being												
Hedonic wellbeing	0.236	<0.001	0.132	0.015	0.194	<0.001	0.199	<0.001	0.172	0.002	0.133	<0.001
Psychological wellbeing	0.376	<0.001	0.581	<0.001	0.518	<0.001	0.526	<0.001	0.532	<0.001	0.493	<0.001
Step 3: Desired future scenarios												
Individualistic Scenario 1	−0.017	0.615	−0.025	0.488	−0.018	0.571	0.101	0.001	−0.010	0.786	0.107	<0.001
Sustainable Scenario 2	−0.051	0.136	0.035	0.336	−0.055	0.105	−0.083	0.007	0.011	0.750	0.024	0.065
	Adj. R^2	Sig.	Adj. R^2	Sig.	Adj. R^2	Sig.	Adj. R^2	Sig.	Adj. R^2	Sig.	Adj. R^2	Sig.
Model 1: Step 1	0.024	0.001	0.041	<0.001	0.076	<0.001	0.032	<0.001	−0.001	0.494	0.062	<0.001
Model 2: Step 1 and 2	0.319	<0.001	0.486	<0.001	0.478	<0.001	0.486	<0.001	0.461	<0.001	0.411	<0.001
Model 3: Step 1, 2 and 3	0.321	0.192	0.487	0.308	0.479	0.230	0.500	<0.001	0.459	0.878	0.421	<0.001
Change in R^2 Model 3	0.001		<0.001		0.001		0.014		−0.002		0.010	

their countries and that people in other countries like Switzerland, Italy, Spain, and South Africa were widely pessimistic. Whereas the economic development and employment opportunities were expected to improve, the most negative prospects and urgent concerns arose with regard to the spreading gap between the rich and the poor, the deterioration of the natural environment, the threats to family life, and the decline in mental health of the population.

Scenarios are images of the future, which could be more or less probable, possible, and desirable. We asked our participants to assess the likelihood of two opposite possible future scenarios portraying a crisis and a flourishing image of the future. A majority of the participants in almost all countries considered the crisis scenario to be more probable than the flourishing scenario, as already noticed in past studies (Brunstad, 2002; Nordensvard, 2014; Rubin, 2002). People in European countries such as Switzerland, Spain, and Poland, but also in South Africa, were much more pessimistic regarding the apparent threat of the crisis scenario and held a weaker belief in a flourishing future. Surprisingly, people in poorer countries like Nigeria and Colombia could held a stronger belief in a flourishing future.

It is particularly noteworthy that the population in Switzerland, the country in our study with the highest GDP per capita, had the grimmest expectations regarding future quality of life and that people in Nigeria, the poorest country in terms of GDP per capita, held the most positive expectations. This can be interpreted in a historical and cultural context. Since the late nineteenth century, Europe was spurred by the belief in a universal economic growth and progress, which was further reinforced during the reconstruction after World War II. Nowadays, people in countries with a high level of prosperity mostly fear a deterioration of their living conditions (Adolph et al., 2016). For example, in countries like Switzerland with a high level of personal safety and low criminality, people fear an increase in insecurity and violence. Economic prosperity and technological progress have been the driving forces in the past decades, but they no longer serve as desirable visions for a better future and do not offer people a higher sense of meaning and purpose, particularly because their negative effects on health, well-being and the natural environment are seen as not tolerable anymore.

Different economic and cultural realities in other countries spur other needs and hopes. People in poorer countries have the wish and belief that their situation may improve. It is perfectly understandable that people in countries such as Nigeria, Colombia, and India long for prosperity and well-being. Furthermore, in recent decades people in many developing countries already experienced positive developments. For example, in Colombia, the peace process to overcome the civil war has occasioned a general economic and social stability. However, this should not obscure the fact that many young people in Africa and Latin America feel deprived from future opportunities.

Long-term expectations towards the future of society and the planet can have significant effects on the level of hope and well-being of the population (Eckersley, 2002). Our results disclosed that the levels of perceived personal hope, hedonic and psychological well-being are moderately high in all investigated countries but that the social well-being of the population is considerably more restrained. Remarkably, participants in non-European countries exhibited significantly higher levels of personal hope than those in European countries. Moreover, whereas some countries like Nigeria, Australia and Colombia, countries which seem to be more optimistic regarding the future quality of life, and less concerned about future crises, showed higher levels of hedonic, psychological, and social well-being, other countries like Italy and Poland displayed the lowest.

In a further step, we found that people who not only believe in a crisis-like future scenario and who were also more sceptical with regard to a flourishing future, especially people in Switzerland, Poland, and Spain, also displayed significantly lower levels of personal hope. Moreover, the impaired belief in a positive future seemed to have more negative effects on hope and social well-being than the expectation of a dreadful future. People in Poland, Italy and Switzerland were especially pessimistic with regard to the future prospects and likewise reported lower levels of perceived hope and all facets of well-being.

A special case worthy to be mentioned separately is South Africa. People in South Africa are as concerned as e.g., Swiss and Italians regarding the dire prospects in their country. They held little belief in the improvement of their quality of life and in a future flourishing society and were concerned regarding future crises. However, despite these pessimistic outlooks, the South African participants seemed able to remain hopeful and enjoy somewhat higher levels of psychological and social well-being comparable to those in Nigeria, Australia, and Colombia. This suggests that people in South Africa may retain sources of hope and well-being that are less available to people in other countries such as Poland, Italy, and Switzerland.

Finally, we want to address the results related to the desirable future scenarios. The first and overall finding is that people in all countries clearly preferred and longed for a social and sustainable future much more than an individualist, competitive and materialistic world, supporting past research (see for example Boulding, 1994; Hicks, 1996). However, in most European countries the gap between the mostly desired sustainable future and the less favored individualist and competitive future is much more pronounced than in other countries like Nigeria, South Africa, and India. People in the latter countries seem to wish to achieve economic and financial prosperity and at the same time protect the environment and preserve social cohesion. In contrast, during the past decades, people in Europe have experienced not only the blessings of economic welfare but also the negative effects of an overly competitive and individualist society.

The sobering finding is that the desire for a better future, be it in materialistic or in ecological and social terms, has only a small impact on perceived hope and well-being. Interestingly, a significant relationship between the wish for a better future and perceived hope was found in Nigeria and South Africa, which are two of the fastest developing countries in Africa. In the European countries, the wish for a social and sustainable future was related to slightly higher levels of hope than the wish for a more competitive and individualistic future. Furthermore, the desire for a sustainable and social future does not spark a stronger feeling of well-being among people, like the desire for more economic wealth and modern technology does in some countries such as Colombia and South Africa. This could indicate that the desire for a social and sustainable future, while inspiring a little bit of hope, does not nurture a sense of meaningfulness, belonging and integration in the social community.

The current mood among people seems to reflect that we have reached a point in history where they feel that things cannot continue to go on like this. Many people, especially in Europe, are uneasy about the direction in which the world is currently heading: Destruction of the natural environment, climate change, natural disasters, wars, political radicalism and the exploitation of the population's mental health due to increasing pressure and competition. At the same time, they feel powerless because they have the impression that they cannot do anything about it. Therefore, the coming decades are generally seen as an age of crises and problems instead of peace and prosperity. These experiences seem to trigger negative feelings of worry and helplessness.

The question, as Snow (2018) formulates it, is whether we want to be a community of hope or of worry. Snow attests that the United States has become a nation of worriers, largely because past administrations have failed to spread social hope. Our societies lack positive and widely accepted images for the future that could provide guidance and direction, as well as the belief that the world's current problems can be solved. Images of the future that merely convey the feeling of more of the same rob people of their passion and enthusiasm for their lives and for the world in general.

Researchers from the fields of Futures Studies and Positive Psychology recognized that it makes little sense to focus only on problems (Slaughter, 1994). According to Hicks (2003), only when a society creates new and powerful pictures of desirable futures, it can begin to mobilize its creative energy again. What the world will look like in the future depends above all on the extent to which we are able to develop positive images of a desirable future. What sustains us are hopes and dreams of a world worth living in. Positive scenarios offer people the vision of an ideal future to work for and emphasize human freedom and dignity. Humans are always free to imagine and strive for a completely different and better world. The goal is to engage in alternative and desirable visions of the future, in the conviction that we must not merely surrender to current constrains and adapt to a bleak future, but actively and responsibly shape it. This requires future designs and concrete goals based on individual and collective values and dreams of a better world. In this sense, collective hope should help to overcome anxiety and apathy, inspiring faith, and trust in the achievability of a better future (Blöser & Stahl, 2019; Braithwaite, 2004; McGeer, 2004; Shade, 2019; Rorty, 2002). This is especially possible within a human community, where people focus on the positive aspects of life, especially on the hope, belief, and trust that even in difficult times, despite problems and disappointments, it is possible to live a better life if we take the appropriate attitude towards it and actively work together to achieve it.

4.5 Limitations

At this point it is necessary to mention a number of limitations of our study. The cross-sectional design of our research impedes us to drive any conclusion about causality. The most likely is the existence of a reciprocal effect. Happy and hopeful people usually hold more optimistic views of the future and vice-versa: positive expectations of the future will foster people's hopefulness and well-being. A further limitation is the lack of representativeness of our samples and of homogeneity across samples. However, due to the dissimilar demographic structures of the national populations, the criteria of representativeness and homogeneity across samples remain in competition with each other. The more representative the individual samples, the lower the homogeneity across samples and vice-versa. The survey was performed via online channels. A certain proportion of people with restricted or no access to online media are excluded from the study. This may especially be the case in samples from developing, non-western countries, where access to internet is often restricted to certain socio-economic groups. From the four goodness to fit indices utilized to test group invariance of the PHS, three revealed adequate results and one (the CFI) did not, however to a small extent.

4.6 Conclusions

In this chapter we extended and examined the definition of hope encompassing the social and long-term future expectations and yearnings of the population. People will hope for a better world once they can develop and manifest desired images of the future and believe that despite current adversities and challenges, a flourishing future could be possible if we trust in our collective capacity to work together towards common ideals and visions. Our findings draw a rather gloomy picture of people's global future prospects, but underscore the strong universal wish for a sustainable, harmonious, just, and cooperative human community. It lies in our hands to encourage and support people to capture this vision and form communities of hope and action to overcome current fears and worries and contribute to the realization of their hoped-for future. For this, we need to develop, implement, and examine hope interventions that not only focus on personal hopes and foster hopefulness at the individual level, but bring people together to join their particular strengths, form a community in which members respect, encourage and support each other and work hand in hand in concrete initiatives and institutions of social hope. By doing so, we will not only build a better future together but also enhance our personal and social well-being in the here and now.

Appendix 4.1: Demographic Structure

Number of Participants, Mean Age and Standard Deviation and GDP Per Capita

	N	%	M_{age}	SD_{age}	GDP per capita in U$S
Australia	474	4.7	47.53	13.05	51,693
Colombia	311	3.1	26.19	8.63	5335
Czech Republic	469	4.6	32.75	15.54	22,932
India	1092	8.7	31.15	12.60	1928
Israel	884	2.7	41.65	14.98	44,169
Italy	272	6.5	41.86	13.78	31,714
Nigeria	665	4.7	32.26	8.47	2097
Poland	481	5.0	31.58	10.82	15,721
Portugal	507	5.6	36.45	14.74	22,176
South Africa	574	5.2	39.27	14.85	5656
Spain	529	38.6	35.19	15.22	27,063
Switzerland	3935	10.7	46.82	15.67	87,097
Total	10,193	100.0	40.04	15.76	

Gender

		Australia	Colombia	Czech Rep.	India	Israel	Italy	Nigeria	Poland	Portugal	*South Africa*	Spain	Switzerland	Total
Male	n	232	151	132	529	262	75	434	140	124	*252*	116	1797	4473
	%	48.9%	48.6%	28.1%	48.4%	29.6%	27.6%	65.3%	29.1%	24.5%	*43.9%*	21.9%	45.7%	41.9%
Female	n	242	160	337	563	622	197	231	341	383	*322*	413	2138	6190
	%	51.1%	51.4%	71.9%	51.6%	70.4%	72.4%	34.7%	70.9%	75.5%	*56.1%*	78.1%	54.3%	58.0%

Marital Status

		Australia	Colombia	Czech Rep.	India	Israel	Italy	Nigeria	Poland	Portugal	*South Africa*	Spain	Switzerland	Total
Still living with my parents	n	20	182	136	469	92	45	112	85	142	106	206	231	1921
	%	4.2%	58.5%	29.0%	42.9%	10.4%	16.5%	16.8%	17.7%	28.0%	18.5%	38.9%	5.9%	18.0%
Single, unmarried	n	41	63	67	140	108	36	295	71	84	82	67	589	1710
	%	8.6%	20.3%	14.3%	12.8%	12.2%	13.2%	44.4%	14.8%	16.6%	14.3%	12.7%	15.0%	16.0%
Living in a partnership but in separate households	n	16	10	44	9	46	33	11	43	17	14	26	314	592
	%	3.4%	3.2%	9.4%	0.8%	5.2%	12.1%	1.7%	8.9%	3.4%	2.4%	4.9%	8.0%	5.6%
Living together in a partnership	n	54	17	70	18	82	60	4	101	65	92	58	719	1420
	%	11.4%	5.5%	14.9%	1.6%	9.3%	22.1%	0.6%	21.0%	12.8%	16.0%	11.0%	18.3%	13.3%
Married	n	298	35	117	428	500	79	228	166	150	224	150	1531	4079
	%	62.9%	11.3%	24.9%	39.2%	56.6%	29.0%	34.3%	34.5%	29.6%	39.0%	28.4%	38.9%	38.2%
Divorced / separated	n	42	4	27	16	45	16	11	14	46	43	21	459	781
	%	8.9%	1.3%	5.8%	1.5%	5.1%	5.9%	1.7%	2.9%	9.1%	7.5%	4.0%	11.7%	7.3%
Widowed	n	3	0	3	12	11	3	4	1	3	13	1	92	162
	%	0.6%	0.0%	1.7%	1.1%	1.2%	1.1%	0.6%	0.2%	0.6%	2.3%	0.2%	2.3%	1.5%

Education

		Australia	Colombia	Czech Rep.	India	Israel	Italia	Nigeria	Poland	Portugal	*South Africa*	Spain	Switzerland	total
Did not finish school	n	4	0	0	4	5	0	1	0	0	6	12	41	79
	%	0.8%	0.0%	0.0%	0.4%	0.6%	0.0%	0.2%	0.0%	0.0%	1.0%	1.1%	1.0%	0.6%
Primary school	n	0	0	16	36	1	18	0	4	1	4	61	190	335
	%	0.0%	0.0%	3.4%	3.3%	0.1%	6.6%	0.0%	0.8%	0.2%	0.7%	5.9%	4.8%	2.9%
Secondary school	n	54	67	287	214	96	54	23	185	147	211	361	1111	3013
	%	11.4%	21.5%	61.2%	19.6%	10.9%	19.9%	3.5%	38.5%	29.0%	32.1%	34.5%	28.2%	26.5%
Professional training / Diploma	n	126	14	0	526	110	69	22	64	226	140	271	2146	4186
	%	40.0%	4.5%	0.0%	48.2%	12.4%	52.7%	3.3%	13.3%	44.6%	24.4%	25.9%	54.5%	36.8%
Tertiary education / University	n	131	230	166	312	672	131	619	228	124	212	349	447	3750
	%	41.6%	74.0%	35.4%	28.6%	76.0%	48.2%	93.1%	47.4%	24.5%	37.1%	66.0%	11.4%	33.0%

Main Activity

		Australia	Colombia	Czech Rep.	India	Israel	Italy	Nigeria	Poland	Portugal	*South Africa*	Spain	Switzerland	Total
In education or training (student)	n	23	178	236	504	150	62	171	144	171	83	216	197	2197
	%	4.9%	57.2%	50.3%	46.2%	17.0%	22.8%	25.7%	29.9%	33.7%	14.5%	40.8%	5.0%	20.6%
Household / raising children	n	16	2	15	118	17	13	7	18	2	16	12	181	432
	%	3.4%	0.6%	3.2%	10.8%	1.9%	4.8%	1.1%	3.7%	0.4%	2.8%	2.3%	4.6%	4.1%
Part-time job	n	77	13	33	57	143	41	102	33	45	73	62	830	1567
	%	16.2%	4.2%	7.0%	5.2%	16.2%	15.1%	15.3%	6.9%	8.9%	12.7%	11.7%	21.1%	14.7%
Fulltime job	n	312	113	155	352	492	126	276	269	260	293	202	1777	4866
	%	65.8%	36.3%	33.0%	32.2%	55.7%	46.3%	41.5%	55.9%	51.3%	51.0%	38.2%	45.2%	45.6%
Unemployed	n	22	5	0	46	28	16	103	7	17	68	13	212	601
	%	4.6%	1.6%	0.0%	4.2%	3.2%	5.9%	15.5%	1.5%	3.4%	11.8%	2.5%	5.4%	5.6%
Retired	n	24	0	30	15	54	14	6	10	12	41	24	738	1002
	%	5.1%	0.0%	6.4%	1.4%	6.1%	5.1%	0.9%	2.1%	2.4%	7.1%	4.5%	18.8%	9.4%

Professional Status

		Australia	Colombia	Czech Rep.	India	Israel	Italy	Nigeria	Poland	Portugal	*South Africa*	Spain	Switzerland	Total
No position in an organization (eg. at school, housekeeping, unemployed, retired)	n	47	63	154	224	101	69	101	32	111	127	136	657	1934
	%	9.9%	20.3%	32.8%	20.5%	11.4%	25.4%	15.2%	6.7%	21.9%	22.1%	25.7%	16.7%	18.1%
In education / training	n	23	101	91	499	110	34	159	147	68	90	98	168	1656
	%	4.9%	32.5%	19.4%	45.7%	12.4%	12.5%	23.9%	30.6%	13.4%	15.7%	18.5%	4.3%	15.5%
Employee	n	150	58	155	242	319	55	162	195	199	138	196	1705	3691
	%	31.6%	18.6%	33.0%	22.2%	36.1%	20.2%	24.4%	40.5%	39.3%	24.0%	37.1%	43.3%	34.6%
Junior / Middle management	n	64	53	32	70	151	16	79	49	71	102	42	729	1543
	%	13.5%	17.0%	6.8%	6.4%	17.1%	5.9%	11.9%	10.2%	14.0%	17.8%	7.9%	18.5%	14.5%
Senior management / Board of directors	n	49	24	6	18	95	21	47	9	22	37	37	275	666
	%	10.3%	7.7%	1.3%	1.6%	10.7%	7.7%	7.1%	1.9%	4.3%	6.4%	7.0%	7.0%	6.2%
Entrepreneur / Business owner	n	141	12	31	39	108	77	117	49	36	80	20	401	1175
	%	29.7%	3.9%	6.6%	3.6%	12.2%	28.3%	17.6%	10.2%	7.1%	13.9%	3.8%	10.2%	11.0%

Religion

		Australia	Colombia	Czech Rep.	India	Israel	Italy	Nigeria	Poland	Portugal	*South Africa*	Spain	Switzerland	Total
Catholic	n	80	163	101	224	8	130	326	308	244	41	288	1100	3052
	%	16 9%	52.4%	21.5%	20.5%	0.9%	47.8%	49.0%	64.0%	48.1%	7.1%	54.4%	28.0%	28.6%
Protestant	n	43	8	11	14	4	0	131	4	10	69	2	796	1135
	%	9.1%	2.6%	2.3%	1.3%	0.5%	0.0%	19.7%	0.8%	2.0%	12.0%	0.4%	20.2%	10.6%
Another Christian church or community	n	66	8	26	25	0	2	155	11	5	265	1	138	929
	%	13 9%	2.6%	5.5%	2.3%	0.0%	0.7%	23.3%	2.3%	1.0%	46..2%	0.2%	3.5%	8.7%
Muslim	n	5	0	0	215	9	1	14	0	2	16	2	71	347
	%	1.1%	0.0%	0.0%	19.7%	1.0%	0.4%	2.1%	0.0%	0.4%	2.8%	0.4%	1.8%	3.3%
Jewish	n	17	0	1	0	496	1	0	0	0	5	0	11	535
	%	3.6%	0.0%	0.2%	0.0%	56.1%	0.4%	0.0%	0.0%	0.0%	0.9%	0.0%	0.3%	5.0%
Hindu	n	14	0	0	533	3	1	0	0	0	8	0	1	568
	%	3.0%	0.0%	0.0%	48.8%	0.3%	0.4%	0.0%	0.0%	0.0%	1.4%	0.0%	0.0%	5.3%
Buddhist	n	9	0	5	0	3	9	0	2	3	1	0	27	60
	%	1.9%	0.0%	1.1%	0.0%	0.3%	3.3%	0.0%	0.4%	0.6%	0.2%	0.0%	0.7%	0.6%
I am a spiritual person outside the traditional world religions	n	95	60	156	37	138	32	28	50	96	92	35	340	1236
	%	20.0%	19.3%	33.3%	3.4%	15.6%	11.8%	4.2%	10.4%	18.9%	16.0%	6.6%	8.6%	11.6%
Without religion or confession	n	121	56	137	24	132	86	4	96	120	48	170	1352	2384
	%	25.5%	18.0%	29.2%	2.2%	14.9%	31.6%	0.6%	20.0%	23.7%	8.4%	32.1%	34.4%	22.4%
Something different	n	24	16	32	20	91	10	7	10	27	29	31	99	419
	%	5.1%	5.1%	6.8%	1.8%	10.3%	3.7%	1.1%	2.1%	5.3%	5.1%	5.9%	2.5%	3.9%

Appendix 4.2: Partial Bivariate Pearson's Correlations Between Future Prospects and Perceived Hope and Well-Being

Appendix 4.2.1: Correlation Coefficients Australia

	Perceived Hope	Hedonic well-being	Psychological well-being	Social well-being
Quality of Life 2040	0.291**	0.179**	0.209**	0.344**
The country's economy	0.219**	0.151**	0.201**	0.276**
Employment prospects	0.217**	0.176**	0.210**	0.307**
Gap between rich and poor	0.197**	0.125**	0.141**	0.251**
Family life	0.212**	0.214**	0.214**	0.338**
Our natural environment	0.274**	0.187**	0.203**	0.309**
The physical health of the population	0.132**	0.104*	0.116*	0.307**
The mental health of the population	0.176**	0.174**	0.197**	0.383**
Substance abuse	0.208**	0.162**	0.165**	0.295**
Crime and violence	0.193**	0.136**	0.187**	0.351**
Racism	0.152**	0.167**	0.142**	0.248**
Justice and equality	0.170**	0.100*	0.118*	0.267**
Expected Crisis Scenario 1	−0.101*	−0.124**	−0.100*	−0.210**
Expected Flourishing Scenario 2	0.187**	0.152**	0.144**	0.280**
Desirable Competitive Scenario 1	0.145**	0.038	0.060	0.103*
Desirable Sustainable Scenario 2	0.037	−0.020	0.010	0.040

Note: **. Correlation is significant at 0.01 level; *. Correlation is significant at 0.05 level; Control variables: Gender, age, marital status, education, main activity and professional status

Appendix 4.2.2: Correlation Coefficients Colombia

	Perceived Hope	Hedonic well-being	Psychological well-being	Social well-being
Quality of Life 2040	0.256**	0.275**	0.294**	0.272**
The country's economy	0.220**	0.231**	0.262**	0.267**
Employment prospects	0.263**	0.201**	0.241**	0.231**
Gap between rich and poor	0.243**	0.261**	0.275**	0.309**

(continued)

	Perceived Hope	Hedonic well-being	Psychological well-being	Social well-being
Family life	0.213**	0.207**	0.299**	0.266**
Our natural environment	0.254**	0.252**	0.286**	0.241**
The physical health of the population	0.217**	0.205**	0.236**	0.242**
The mental health of the population	0.218**	0.200**	0.259**	0.321**
Substance abuse	0.125*	0.092	0.166**	0.187**
Crime and violence	0.144*	0.211**	0.253**	0.200**
Racism	0.103	0.155**	0.170**	0.122*
Justice and equality	0.226**	0.179**	0.214**	0.241**
Expected Crisis Scenario 1	−0.146*	−0.152**	−0.101	−0.161**
Expected Flourishing Scenario 2	0.309**	0.306**	0.341**	0.369**
Desirable Competitive Scenario 1	0.118*	0.159**	0.169**	0.265**
Desirable Sustainable Scenario 2	0.072	0.043	0.059	−0.029

Note: **. Correlation is significant at 0.01 level; *. Correlation is significant at 0.05 level; Control variables: Gender, age, marital status, education, main activity and professional status

Appendix 4.2.3: Correlation Coefficients Czech Republic

	Perceived Hope	Hedonic well-being	Psychological well-being	Social well-being
Quality of Life 2040	0.151**	0.132**	0.156**	0.244**
The country's economy	0.127**	0.099*	0.098*	0.183**
Employment prospects	0.169**	0.158**	0.179**	0.223**
Gap between rich and poor	0.192**	0.112*	0.096*	0.146**
Family life	0.017	0.073	0.097*	0.158**
Our natural environment	0.233**	0.138**	0.171**	0.210**
The physical health of the population	0.079	0.070	0.086	0.116*
The mental health of the population	0.181**	0.144**	0.165**	0.201**
Substance abuse	0.065	0.023	−0.005	0.066
Crime and violence	0.096*	0.039	0.067	0.165**
Racism	0.119*	0.071	0.065	0.087
Justice and equality	0.148**	0.085	0.061	0.135**
Expected Crisis Scenario 1	−0.149**	−0.151**	−0.140**	−0.231**
Expected Flourishing Scenario 2	0.127**	0.183**	0.219**	0.319**

(continued)

	Perceived Hope	Hedonic well-being	Psychological well-being	Social well-being
Desirable Competitive Scenario 1	−0.040	0.041	0.029	0.032
Desirable Sustainable Scenario 2	0.106*	−0.024	0.010	−0.002

Note: **. Correlation is significant at 0.01 level; *. Correlation is significant at 0.05 level; Control variables: Gender, age, marital status, education, main activity and professional status

Appendix 4.2.4: Correlation Coefficients India

	Perceived Hope	Hedonic well-being	Psychological well-being	Social well-being
Quality of Life 2040	0.185**	0.078**	0.175**	0.191**
The country's economy	0.088**	0.113**	0.154**	0.177**
Employment prospects	0.066*	0.095**	0.109**	0.196**
Gap between rich and poor	0.116**	0.081**	0.076*	0.152**
Family life	0.138**	0.090**	0.177**	0.245**
Our natural environment	0.051	0.166**	0.120**	0.173**
The physical health of the population	0.121**	0.132**	0.181**	0.256**
The mental health of the population	0.126**	0.136**	0.176**	0.271**
Substance abuse	0.031	0.068*	0.148**	0.180**
Crime and violence	0.055	0.141**	0.108**	0.211**
Racism	0.032	0.015	0.100**	0.198**
Justice and equality	0.041	0.115**	0.161**	0.260**
Expected Crisis Scenario 1	−0.018	0.050	−0.063*	−0.165**
Expected Flourishing Scenario 2	0.044	0.137**	0.128**	0.182**
Desirable Competitive Scenario 1	0.009	0.151**	0.115**	0.139**
Desirable Sustainable Scenario 2	0.138**	0.149**	0.174**	0.100**

Note: **. Correlation is significant at 0.01 level; *. Correlation is significant at 0.05 level; Control variables: Gender, age, marital status, education, main activity and professional status

Appendix 4.2.5: Correlation Coefficients Israel

	Perceived Hope	Hedonic well-being	Psychological well-being	Social well-being
Quality of Life 2040	0.344**	0.258**	0.236**	0.410**
The country's economy	0.311**	0.259**	0.252**	0.389**
Employment prospects	0.299**	0.267**	0.232**	0.361**
Gap between rich and poor	0.320**	0.239**	0.208**	0.410**
Family life	0.284**	0.238**	0.256**	0.310**
Our natural environment	0.304**	0.249**	0.225**	0.367**
The physical health of the population	0.249**	0.251**	0.239**	0.318**
The mental health of the population	0.367**	0.332**	0.307**	0.401**
Substance abuse	0.164**	0.168**	0.163**	0.265**
Crime and violence	0.286**	0.207**	0.197**	0.349**
Racism	0.290**	0.203**	0.192**	0.391**
Justice and equality	0.315**	0.233**	0.194**	0.403**
Expected Crisis Scenario 1	−0.238**	−0.150**	−0.144**	−0.285**
Expected Flourishing Scenario 2	0.344**	0.271**	0.240**	0.339**
Desirable Competitive Scenario 1	−0.051	0.032	0.020	0.046
Desirable Sustainable Scenario 2	0.050	0.045	0.055	0.044

Note: **. Correlation is significant at 0.01 level; *. Correlation is significant at 0.05 level; Control variables: Gender, age, marital status, education, main activity and professional status

Appendix 4.2.6: Correlation Coefficients Italy

	Perceived Hope	Hedonic well-being	Psychological well-being	Social well-being
Quality of Life 2040	0.223**	0.158**	0.138*	0.250**
The country's economy	0.255**	0.131*	0.149*	0.218**
Employment prospects	0.321**	0.158**	0.158**	0.226**
Gap between rich and poor	0.272**	0.209**	0.175**	0.293**
Family life	0.196**	0.121*	0.124*	0.209**
Our natural environment	0.252**	0.244**	0.190**	0.263**
The physical health of the population	0.212**	0.182**	0.179**	0.284**
The mental health of the population	0.281**	0.215**	0.216**	0.319**

(continued)

	Perceived Hope	Hedonic well-being	Psychological well-being	Social well-being
Substance abuse	0.159**	0.047	0.079	0.152*
Crime and violence	0.247**	0.179**	0.181**	0.245**
Racism	0.208**	0.118	0.109	0.256**
Justice and equality	0.201**	0.162**	0.212**	0.279**
Expected Crisis Scenario 1	−0.213**	−0.171**	−0.190**	−0.253**
Expected Flourishing Scenario 2	0.291**	0.162**	0.281**	0.327**
Desirable Competitive Scenario 1	0.052	0.135*	0.157*	0.126*
Desirable Sustainable Scenario 2	0.026	0.030	0.015	−0.085

Note: **. Correlation is significant at 0.01 level; *. Correlation is significant at 0.05 level; Control variables: Gender, age, marital status, education, main activity and professional status

Appendix 4.2.7: Correlation Coefficients Nigeria

	Perceived Hope	Hedonic well-being	Psychological well-being	Social well-being
Quality of Life 2040	0.188**	0.158**	0.108**	0.175**
The country's economy	0.170**	0.152**	0.105**	0.230**
Employment prospects	0.186**	0.147**	0.103**	0.220**
Gap between rich and poor	0.160**	0.127**	0.090*	0.232**
Family life	0.183**	0.178**	0.173**	0.245**
Our natural environment	0.198**	0.160**	0.134**	0.235**
The physical health of the population	0.192**	0.170**	0.148**	0.230**
The mental health of the population	0.209**	0.164**	0.161**	0.246**
Substance abuse	0.156**	0.123**	0.108**	0.203**
Crime and violence	0.147**	0.132**	0.106**	0.228**
Racism	0.183**	0.150**	0.128**	0.215**
Justice and equality	0.177**	0.130**	0.103**	0.231**
Expected Crisis Scenario 1	0.063	−0.028	0.076	−0.042
Expected Flourishing Scenario 2	0.153**	0.131**	0.171**	0.181**
Desirable Competitive Scenario 1	0.132**	0.089*	0.149**	0.042
Desirable Sustainable Scenario 2	0.186**	0.139**	0.155**	0.033

Note: **. Correlation is significant at 0.01 level; *. Correlation is significant at 0.05 level; Control variables: Gender, age, marital status, education, main activity and professional status

Appendix 4.2.8: Correlation Coefficients Poland

	Perceived Hope	Hedonic well-being	Psychological well-being	Social well-being
Quality of Life 2040	0.311**	0.268**	0.294**	0.317**
The country's economy	0.287**	0.265**	0.299**	0.325**
Employment prospects	0.304**	0.227**	0.271**	0.269**
Gap between rich and poor	0.225**	0.214**	0.245**	0.300**
Family life	0.192**	0.141**	0.193**	0.265**
Our natural environment	0.240**	0.182**	0.243**	0.271**
The physical health of the population	0.241**	0.188**	0.262**	0.332**
The mental health of the population	0.330**	0.253**	0.288**	0.356**
Substance abuse	0.125**	0.117*	0.153**	0.267**
Crime and violence	0.213**	0.138**	0.237**	0.263**
Racism	0.219**	0.171**	0.158**	0.213**
Justice and equality	0.252**	0.216**	0.221**	0.320**
Expected Crisis Scenario 1	−0.222**	−0.220**	−0.240**	−0.348**
Expected Flourishing Scenario 2	0.265**	0.199**	0.270**	0.387**
Desirable Competitive Scenario 1	−0.007	0.025	0.007	−0.033
Desirable Sustainable Scenario 2	0.092*	0.030	0.074	0.093*

Note: **. Correlation is significant at 0.01 level; *. Correlation is significant at 0.05 level; Control variables: Gender, age, marital status, education, main activity and professional status

Appendix 4.2.9: Correlation Coefficients Portugal

	Perceived Hope	Hedonic well-being	Psychological well-being	Social well-being
Quality of Life 2040	0.232**	0.177**	0.165**	0.315**
The country's economy	0.249**	0.196**	0.158**	0.246**
Employment prospects	0.244**	0.188**	0.138**	0.242**
Gap between rich and poor	0.215**	0.202**	0.145**	0.197**
Family life	0.239**	0.208**	0.172**	0.251**
Our natural environment	0.160**	0.130**	0.091*	0.182**
The physical health of the population	0.205**	0.213**	0.174**	0.244**
The mental health of the population	0.221**	0.238**	0.182**	0.255**
Substance abuse	0.137**	0.145**	0.080	0.169**

(continued)

	Perceived Hope	Hedonic well-being	Psychological well-being	Social well-being
Crime and violence	0.124**	0.138**	0.079	0.175**
Racism	0.138**	0.154**	0.105*	0.186**
Justice and equality	0.214**	0.188**	0.153**	0.240**
Expected Crisis Scenario 1	−0.153**	−0.102*	−0.073	−0.205**
Expected Flourishing Scenario 2	0.249**	0.153**	0.152**	0.300**
Desirable Competitive Scenario 1	0.065	0.017	0.038	0.004
Desirable Sustainable Scenario 2	0.112*	0.174**	0.176**	0.069

Note: **. Correlation is significant at 0.01 level; *. Correlation is significant at 0.05 level; Control variables: Gender, age, marital status, education, main activity and professional status

Appendix 4.2.10: Correlation Coefficients South Africa

	Perceived Hope	Hedonic well-being	Psychological well-being	Social well-being
Quality of Life 2040	0.387**	0.266**	0.194	0.384**
The country's economy	0.398**	0.289**	0.178	0.250*
Employment prospects	0.365**	0.247*	0.167	0.274**
Gap between rich and poor	0.237*	0.253*	0.141	0.227*
Family life	0.291**	0.404**	0.366**	0.372**
Our natural environment	0.100	0.095	0.011	0.249*
The physical health of the population	0.309**	0.312**	0.223*	0.272**
The mental health of the population	0.263**	0.234*	0.130	0.260*
Substance abuse	0.111	0.221*	0.214*	0.226*
Crime and violence	0.274**	0.277**	0.147	0.293**
Racism	0.181	0.206*	0.124	0.163
Justice and equality	0.189	0.240*	0.165	0.225*
Expected Crisis Scenario 1	−0.199	−0.165	−0.163	−0.338**
Expected Flourishing Scenario 2	0.198	0.070	0.062	0.212*
Desirable Competitive Scenario 1	0.100	0.130	0.075	0.105
Desirable Sustainable Scenario 2	−0.045	0.106	0.130	0.133

Note: **. Correlation is significant at 0.01 level; *. Correlation is significant at 0.05 level; Control variables: Gender, age, marital status, education, main activity and professional status

Appendix 4.2.11: Correlation Coefficients Spain

	Perceived Hope	Hedonic well-being	Psychological well-being	Social well-being
Quality of Life 2040	0.233**	0.201**	0.200**	0.263**
The country's economy	0.310**	0.265**	0.257**	0.336**
Employment prospects	0.321**	0.284**	0.269**	0.333**
Gap between rich and poor	0.273**	0.242**	0.204**	0.321**
Family life	0.229**	0.220**	0.205**	0.301**
Our natural environment	0.284**	0.249**	0.218**	0.315**
The physical health of the population	0.173**	0.210**	0.125**	0.236**
The mental health of the population	0.278**	0.291**	0.232**	0.326**
Substance abuse	0.182**	0.186**	0.163**	0.230**
Crime and violence	0.301**	0.252**	0.215**	0.297**
Racism	0.238**	0.264**	0.206**	0.284**
Justice and equality	0.262**	0.242**	0.220**	0.312**
Expected Crisis Scenario 1	−0.134**	−0.150**	−0.119**	−0.172**
Expected Flourishing Scenario 2	0.294**	0.255**	0.267**	0.365**
Desirable Competitive Scenario 1	0.033	0.000	0.016	−0.004
Desirable Sustainable Scenario 2	0.084	0.119**	0.068	0.069

Note: **. Correlation is significant at 0.01 level; *. Correlation is significant at 0.05 level; Control variables: Gender, age, marital status, education, main activity and professional status

Appendix 4.2.12: Correlation Coefficients Switzerland

	Perceived Hope	Hedonic well-being	Psychological well-being	Social well-being
Quality of Life 2040	0.266**	0.189**	0.186**	0.347**
The country's economy	0.181**	0.147**	0.142**	0.273**
Employment prospects	0.234**	0.203**	0.193**	0.318**
Gap between rich and poor	0.210**	0.161**	0.167**	0.282**
Family life	0.197**	0.184**	0.168**	0.248**
Our natural environment	0.199**	0.142**	0.152**	0.272**
The physical health of the population	0.185**	0.145**	0.147**	0.255**
The mental health of the population	0.242**	0.179**	0.166**	0.322**
Substance abuse	0.133**	0.098**	0.081**	0.196**

(continued)

	Perceived Hope	Hedonic well-being	Psychological well-being	Social well-being
Crime and violence	0.196**	0.134**	0.144**	0.279**
Racism	0.150**	0.107**	0.117**	0.211**
Justice and equality	0.209**	0.171**	0.167**	0.283**
Expected Crisis Scenario 1	−0.194**	−0.115**	−0.102**	−0.263**
Expected Flourishing Scenario 2	0.244**	0.169**	0.161**	0.315**
Desirable Competitive Scenario 1	0.102**	0.072**	0.089**	0.154**
Desirable Sustainable Scenario 2	0.043**	0.009	0.030	0.008

Note: **. Correlation is significant at 0.01 level; *. Correlation is significant at 0.05 level; Control variables: Gender, age, marital status, education, main activity and professional status

References

Adolph, D., Schneider, S., & Margraf, J. (2016). German anxiety barometer—clinical and everyday-life anxieties in the general population. *Frontiers in Psychology, 7*(1344), 1–12. https://doi.org/10.3389/fpsyg.2016.01344

Baumeister, R. F., Maranges, H. M., & Sjåstad, H. (2018). Consciousness of the future as a matrix of maybe: Pragmatic prospection and the simulation of alternative possibilities. *Psychology of Consciousness: Theory, Research, and Practice, 5*(3), 223. https://doi.org/10.1037/cns0000154

Bell, W. (1996). *An overview of futures studies* (pp. 28–56). Foundations.

Bell, W. (1997). The purposes of Futures Studies. *The Futurist, 31*(6), 42–45.

Bell, W. (2003). *Foundations of futures studies. History, purposes, and knowledge* (Vol. 1). Transaction Publishers.

Bell, W. (2004). Humanity's Common Values Seeking a Positive Future. *The Futurist, 38*(5), 30.

Bell, W. (2009). *Foundations of futures studies: History, purposes, knowledge. Volume I: Human science for a New Era.* Transaction Publishers.

Blöser, C., & Stahl, T. (2019). An Introduction. In C. Blöser & T. Stahl (Eds.), *The Moral Psychology of Hope* (pp. 1–11). Rowman & Littlefield International.

Boulding, E. (1994). Image and Action in Peace Building. In D. Hicks (Ed.), *Preparing for the Future: Notes & Queries for Concerned Educators* (pp. 61–84). Adamantine Press. https://doi.org/10.1111/j.1540-4560.1988.tb02061.x

Braithwaite, V. (2004). Collective hope. *The Annals of the American Academy of Political and Social Science, 592*(1), 6–15.

Brunstad, P. O. (2002). Longing for belonging: Youth culture in Norway. In J. Gidley, N. Ingwersen, & S. Inayatullah (Eds.), *Youth futures: Comparative research and transformative visions* (pp. 143–154). Greenwood Publishing Group.

Chen, F. F. (2007). Sensitivity of goodness of fit indexes to lack of measurement invariance. *Structural Equation Modeling: A Multidisciplinary Journal, 14*(3), 464–504. https://doi.org/10.1080/10705510701301834

Dator, J. (1996). Futures Studies as Applied Knowledge. In R. Slaughter (Ed.), *New Thinking for a New Millennium* (pp. 105–115). Routledge.

Delle Fave, A. (2020). Eudaimonic and hedonic happiness. In F. Maggino (Ed.), *Encyclopedia of quality of life and well-being research* (pp. 1–7). Springer International Publishing.

Delle Fave, A., Brdar, I., Freire, T., Vella-Brodrick, D., & Wissing, M. P. (2011). The eudaimonic and hedonic components of happiness: Qualitative and quantitative findings. *Social Indicators Research, 100*(2), 185–207. https://doi.org/10.1007/s11205-010-9632-5

Delle Fave, A., Brdar, I., Wissing, M. P., Araujo, U., Castro Solano, A., Freire, T., Hernández-Pozo, M., Jose, T., Martos, T., Nafstad, H., Nakamura, J., Singh, K., & Soosai-Nathan, L. (2016). Lay definitions of happiness across nations: The primacy of inner harmony and relational connectedness. *Frontiers in Psychology, 7*, 30–52. https://doi.org/10.3389/fpsyg.2016.00030

Delle Fave, A., & Soosai-Nathan, L. (2014). Meaning as inter-connectedness: theoretical perspectives and empirical evidence. *Journal of Psychology in Africa, 24*(1), 33–43. https://doi.org/10.1080/14330237.2014.904090

Delle Fave, A., Wissing, M., Brdar, I., Vella-Brodrick, D., & Freire, T. (2013). Cross-cultural perceptions of meaning and goals in adulthood: Their roots and relations with happiness. In A. S. Waterman (Ed.), *The best within us: Positive psychology perspectives on eudaimonia* (pp. 227–247). American Psychological Association. https://doi.org/10.1037/14092-012

Diener, E. (2000). Subjective well-being: The science of happiness and a proposal for a national index. *American Psychologist, 55*(1), 34–43. https://doi.org/10.1037/0003-066X.55.1.34

Eckersley, R. (1999). Dreams and expectations: Young people's expected and preferred futures and their significance for education. *Futures, 31*(1), 73–90. https://doi.org/10.1016/S0016-3287(98)00111-6

Eckersley, R. (2002). Future visions, social realities, and private lives: Young people and their personal well-being. In J. Gidley, N. Ingwersen, & S. Inayatullah (Eds.), *Youth futures: Comparative research and transformative visions* (pp. 31–42). Greenwood Publishing Group.

Eckersley, R., Cahill, H., Wierenga, A., & Wyn, J. (2007). *Generations in dialogue about the future: The hopes and fears of young Australians*. Canberra: Australia 21 Ltd. Melbourne: Australian Youth Research Centre.

Gidley, J. M., & Hampson, G. P. (2005). The evolution of futures in school education. *Futures, 37*(4), 255–271.

Grund, J., & Brock, A. (2019). Why we should empty Pandora's box to create a sustainable future: Hope, sustainability and its implications for education. *Sustainability, 11*(3), 893. https://doi.org/10.3390/su11030893

Gutiérrez, G. (2001). *A theology of liberation*. SCM Press.

Hickman, C. (2020). We need to (find a way to) talk about . . . Eco-anxiety. *Journal of Social Work Practice, 34*(4), 411–424. https://doi.org/10.1080/02650533.2020.184416

Hicks, D. (1996). Retrieving the dream: how students envision their preferable futures. *Futures, 28*(8), 741–749. https://doi.org/10.1016/0016-3287(96)00032-8

Hicks, D. (2003). *Lessons for the future: The missing dimension in education*. Routledge. https://doi.org/10.4324/9780203219331

Hicks, D. (2012). The future only arrives when things look dangerous: Reflections on futures education in the UK. *Futures, 44*(1), 4–13. https://doi.org/10.1016/j.futures.2011.08.002

Holden, C. (2002). Citizens of the New Century: Perspectives from the United Kingdom. In J. Gidley & S. Inayatullah (Eds.), *Youth Futures – Comparative Research and Transformative Visions* (pp. 131–142). Praeger.

Hu, L. T., & Bentler, P. M. (1999). Cutoff criteria for fit indexes in covariance structure analysis: Conventional criteria versus new alternatives. *Structural Equation Modeling: A Multidisciplinary Journal, 6*(1), 1–55. https://doi.org/10.1080/10705519909540118

Inayatullah, S. (2000). *Alternative futures: Methodology, society, macrohistory and the long-term future*. Tamkang Chair Lecture Series.

Inayatullah, S. (2002). Youth, scenarios, and metaphors of the future. In J. Giddley & S. Inayatullah (Eds.), *Youth futures: comparative research and transformative visions* (pp. 229–236). Greenwood Publishing Group.

Keyes, C. L. (2002). The mental health continuum: From languishing to flourishing in life. *Journal of Health and Social Behavior, 43*(2), 207–222. https://doi.org/10.2307/3090197

Keyes, C. L. (2014). Happiness, flourishing, and life satisfaction. In W. C. Cockerham, R. Dingwall, & S. R. Quah (Eds.), *The Wiley Blackwell encyclopedia of health, illness, behavior, and society* (pp. 747–751). John Wiley & Sons. https://doi.org/10.1002/9781118410868.wbehibs454

Keyes, C. L., & Haidt, J. (2010). Flourishing. In I. B. Weiner & W. E. Craighead (Eds.), *The Corsini encyclopedia of psychology* (Vol. 4, pp. 99–107). John Wiley & Sons.

Keyes, C. L., Wissing, M., Potgieter, J. P., Temane, M., Kruger, A., & Van Rooy, S. (2008). Evaluation of the mental health continuum–short form (MHC–SF) in setswana-speaking South Africans. *Clinical Psychology & Psychotherapy, 15*(3), 181–192. https://doi.org/10.1002/cpp.572

Kleist, N., & Jansen, S. (2016). Introduction: Hope over time—Crisis, immobility and future-making. *History and Anthropology, 27*(4), 373–392. https://doi.org/10.1080/02757206.2016.1207636

Krafft, A. M., Guse, T., & Maree, D. (2021). Distinguishing perceived hope and dispositional optimism: Theoretical foundations and empirical findings beyond future expectancies and cognition. *Journal of Well-Being Assessment*, 1–27. https://doi.org/10.1007/s41543-020-00030-4.

Krafft, A. M., Martin-Krumm, C., & Fenouillet, F. (2019, April 1). Adaptation, further elaboration, and validation of a scale to measure hope as perceived by people. *Assessment.* https://doi.org/10.1177/1073191117700724.

Lomas, T., Waters, L., Williams, P., Oades, L. G., & Kern, M. L. (2021). Third wave positive psychology: Broadening towards complexity. *The Journal of Positive Psychology, 16*(5), 660–674. https://doi.org/10.1080/17439760.2020.1805501

Marsh, H. W. (1994). Confirmatory factor analysis models of factorial invariance: A multifaceted approach. *Structural Equation Modeling, 1*, 5–34. https://doi.org/10.1080/10705519409539960

Marsh, H. W., Balla, J. R., & Hau, K. (1996). An evaluation of incremental fit indices: A clarification of mathematical and empirical properties. In G. A. Marcoulides & R. E. Schumacker (Eds.), *Advanced structural equation modeling: Issues and techniques* (pp. 315–353). Lawrence Erlbaum.

Marujo, H. A., & Neto, L. M. (Eds.). (2014). *Positive Nations and Communities: Collective, Qualitative, and Cultural-Sensitive Processes in Positive Psychology*. Springer.

Marujo, H. Á., Velez, M. J., Gonçalves, S. P., Neto, L. M., Krafft, A. M., & Casais, M. (2021). The value of hope: Validation of the perceived hope scale in the Portuguese population. *Current Psychology*, 1–9. https://doi.org/10.1007/s12144-021-02115-6.

Massimini, F., & Delle Fave, D. A. (2000). Individual development in a bio-cultural perspective. *American Psychologist, 55*(1), 24–33. https://doi.org/10.1037/0003-066X.55.1.24

McGeer, V. (2004). The art of good hope. *The Annals of the American Academy of Political and Social Science, 592*(1), 100–127. https://doi.org/10.1177/0002716203261781

Nordensvard, J. (2014). Dystopia and disutopia: Hope and hopelessness in German pupils' future narratives. *Journal of Educational Change, 15*(4), 443–465. https://doi.org/10.1007/s10833-014-9237-x

Oettingen, G. (2012). Future thought and behaviour change. *European Review of Social Psychology, 23*, 1–63. https://doi.org/10.1080/10463283.2011.643698

Polak, F. (1961/1973). The Image of the Future, translated from the Dutch and abridged by Elise Boulding. : Jossey-Bass/Elsevier.

Rorty, R. (1998). *Achieving our country*. Harvard University Press.

Rorty, R. (1999). *Philosophy and social hope*. Penguin Books.

Rorty, R. (2002). Hope and the future. *Peace Review, 14*(2), 149–155. https://doi.org/10.1080/10402650220140166

Rubin, A. (2002). Reflections upon the late-modern transition as seen in the images of the future held by young Finns. In J. Gidley, N. Ingwersen, & S. Inayatullah (Eds.), *Youth futures: Comparative research and transformative visions* (pp. 99–110). Greenwood Publishing Group.

Ryan, R. M., & Deci, E. L. (2001). On happiness and human potentials: A review of research on hedonic and eudaimonic well-being. *Annual Review of Psychology, 52*, 141–166. https://doi.org/10.1146/annurev.psych.52.1.141

Ryff, C. D. (1989). Happiness Is Everything, or Is It? Explorations on the Meaning of Psychological Well-Being. *Journal of Personality and Social Psychology, 57*, 1069–1081. https://doi.org/10.1037/0022-3514.57.6.1069

Ryff, C. D., & Keyes, C. L. M. (1995). The Structure of Psychological Well-Being Revisited. *Journal of Personality and Social Psychology, 69*, 719–727. https://doi.org/10.1037/0022-3514.69.4.719

Ryff, C. D., & Singer, B. H. (2008). Know thyself and become what you are: A eudaimonic approach to psychological well-being. *Journal of Happiness Studies, 9*, 13–39. https://doi.org/10.1007/s10902-006-9019-0

Scheier, M. E., & Carver, C. S. (1987). Dispositional optimism and physical well-being: The influence of generalized outcome expectancies on health. *Journal of Personality, 55*(2), 169–210. https://doi.org/10.1111/j.1467-6494.1987.tb00434.x

Scioli, A., Ricci, M., Nyugen, T., & Scioli, E. R. (2011). Hope: Its nature and measurement. *Psychology of Religion and Spirituality, 3*(2), 78–97. https://doi.org/10.1037/a0020903

Searle, K., & Gow, K. (2010). Do concerns about climate change lead to distress? *International Journal of Climate Change Strategies and Management, 2*(4), 362–379. https://doi.org/10.1108/17568691011089891

Seligman, M. E. (1990). *Learned optimism: How to change your mind and your life*. Vintage Books.

Seligman, M. E., Peter Railton, P., Baumeister, R., & Sripada, C. (2016). *Homo prospectus*. Oxford University Press.

Shade, P. (2019). Shame, Hope, and the Courage to Transgress. In R. Green (Ed.), *Theories of Hope: Exploring Alternative Affective Dimensions of Human Experience* (pp. 47–70). Rowman & Littlefield.

Slaughter, R. A. (1994). Changing Images of Futures in the 20th Century. In D. Hicks (Ed.), *Preparing for the Future – Notes & Queries for Concerned Educators* (pp. 39–59). Adamantine Press Ltd..

Slaughter, R. (2002). From rhetoric to reality: The emergence of futures into the educational mainstream. In J. Giddley & S. Inayatullah (Eds.), *Youth futures: Comparative research and transformative visions* (pp. 175–186). Greenwood Publishing Group.

Slezackova, A., Prošek, T., Malatincová, T., & Krafft, A. M. (2020). Psychometrické vlastnosti české verze Škály prožívané naděje: faktorová struktura a vnitřní konzistence [Psychometric characteristics of the Czech version of The Perceived Hope Scale: Factor structure and internal consistency]. *Československá psychologie/Czechoslovak Psychology, 64*(3), 288–305.

Snow, N. E. (2018). Hope as a democratic civic virtue. *Metaphilosophy, 49*(3), 407–427. https://doi.org/10.1111/meta.12299

Snyder, C. R. (1994). *The psychology of hope: You can get there from here*. Simon & Schuster.

Stahl, T. (2019). Political hope and cooperative community. In C. Blöser & T. Stahl (Eds.), *2019* (pp. 265–283). The Moral Psychology of Hope.

Stewart, C. (2002). Re-Imagining Your Neighborhood: a Model for Futures Education. In G. Gidley, I. Inayatullah, & S. (Eds.), *Youth futures: comparative research and transformative visions* (pp. 187–196). Greenwood Publishing Group.

Stitzlein, S. (2019). Pragmatist Hope. In C. Blöser & T. Stahl (Eds.), *2019* (pp. 93–112). The Moral Psychology of Hope.

Toffler, A. (1974). *Learning for tomorrow: The role of the future in education*. Random House Inc.
Vandenberg, R. J., & Lance, C. E. (2000). A review and synthesis of the measurement invariance literature: Suggestions, practices, and recommendations for organizational research. *Organizational Research Methods, 3*(1), 4–70. https://doi.org/10.1177/109442810031002
Wissing, M. P. (2018). Embracing well-being in diverse contexts: The third wave of positive psychology. In *Invited Address at the First Africa Positive Psychology Conference, Potchefstroom, South Africa*, (Potchefstroom: FAPPC). https://doi.org/10.1007/978-3-030-85924-4_1.
Wissing, M. P. (2022). Beyond the "Third Wave of Positive Psychology": Challenges and Opportunities for Future Research. *Frontiers in Psychology, 12*(January), 1–20. https://doi.org/10.3389/fpsyg.2021.795067

Andreas Krafft holds a doctoral degree in Management Sciences at the University of St. Gallen (Switzerland) with special focus on Organizational Psychology, Culture and Development. He has academic specializations in Social Psychology of Organizations, Work and Health Psychology as well as Positive Psychology from the University of Zürich. Andreas is associate researcher for Futures Studies and lecturer at the Institute of Systemic Management and Public Governance at the University of St. Gallen. Furthermore, he teaches at the University of Zürich in the field of Work and Health, at the Master of Applied Positive Psychology at the University of Lisbon, Portugal, as well as at the Master of Futures Studies from the Free University Berlin. He is co-president of swissfuture, the Swiss Society for Futures Studies, member of the executive board of SWIPPA (the Swiss Positive Psychology Association) and of the DACH-PP (German speaking Association of Positive Psychology). Since many years he leads the International Research Network of the Hope Barometer.

Dr JohnBosco Chika Chukwuorji is a Senior Lecturer at the Department of Psychology, University of Nigeria, Nsukka. He was a Fulbright scholar and visiting researcher at Cleveland State University Cleveland, Ohio USA (2019-2020). He holds a PhD in clinical psychology obtained from the University of Nigeria Nsukka. As a research fellow in the Center for Translational and Implementation Research (CTAIR), University of Nigeria Nsukka, he is a core team member in the use of implementation science to enhance the effectiveness and quality of healthcare services in Nigeria. His research is focused on finding innovative approaches to provide quality mental healthcare for people living with challenging health conditions, forcibly displaced persons, justice-involved individuals, underserved communities and the general population. In addition to being the Editor of Nigerian Journal of Psychological Research, he is associate editor of three Journals (Fulbright Chronicles, Nigerian Journal of Psychology, Journal of International Politics & Development Studies) and editorial board member of four journals (BMC Psychology, Journal of Child & Adolescent Trauma, CPQ Women and Child Health, Journal of Psychology and Allied Disciplines).

Dr Rajneesh Choubisa is Associate Professor of Psychology in the Department of Humanities and Social Sciences at Birla Institute of Technology and Science, (BITS) Pilani, Pilani Campus, India. He is a behavioral scientist by training and specializes in Positive Psychology from IIT Delhi. He has carried out meaningful research in the area of positive psychological measurement, positive organizational psychology and well-being promotion. He has rendered his expertise for reviewing projects at the European Commission's Institute of Advance Studies, among others. He is actively providing his expertise in the capacity of reviewer and academic editor for many top quality journals in the field. As an Indian collaborator of the Hope Barometer project, he has keen interest in exploring positive psychological variables theoretically, and also testing the practicability of these variables through customized, theory-driven, tailor-made programs and interventions.

Dr. Stella Conte is professor at the University of Cagliari, Italy. She is a member of the Italian Association of Psychology (A.I.P., Experimental Session) and of the Italian Association of Ethology. She is a referee for "Psychological Research" and "International Journal of Psychology". Her main research interest focuses on the following areas: the methodological issues of research on cognitive activity in human and animal: Vigilance and Attention, Language, Perception and Memory, as well as Cooperative Learning, Ethological studies of gulls, BFC and changes after treatment in children and adults and Theater therapy in adults and children. She has been the Scientific Responsible of a number of research projects: 2020 Creation of Help Desk for the Prevention of New Technology Addictions Foundation. She is the author of 180 scientific works, including monographies, chapters of books, scientific papers and proceedings published in national and international Journals.

Valle Flores-Lucas is Associate Professor at Valladolid University, in the psychology department. She led the Postgraduate course on Positive Psychology and Humour sense at Valladolid University. Her research work has been centred on two main research lines: developmental language and communication disorders. In the last years, she started another research line in the field of Positive Psychology mainly in the study of hope and its relations with other positive strengths and its applications on education. She is member of the Spanish Positive Psychology Society.

Dr. Tharina Guse is a counselling psychologist and obtained an MA (Counselling Psychology) degree from the Potchefstroom University (now North-West University) in 1989. She was in full-time private practice for the next 15 years providing psychotherapy for children, adolescents and adults. In 2003 she obtained her PhD (Psychology) from Potchefstroom University. She returned to academia in 2005 and joined the University of Johannesburg. Since April 2018 she is a professor and Head of the Department of Psychology at the University of Pretoria. Currently she serves on the Professional Board for Psychology of the Health Professions Council of South Africa (HPCSA). She is also President of the recently founded South African Positive Psychology Association (SAPPA). Her research focuses are on positive psychology in general and in particular on psychosocial well-being, positive psychology interventions and psychological strengths such as hope and gratitude. Closely aligned with this broad focus she also conducts research on the application of hypnosis for the promotion of mental health and well-being.

Dr hab. Elżbieta Kasprzak, psychologist, professor at the Kazimierz Wielki University in Bydgoszcz, Poland. Researcher of the determinants of careers and their consequences for the well-being of employees. An important area of her scientific interests are various aspects of positive functioning at work, job satisfaction, hope and passion at work, as well as the conditions and effects of job crafting and proactivity at work. Since 2015 she has been participating in the international research network of the Hope Barometer.

Helena Agueda Marujo has a PhD in Psychology. She is Associate Professor at the Instituto Superior de Ciências Sociais e Politicas of the University of Lisbon, where she holds the positions of Executive Coordinator of Masters and PhDs programs in Development Human Resources Policies; of Scientific Coordinator of the Postgraduate Degree in Applied Positive Psychology; of researcher at the Centre for Administration and Public Policy (CAPP); and of member of the Ethics Committee. She is the Coordinator of the UNESCO Chair in Education for Global Peace Sustainability at the University of Lisbon. Helena is a member of the Advisory Board of the International Positive Psychology Association and of the Board of Directors of the European Positive Psychology Network.

Dr. Chitra S. Nair started her career as Assistant Professor of Sociology at Government K.N.M. College, Thiruvananthapuram under University of Kerala in 2015. Her ongoing research focuses on positive psychology, improving quality of life and happiness of the marginalized, social exclusion and human rights issues, life course of centenarians and understanding the indigenous approaches to "Healthy Ageing". Her social engagements include advocacy for aged and women through local self-governments, NGOs, student level interventions, industrial partners and academic institutions. Her ongoing engagements include the Major Research Project from National Commission for Women, India to conduct research study titled 'Reproductive Rights and Choices of Fisher Women in Coastal Kerala—an Ethnographic Enquiry' and the Minor Research Project from Indian Council for Social Science Research for the research study on Intimate Partner Violence.

Dr. Dorit Redlich-Amirav is an occupational therapist who works in the field of hope and mental health, mainly with family members. She completed her doctoral studies in the Department of Rehabilitation Medicine at the University of Alberta, Edmonton, Canada. Hope in mothers of adult children with mental illness in an environment of socio-political conflict. She teaches in the field of hope and mental health in the school of health professions at Tel Aviv University. On the subject of hope, she teaches a 'Circle of Hope' course at Levinsky-Wingate Academic Center and at the Ono Academic Campus. In addition, she leads the Hope Index project in Israel.

Dr. Mark Sinclair is an experienced educator, governance and technology professional. Dr Sinclair's career spans multi-sector education; corporate advisory at KPMG and AT Kearney and IT strategy (banking & public sectors). Dr. Sinclair has advised senior executives at over 100 organizations in a broad range of industries throughout Australia, Southeast Asia and the Middle East, helped establish a successful technology start-up and, over the last 20 years, overseen the development of an Education College that has provided education to 100,000 students.

Alena Slezackova, Ph.D., is an Associate Professor of Psychology and a Vice Head of the Dept. of Psychology and Psychosomatics, Faculty of Medicine, Masaryk University, in Brno, Czech Republic. Her scientific interests include mainly hope, mental health, and well-being. She also has a special interest in the research and practice of mindfulness. Alena is a founder and director of the Czech Positive Psychology Centre (CPPC), a member of the Advisory Council of the International Positive Psychology Association (IPPA), and a member of the Executive Board of the European Network for Positive Psychology (ENPP). She has been a member of several international research projects, and she serves on the editorial boards of five academic psychological journals. Alena is the author of the first comprehensive monograph on positive psychology in the Czech language and dozens of scientific publications in positive psychology and health psychology.

Dr Patryk Stecz, a psychologist, is an assistant professor at the Institute of Psychology, University of Lodz, Poland. From 2014-2017 and 2021-2025, he was elected to the Executive Board of the Polish Suicidology Association. Dr Stecz completed his Ph.D. at the Medical University of Lodz. He published approx. 40 scientific works related to applied clinical psychology (attitudes towards suicide, positive suicidology, religious coping, well-being predictors in clinical and non-clinical populations, risk behavior in students with visual impairment, studies on hope). Dr Stecz has been serving psychological support at the Academic Counseling Centre (Technical University of Lodz) for students and employees with disabilities and special needs since 2008. Dr Stecz was aged 31 when he received the Medical University Rector's Scientific Award. Currently he is finishing a four-year post-graduate Clinical Psychology Specialization Program (Center of Postgraduate Medical Education).

Olga Varsos is the co-Author of the POWER Coaching and the GOAL Models, with extensive experience in executive, adult, homeless and at-risk youth coaching. These leading programs are used extensively in Australia and internationally in the not-for-profit, education, community, and indigenous youth sectors, focusing on instilling hope to establish goals to help ensure positive lasting change. Olga started her career as a social worker, firstly in the health sector before moving to project managing service delivery in the community sector. Olga has post graduate degrees in Social Work, Human Resources and is an accredited EQ Practitioner.

Eduardo Wills Herrera is an organizational and well-being scholar and has developed his academic career at Universidad de Los Andes in Bogotá Colombia where he has been Director and full professor at the Interdisciplinary Center for Development Studies (CIDER) and full professor at the Management School where he was Director of the Ph.D. program. He earned a Ph.D. in Organizational behavior from Tulane University, New Orleans, and a Master's in Development Studies from the Institute of Social Studies ISS at The Hague. His research is related to exploring Subjective Well-being as an indicator of development and quality of life in countries and as an indicator of the flourishing of people in organizations. He contributed as the director of Plan Nacional de Rehabilitación, PNR, and was Director of the Mission for State Moralization and efficiency at the Presidency of the Republic of Colombia.

Chapter 5
Worldviews and Basic Beliefs of Hope

Andreas M. Krafft, Tharina Guse, Elżbieta Kasprzak, Dorit Redlich-Amirav, and Patryk Stecz

Abstract To further elaborate on the concept of hope outlined in Chap. 2, the purpose of this contribution is to investigate the role of basic beliefs and worldviews in sustaining the general perception of hope in different cultures. We begin by introducing the theoretical concepts about the nature of basic beliefs and worldviews, especially with regard to a future-oriented thinking. Employing the Perceived Hope Scale, the Dispositional Hope Scale, the Assumptive Worldviews, and several variables of subjective and psychological well-being, we investigate the levels and predictors of hope in six distinct samples of the Hope Barometer 2017 (N = 6548). Our findings support the notion of hope as a multidimensional phenomenon with certain universal features across cultures while recognizing that people in different cultures experience hope based on specific worldviews, independently from the nation's economic wealth.

A. M. Krafft (✉)
Institute of Systemic Management and Public Governance, University of St. Gallen, St. Gallen, Switzerland
e-mail: andreas.krafft@unisg.ch

T. Guse
Department of Psychology, University of Pretoria, Pretoria, South Africa

E. Kasprzak
Department of Work and Organisational Psychology, Institute of Psychology, Kazimierz Wielki University of Bydgoszcz, Bydgoszcz, Poland

D. Redlich-Amirav
Sackler Faculty of Medicine, Tel Aviv University, Tel Aviv-Yafo, Israel

P. Stecz
Department of Clinical Psychology and Psychopathology, Institute of Psychology, University of Łódź, Łódź, Poland

A. M. Krafft et al. (eds.), *Hope across cultures*, Cross-Cultural Advancements in Positive Psychology 14, https://doi.org/10.1007/978-3-031-24412-4_5

5.1 Introduction

The orthodox conceptualization of hope in philosophy maintains that the phenomenon of hope is constituted by a wish or desire for some good and the belief in the possibility of its realization. According to current philosophical debates, these two aspects seem to be necessary but not sufficient elements of hope (Milona, 2020). The model developed in Chap. 2 is based on this standard account and incorporates additional elements coming from current philosophical and psychological studies (Bovens, 1999; Meirav, 2009; Milona, 2019; Krafft & Walker, 2018a, 2018b; Scioli & Biller, 2009). Hope is therefore composed by a wish or desire for a valuable good or goal, the belief that its realization is possible, the awareness of difficulties, obstacles and setbacks and the trust in our own and other resources that helps us to overcome such obstacles and nourishes our willpower.

This chapter is dedicated to exploring the second domain of this hope concept, which is the role basic beliefs play in sustaining and fostering hope. According to philosophical considerations that are supported by empirical evidence from psychological studies, hope is distinct from optimism in the sense that the hoping person believes in an even small possibility of attaining a certain wish, whereas to be optimistic, the outcome has to be retained as rather or highly probable (Bruininks & Malle, 2005; Krafft et al., 2021; Miceli & Castelfranchi, 2010; Scioli et al., 1997). Fundamentally, whereas future expectations, on which the concepts of dispositional hope (Snyder, 2002) and optimism (Scheier et al., 2001) are based, are grounded on rational considerations, hope is basically related to personal beliefs (Leung et al., 2009). In a broader sense, hope is anchored in the belief that the future will provide new possibilities and current situations can (but not necessarily will) change for the better.

The belief in the possibility (or impossibility) of a desired outcome is largely of subjective nature. One hundred years ago, most people would have considered the idea of traveling to the moon as ridiculous. In past epochs, the abolishment of slavery, the equality of rights for men and women or the marriage of homosexual couples were rendered unthinkable. However, over time certain people began to believe that change is possible, that things previously considered to be impossible can be achieved. Based on this belief, they engaged themselves to fulfill their visions. Today, many of these ideas are a self-evident reality in many countries.

We are confronted daily with questions such as when, how and why do people believe in the even slight possibility of a certain outcome? For example: Why does someone believe in the possibility of recovering from a chronic illness? When does a person believe in the possibility of getting a new job during an economic crisis at the age of 60? How do parents believe that their child will successfully complete high school, despite current troubles during adolescence? The answers to these and similar questions will depend not only on objective facts but also on individual and collective beliefs and worldviews, something we will explore in the following sections.

Several researchers in psychology have incorporated personal and cultural beliefs in the study of hope (see Averill et al., 1990; Averill & Sundararajan, 2005; Scioli & Biller, 2009; Tennen et al., 2002). These authors maintained that the nature of hope must be understood in the context of the cultures in which the term is embedded. Further, they emphasized a variety of dimensions and experiences such as social trust, positive emotions, and spiritual faith, above cognition, self-mastery, and personal control. In our study, we would like to follow and further develop this tradition by investigating in more detail the role of basic beliefs and cultural characteristics in the experience of hope.

5.2 Theoretical Background

5.2.1 Basic Beliefs and the Role and Nature of Worldviews

All human beings have basic beliefs, assumptions and attitudes that guide their perceptions about the world and themselves as well as their behavior (Allport, 1955). These fundamental beliefs and assumptions tend to be coherently structured in belief systems, narratives, and attitudes towards life, which are condensed in individual and collective worldviews. Kant was one of the first philosophers who used the term "worldview" (in German "Weltanschauung") to describe a person's broad outlook to the world (Kant, 1790/1987 in Nilsson, 2013). More than 100 years later, two other German Philosophers, Wilhelm Dilthey (1890/1957) and Karl Jaspers (1919), formulated a comprehensive theory of the nature, purpose, and development of worldviews as a fundamental philosophy of life.

According to Dilthey (1890/1957), worldviews are the attempt to explain "the riddle of life". The paradox of worldviews is that they are anchored in daily experiences and at the same time focus on things that transcend the observable world. Worldviews, as a set of basic beliefs, assumptions, and values, are especially relevant when one is confronted with the unknown, where uncertainties and inconsistencies arise, where we feel an urge to explain the inexplicable. As soon as our daily knowledge and understanding encounters limits, higher forms of understanding develop. In a world full of uncertainties and inconsistencies, we develop theories why things are the way they are. We form a picture of reality as we experience and imagine it. In order to understand the sometimes incomprehensible, we think about reasons and create an explanation of the nature of the world and ourselves (Koltko-Rivera, 2004).

Over the past decades, the topic of worldviews, basic beliefs and assumptions has attracted the attention of scientists and researchers in several areas of psychology (Nilsson, 2013; Janoff-Bulman, 1992; Koltko-Rivera, 2004; Ibrahim, 1984, 1985, 2003; Clifton et al., 2019). Although there is still no unifying psychological theory of worldviews and basic beliefs, all dedicated authors agree on the fundamental role of these phenomena in our psychological processes. Worldviews are formed by basic believes and assumptions about the world and the social environment that are intimately connected to cognition, emotions, and behavior (Koltko-Rivera, 2004).

Worldviews are also consistent narratives that connect the past, the present and the future in a coherent way. The definition of Koltko-Rivera is especially suitable to understand the role of worldviews in studying future expectations and hope:

> *A worldview is a way of describing the universe and life within it, both in terms of what is and what ought to be. A given worldview is a set of beliefs that includes limiting statements and assumptions regarding what exists and what does not (either in actuality, or in principle), what objects or experiences are good or bad, and what objectives, behaviors, and relationships are desirable or undesirable. A worldview defines what can be known or done in the world, and how it can be known or done. In addition to defining what goals can be sought in life, a worldview defines what goals should be pursued. Worldviews include assumptions that may be unproven, and even unprovable, but these assumptions are superordinate, in that they provide the epistemic and ontological foundations for other beliefs within a belief system.* (Koltko-Rivera, 2004, p. 4).

5.2.2 Worldviews, the Self, and Hope for the Future

Dilthey's (1890/1957) pioneering and systematic philosophy of worldviews has the purpose to explain the enigma of life itself. The possession of worldviews is a condition underlying human life. The meaning and nature of life can only be grasped through our worldviews that give answers to questions such as: Who am I? Why do I exist? What am I supposed to do in this world? The structural elements of worldviews are concordant with the three elements of the human experience, i.e., cognition, emotion and will. The cognitive picture of the world and oneself is laden with affective value. Objects and experiences are perceived as friendly or harmful and valued as worthy or unworthy. At the meta-level, the person develops the supreme concept of the highest good and value of life and defines the ideal of how to live one's personal life. This results in a comprehensive life plan including personal and social goals, principles, and norms of action to shape one's future (Aerts et al., 1994).

Therefore, from a psychological perspective, worldviews are not only a set of basic beliefs and assumptions that describe reality or lenses with which the individual looks at the world. Worldviews are much more than that. They are embedded in the individual's psychological structure and become an integral part of his/her personality in terms of cognition, volition, affect, and behavior (Nilsson, 2014). Worldviews not only define how we see the world but also who we are, how we feel, think and act. Our fundamental perspective on life, of how we conceive the world and ourselves, the meaning and the reality of life, all our existence is rooted in our worldviews (Ibrahim & Heuer, 2016).

Fundamental assumptions about the world and ourselves have an impact on the way a person anticipates future events (Kelly, 1955). People's thoughts, emotions and judgements are strongly influenced by their beliefs about what will or can happen. Since different people can have different worldviews, they will also differ from each other in the way they assess present and future reality (Koltko-Rivera,

2004). Beck (1974), for example, demonstrated how beliefs about the self (e.g., "I'm worthless"), the self's future (e.g., "My future seems dark."), and the external environment create a sense of hopelessness that plays a fundamental role in the emergence of depression.

Janoff-Bulman (1992) developed a model of generalized fundamental assumptions about the nature and meaningfulness of the world and oneself as a requirement for optimal human functioning. Reverting to Erikson's first developmental stage in early childhood, she argued that the child's view of self, world, and the connection between both originates in early preverbal interactions with the caregivers. For Erikson (1998), hope is the first basic virtue emerging from the positive development in the conflict between anxiety and trust, which leaves a lasting tendency in the child to believe in fulfilling his/her existential needs despite the distress and anger associated with them. This basic trust and hope become part of human identity, a basic sense of order and consistency between past, present, and future, maintained throughout life. Based on such experiences, the infant continues to establish positive expectations about the world, the nature of other people, of the own self, and the future.

These fundamental assumptions of hope and trust are the basis for personal growth and development. Janoff-Bulman refers to an episode in William James' life, where hope and confidence in himself were the keys to overcome fear and mistrust:

> *In this case (and it is one of an immense class) the part of wisdom clearly is to believe what one desires... There are then cases when faith creates its own verification. Believe, and you shall be right, for you shall save yourself; doubt, and you shall be right, for you shall perish. The only difference is that to believe is greatly to your advantage.* (James, 1962, cited in Janoff-Bulman, 1992, p. 24).

5.2.3 Types of Worldviews

Authors in many disciplines such as philosophy, anthropology and psychology have identified primal basic beliefs and fundamental assumptions that converge in certain typical worldviews. For example, Rokeach (1968) distinguished between existential beliefs (things are true or false), evaluative beliefs (the judgement of good or bad), and prescriptive beliefs (states, goals or actions that are considered desirable or undesirable). One basic belief concerns the quality and basic character of human nature as good or evil (Wrightsman, 1962). In daily life, people tend to generalize from their experiences and believe in the goodness and kindness of people, or, alternatively, that people are essentially self-centered and selfish. Those who believe in altruism believe that people sincerely care and will help others in need and give them hope. Another belief is aligned with the self-concept and relationships with other people. Triandis (1995) highlights the importance of the individualist-collectivist orientations in establishing the self-concept, personal goals, and preferred actions.

Some beliefs are related to the future consequences of current actions. A widely held belief is that of a just (or unjust) world, i.e., the belief that people usually get what they deserve (e.g., life blesses good people and punishes the bad) (Lerner, 1980). An alternative assumption is that of randomness, meaning that things happen by chance without any logic or meaning. Another basic belief is related to what Rotter (1966) denominated locus of control: the individual's perception of the underlying main causes of events in life. A person-centered worldview will rely on the agency, ability, and efforts of the individual to master life challenges. The external locus of control is the belief in external forces not only in terms of powerful others but also in terms of luck, fate, destiny, etc.

One of the most fundamental attitudes or moods of life, as Dilthey (1890/1957) called them, is that of optimism and pessimism (Ibrahim & Heuer, 2016). The optimistic worldview is based on the assumption that more positive than negative things will happen to oneself (Carver & Scheier, 2014). This belief nurtures a sense of confidence and fosters a positive expectation about the future. The opposite is the pessimistic worldview, where one expects more negative than positive things to happen in one's life. People with a pessimistic basic attitude not only perceive the world as threatening but also tend to create a negative self-evaluation of themselves (Ibrahim, 1993).

Further types of basic beliefs are related to a religious or spiritual vs. a materialistic worldview. Huber and Huber (2012) as well as Zinnbauer and Pargament (2005), among others, have studied how the centrality of religious/spiritual beliefs and experiences affect the individual's attitudes, cognitions, affects, and behaviors. For example, religious and spiritual beliefs can consider the world and the universe to be an interconnected unity guided by a Divine Being or consciousness with which people on earth should live in harmony. In this case, hope is directed to something greater than oneself or the material world, transcending the physical reality, both in terms of what religious people ultimately hope for (e.g., the communion with the Divine) and the sources of their hope (e.g., the loving kindness of an almighty Divine Power). Despite their basic transcendent character, these kinds of beliefs have a strong impact on the expectations, decisions and behaviors of people in the here and now.

5.2.4 Worldviews and Culture

Every person experiences life differently, and at the same time, there are certain aspects of life grounded in habits, traditions, and norms that are common to society and give people an inherent psychic order or epistemic certainty. For Dilthey (1890/1957), worldviews always emerge within a historical and cultural context. From a social constructivist perspective, worldviews are culturally transmitted in order to give a sense of coherence to people's experiences (Berger & Luckmann, 1966). Through socialization within a socio-historical and family context, shared worldviews transmit a sense of meaning, stability, and security to its members. Many researchers have studied the cultural differences in cognition, values and basic beliefs and have demonstrated that culture has a great impact on cognition, emotions and behavior (Lonner & Adamopoulos, 1997; Hong et al., 2000).

Culture has been defined as a "shared set of beliefs, attitudes, norms, values, and behaviors organized around a central theme and found among speakers of one language, in one time period, and in one geographic region." (Triandis, 1997, p. 443). People of the same culture perceive and judge things and act in a similar way. Every culture includes a certain approach to the world and to life. This means that cultural beliefs about how things are and how they should be are constituent of the individual's perception and volition (Miller, 1999). Therefore, worldviews can be seen as socially shared meaning and belief systems that can originate from religions, philosophies, scientific paradigms, political ideologies, and a certain "Zeitgeist" or spirit of a community. Through the influence of culture, many assumptions and beliefs are taken for granted without conscious deliberation (Nilsson, 2013).

Some authors even talk about a collective or cultural mentality, mood or identity that combine the past, the present and the future, generating strong and long-lasting basic attitudes toward individual and social realities such as family, happiness, work, the economy etc. (Dana, 1993; Ibrahim & Heuer, 2016). Therefore, basic beliefs combine the way in which reality is interpreted with a sense of the possible. The meaning of the current reality and the sense of future possibilities are closely intertwined. For Dilthey (1890/1957), our task is to open up our spaces of experience as well as our horizons of future possibilities in order to broaden our worldviews and foster personal and social development and growth.

It is important to remark that cultural identities are seldom completely homogeneous and free of inner tensions. Within a dominant culture, a variety of ethnic, religious, sexual, educational, professional, social and regional subcultures can emerge. These subcultures can share a set of basic assumptions and beliefs but also develop alternative perspectives, attitudes, values, and goals that can even contradict the dominant worldviews (Ibrahim et al., 2001). Thanks to these processes, cultures and worldviews are not rigid but in continuous evolution. New life experiences, ideas, and wishes contribute from time to time to an inner renewal of social and personal beliefs and worldviews (Naugle, 2002).

5.2.5 *Basic Beliefs and Science*

Both the everyday experiences and expectations of laypersons as well as philosophical and scientific theories and concepts with their own views on reality and their preferred methods are driven by basic assumptions, beliefs, and worldviews (Dilthey, 1890/1957). Answers to the question about the nature and role of human agency, personality, virtues, free will etc., are embedded in dominant and alternative worldviews. The variety of philosophical systems and psychological disciplines that intend to find the best explanation for human motives and behavior is always a product of a socio-historical context of dominant beliefs, values, and interests.

This is also the case for all disciplines studying the phenomenon of hope from so many different angles, such as the religious, the cognitive, the philosophical, the cultural and the affective among others (Eliott, 2005). Since hope is not a material good or objective fact but an existential inner reality expressed by experiences, feelings, emotions, thoughts, beliefs, wishes, and values, no single theory could claim universal validity to describe such a complex phenomenon. The goal should be to expand our view by studying hope from different angles and with different lenses and to try to integrate as much as possible a variety of (sometimes contradicting) ideas and approaches.

To do so, we should overcome the dualistic either-or-thinking and replace it by a both-and-attitude, with which we can accept and integrate different worldviews into a larger framework. This does not mean that, for practical reasons, we should not focus on one or the other aspect of hope, for example, in order to design effective interventions for specific settings and purposes. However, if the aim is to understand hope in its different facets and contexts, we should elaborate a much more open and comprehensive epistemological, ontological and methodological research program, at the same time acknowledging that every approach will always have its strengths and limitations.

5.2.6 Assessing Worldviews and Basic Assumptions

Janoff-Bulman (1992) investigated how people react to existential life experiences and developed a theory and research instrument to understand better and evaluate implicit basic assumptions. In her view, the psychological mechanisms that occur in extreme situations can tell us a lot about the psychology of worldviews in our daily life. In our opinion, this is particularly true for the study of hope since hope emerges especially in critical life situations. Janoff-Bulman postulated that we usually operate on largely taken for granted fundamental assumptions about the external world and ourselves. These basic assumptions are theories and working models that guide our thoughts, emotions, and behaviors, especially in anticipating or expecting what will happen in the future. She proposed that abstract beliefs belonging to three primary categories are at the core of our basic assumptions: The benevolence of the external world, our self-worth, and the meaningful relationship between them.

The first assumption is that of the belief in the *benevolence of the world*. In general terms, people believe that good things are prevalent over negative events. Most of us believe that the world is a good place to live and that people are basically kind, helpful, and caring. The more positive the assumptions regarding the external world are, the lower is the experience of distress and the higher that of subjective well-being (Janoff-Bulman, 1992; Joseph & Linley, 2005).

The second category of basic assumptions is related to the *meaningfulness of the world*. We usually tend to believe that what happens to us and to other people makes sense. Especially in Western cultures, people used to believe in the moral principle of justice and the possibility of controlling desired outcomes. For example, whereas good people will engage in good actions and therefore experience good things, bad people who harm others will merit bad things occurring to them. This means that what happens in the world and to ourselves can be influenced by our own behavior. The belief in justice and control creates a sense of order and coherence. The opposite belief is that of chance. If events occur at random, they will lack any meaning and instill a sense of helplessness since there is nothing one can do to promote or avoid them.

The third fundamental assumption is that of *self-worth*, which comprises three dimensions. The first dimension involves a global evaluation of the self. Most people perceive themselves as good, decent, and therefore worthy individuals with sound self-esteem. The second dimension refers to the appropriateness and effectiveness of one's actions. In general, we see ourselves engaging in responsible and competent actions and lastly being in control of our life. The third belief is that of luck or misfortune. Sometimes we are not able to control what happens to us. Despite this insufficient control, we can somehow feel protected from misfortune (or not).

Following the qualities of basic beliefs as culturally laden phenomena, we assume that the historical and cultural context may have an impact on the categories and dimensions of basic assumptions and that there could be different associations with the perception of hope. In individualistic cultures, people seem to be rather optimistic about their own lives but far less optimistic about the political and social environment (Janoff-Bulman, 1992). Furthermore, many Western cultures emphasize the principles of personal responsibility, control, and merit. In other cultures, a meaningful world is one governed by collective goals or religious beliefs. In such cultures, control does not rest on the individual but on the community or on a benevolent and almighty Deity responsible for rewarding or punishing people on earth. The role of the family, the characteristics of the education system, and the quality of social practices can have a huge impact on people's basic assumptions as well as on the quality and the sources of hope.

5.3 The Present Study

5.3.1 Objectives

The main purpose of this study is to investigate the role of basic beliefs and assumptions in connection to the perception of hope in different cultures. For this purpose, we employ six national samples of the Hope Barometer collected in November 2017 and compare the levels and relationships of hope with basic assumptions about the world and oneself. One central research question is whether levels of hope in different countries are related to similar or different fundamental assumptions about the world and oneself beyond subjective and psychological well-being. With this, we intend to identify the main pillars and the nomological network of hope finding similarities and differences between the countries. Broadly, we would be able to identify possible universal features of hope as well as culture-specific characteristics.

5.3.2 *Participants*

We analyzed six selected sub-samples of the Hope Barometer collected in November 2017 with participants from the following countries and regions: German-speaking Switzerland (N = 3306), French-speaking Switzerland (N = 1308), Germany (N = 840), South Africa (N = 427), Israel (N = 477), and Poland (N = 190). The questionnaires were provided in German (Switzerland and Germany), French (Switzerland), English (South Africa), Hebrew (Israel), and Polish (Poland). Appendix 5.1 displays the demographic structure of the samples by gender, age, marital status, education, main activity, professional status, and religion. These countries were selected taking into account the best possible comparability between samples. The samples included participants from a wide age range, with the youngest participants in Israel and South Africa and the oldest in Germany. The age structure reflects the existing median age of the analyzed countries in a satisfactory way (Switzerland $MED_{age} = 43$, Germany $MED_{age} = 48$, South Africa $MED_{age} = 28$, Israel $MED_{age} = 31$, Poland $MED_{age} = 42$) (World Data retrieved from the Internet 22.12.2021).

In terms of gender, the total sample had a good distribution of 43.1% men and 56.9% women. The Israeli and the South African samples had a pronounced bias towards female participants. In order to improve the comparability among countries, therefore, we weighted all cases by gender.

The participants varied in terms of additional demographic characteristics. In comparison to the other countries, Germany and Poland included slightly more married people, and the Israeli sample somewhat more single participants. In terms of education, it was difficult to find a common structure due to the very different national education systems. Switzerland and Germany are well known for their unique dual vocational training system, which is barely known in other countries. Consequently, the Swiss and German samples include a larger number of participants with vocational training, whereas the other countries had more participants with tertiary and university education. Furthermore, the Israeli and the South African samples comprised (due to the age structure) a larger number of people in education or training.

There were noteworthy differences regarding religious denomination. Poland had the largest number of Catholic participants, while Germany had the largest, and South Africa had the lowest number of atheists or agnostics. In Israel, one third of the participants denominated themselves as Jewish, roughly 20% as spiritual persons without religion, about 23% as atheists/agnostics, and 20% as something different. In South Africa, a majority (more than one third) belonged to a Christian church other than the traditional Catholic and Protestant, and one-fifth declared to be spiritual but not to belong to an institutionalized religion. A peculiarity of South Africa is its heterogeneity in terms of ethnic groups. From the 427 participants in our survey, 247 (57.8%) were White, 145 (34.0%) Black, 20 (4.7%) Indian, and 9 (2.1%) colored (a South African census category for persons of mixed race).

Even though the samples are not strictly representative of the general population (which will be one of the limitations of our study), they comprise a satisfactory variety of people with different demographic backgrounds. The heterogeneity of the samples reflects the different socio-demographic structures of the individual countries and should be taken into account when interpreting results.

5.3.3 *Procedure and Instruments*

Data collection was performed through the annual online survey of the Hope Barometer in November 2017. Participants were recruited through newspapers via online advertisement, social media and e-mails. No incentives were offered. The inclusion criterion was a minimum age of 18. We used four categories of instruments to measure (1) general hope, (2) subjective well-being, (3) psychological well-being, and (4) basic beliefs about the world and oneself.

5.3.3.1 Instruments to Measure Hope

Perceived Hope Scale

To measure the general level of hope we used the Perceived Hope Scale (PHS) developed by Krafft et al. (2019, 2021). The PHS was developed as a self-rating instrument to avoid any cultural bias regarding the nature and the quality of hope. Therefore, the PHS does not measure future expectations of goal attainment, nor different dimensions of hope, but the level and experience of hope as directly perceived by people, without enquiring about their roots and sources. The PHS is a unidimensional measure including six positively worded items to be rated on a 6-point Likert scale ranging from 0 (strongly disagree) to 5 (strongly agree). The six items cover the general level of hope (e.g., "I feel hopeful"), the belief in the fulfillment of one's hopes, whether hope outweighs anxiety and improves the quality of one's life and if one can remain hopeful even in difficult times. In the current study the six items achieved a high internal consistency in all samples with Cronbach alpha values between $\alpha = .89$ and $\alpha = .91$.

To assess the self-centered and cognitive dimension of hope, we included the two sub-scales of agency and pathways proposed by Snyder et al. (1991).

Agency

Agency refers to the willpower and motivation that is needed to achieve one's goals. Snyder (2000) also speaks of purposeful mental energy and determination. It is the personal expectation that one can effectively achieve the things that seem important to oneself. The Agency sub-scale consists of four items scored on a 6-point scale from 0 (strongly disagree) to 5 (strongly agree). In our samples, Cronbach's alpha reliability coefficients ranged between $\alpha = 0.80$ and $\alpha = 0.86$.

Pathways

Pathways thinking is the perception and belief regarding one's own abilities to find possible ways to achieve goals, especially when obstacles and difficulties occur on the way to the goal. It involves an attitude of self-confidence in the sense of "I will find a way out of this problem and reach my goal". The four items are scored on a 6-point scale from 0 (strongly disagree) to 5 (strongly agree). Internal consistency coefficients ranged between $\alpha = 0.82$ and $\alpha = 87$.

5.3.3.2 Instruments to Measure Subjective Well-being

Subjective well-being comprises a cognitive and an emotional dimension.

Life-Satisfaction Scale

The Satisfaction with Life Scale (SLS) assesses the global level of satisfaction with one's own life, defined as the assessment of life circumstances in comparison to one's expectations (Diener et al., 1985). It assesses the cognitive dimension of subjective well-being. The SLS consists of 5 items scored on a 7-point scale from 1 (strongly disagree) to 7 (strongly agree). Cronbach alpha values in our study ranged between $\alpha = 0.87$ and $\alpha = 0.92$.

Scale for Positive and Negative Emotions (SPANE)

To measure positive and negative emotions we administered the 12 items scale designed by Diener et al. (2010). The participants were asked to think about what they have been doing and experiencing during the past 4 weeks and to score six positive and six negative feelings on a 5-point scale from 1 (very rarely or never) to 5 (very often or always). The internal consistency ranged from $\alpha = 0.90$ to $\alpha = 0.95$ for positive emotions and from $\alpha = 0.86$ to $\alpha = 0.90$ for negative emotions.

5.3.3.3 Instruments to Measure Psychological Well-being

To measure psychological well-being we used three variables assessing meaning in life, altruism (helping others) and harmony in life.

Meaning in Life

One central domain of psychological well-being is determined by the experience that one's life has meaning and purpose. We measured this dimension with the presence of meaning in life sub-scale of the Meaning in Life Questionnaire (Steger et al., 2006). The items were scored on a 7-point Likert scale from 1 (strongly disagree) to 7 (strongly agree) and showed a very good internal consistency between $\alpha = 0.85$ and $\alpha = 0.91$.

Helping Others

Helping others is a pro-social attitude and behavior that positively correlates with empathy, social responsibility and altruism, and negatively correlates with selfishness. We measured this attitude with a short-form of the Helping Attitude Scale (Nickell, 1998), employing 7 items with a 5-point scale from 1 to 5. Cronbach alpha reliability was also high in all samples, ranging between $\alpha = 0.87$ and $\alpha = 0.91$.

Harmony in Life

Kjell et al. (2016) have recently developed the Harmony in Life Scale to measure psychological experiences of inner balance, peace of mind, calm, and unity. The authors highlight the concept of harmony in life as being related to a holistic worldview that incorporates a more balanced and flexible approach to personal well being (e.g., "Most aspects of my life are in balance"). The five items are scored on a 7-point scale from 1 (strongly disagree) to 7 (strongly agree) and displayed good internal reliability of between $\alpha = 0.88$ and $\alpha = 0.93$.

5.3.3.4 Instruments to Measure Basic Beliefs and Assumptions about Oneself and the World

The *World Assumptions Scale* (WAS) of Janoff-Bulman (1989) consists of 32 items describing basic assumptions about the world and oneself. According to the theory, there are three basic categories and eight dimensions of such assumptions: (1) assumptions about the goodness of the world and of people (which are merged into one variable); (2) assumptions about the meaningfulness of what is happening in this world with the dimensions justice, controllability and randomness; and (3) assumptions about oneself including self-worth, self-control, and luck. Respondents are asked to respond to them on a 6-point Likert scale from 0 (strongly disagree) to 5 (strongly agree). The scale includes seven sub-scales:

Benevolence. The benevolence of the world and of people addresses the belief that the world is a good place and that most people are basically good, friendly, and caring. Janoff-Bulman (1992) and other researchers (Elklit et al., 2007) recognized that the eight items load on one single factor, which was also the case in our samples. Cronbach's alpha internal reliability of the eight items ranged from $\alpha = 0.83$ to $\alpha = 0.87$.

Justice. The first dimension of a meaningful world is the belief in an implicit justice on earth. People who do good will also receive something good in return. People who do bad things will have to bear the consequences of their actions. The internal reliability coefficients of the four items ranged from $\alpha = 0.70$ to $\alpha = 0.78$.

Controllability. One can be more or less convinced of the controllability or manageability of events. Through their own behavior, people can "control" the world and the events in it if they do the right things. Alpha coefficients of the four items ranged from $\alpha = 0.74$ to $\alpha = 0.76$.

Randomness. The third assumption regarding a sense of meaningfulness concerns the degree of randomness or coincidence with which certain things seem to happen. When events happen purely by chance, one will feel at the mercy of them and there will hardly be anything that can be done for or against them. The internal consistency displayed by the four items was at an acceptable level from $\alpha = 0.65$ to $\alpha = 0.73$.

Self-worth. The first assumption about oneself concerns one's own self-worth or self-esteem, which is the extent to which people perceive themselves as good, lovable and decent individuals, or on the contrary as unworthy, bad and guilty. In our study, alpha coefficients for the four items ranged between $\alpha = 0.74$ and $\alpha = 0.79$.

Self-control. The second belief about oneself is the concept of self-control, defined as the perception that the person is doing the right things in life and that he or she is in control of his/her life. It addresses the degree to which one views oneself as engaging in right behaviors to control outcomes. The internal consistency of the four items was at an acceptable level between $\alpha = 0.64$ and $\alpha = 0.71$.

Luck. The third basic assumption regarding oneself refers to the perception that one has good or bad luck in life. This entails the belief that one is somehow protected from negative forces from the outside world. The four items of this subscale reached good reliability coefficients from $\alpha = 0.79$ to $\alpha = 0.87$.

Religiosity. Not covered by the WAS but nonetheless an important dimension of basic beliefs is the centrality of religiosity in one's life. To measure it, we employed the short-form of the Santa Clara Strength of Religious Faith Questionnaire (SCSRFQ) (Plante & Boccaccini, 1997; Storch et al., 2004). Individuals with strong religious faith pray and go to church regularly, find meaning and purpose and take decisions guided by their faith, and enjoy being with others who share their faith (Plante & Boccaccini, 1997). The five items to be scored on a 4-point scale (1 to 4) revealed an excellent internal consistency between $\alpha = 0.90$ and $\alpha = 0.94$.

5.3.4 Data Analysis

For the statistical analyses, we used IBM SPSS and AMOS version 27.0. In order to be able to compare mean values between countries, it is advisable to test the invariance of the employed measure between groups. Therefore, by means of multi-group CFA we tested group invariance between all samples for the six items of the Perceived Hope Scale, the main construct and instrument used to assess the general level of hope. Data analyses were then performed in three steps:

Step 1: Firstly, mean values (and standard deviations) were calculated for perceived hope and all well-being and basic assumption variables. We then compared data between samples using univariate and multivariate analysis of variance (ANOVA). To improve the comparability of the samples, we weighted the cases by gender.

Step 2: Through partial bivariate correlations we analyzed the relationships between the well-being variables, the dimensions of basic beliefs, and perceived hope (after controlling for demographic variables) and compared selected results between samples via correlation comparisons (Steiger, 1980).

Step 3: Afterwards we performed multiple regressions to predict perceived hope. Following the theoretical considerations of worldviews, we expected that basic assumptions and beliefs about the world and oneself will constitute an additional set of predictors resulting in higher R^2 values of explained variance in perceived hope, but that the effects could vary between countries. This could be the case beyond demographic variables (gender, age, marital status, education, main activity and professional status), subjective well-being, and psychological well-being. Therefore, we compared the effects of predictive power and explained variance and identified similarities and differences between samples.

5.3.5 Results

5.3.5.1 Group Invariance of the PHS

In order to be able to compare mean values of the PHS and relate them to other variables, we tested invariance using all six national samples. Table 5.1 exhibits the results of the multi-group CFA including the fit indices for the general sample followed by the four models to test different types of invariance. The overall fit indices for the total sample revealed that the one-factor model achieved a good

Table 5.1 Multi-group CFA and analysis of group invariance for the perceived hope scale

	X^2	*df*	CFI	TLI	RMSEA	SRMR
Total sample (N = 6548)	211.34	9	0.991	0.985	0.059	0.017
Country/sample invariance						
Configurational invariance (equal form)	1131.00	126	0.954	0.967	0.035	0.029
Metric invariance (equal loadings)	1151.30	131	0.954	0.968	0.035	0.028
Scalar invariance (equal intercepts)	1534.85	137	0.936	0.958	0.039	0.028
Strict invariance (equal residuals)	1799.04	144	0.925	0.953	0.042	0.037

Note: *CFA* Confirmatory Factor Analysis, *CFI* Comparative fit index, *TLI* Tucker-Lewis index, *RMSEA* Root mean square error of approximation, *SRMR* Standardized root mean residual

model fit (CFI and TLI > 0.95, RMSEA and SRMR < 0.08) (Hu & Bentler, 1999). The equal form used as baseline model also provided a good fit to the data, suggesting reasonable support for configurational invariance across the groups. Likewise, all indices comparing the further models with the baseline model were under the threshold values recommended by the literature (Chen, 2007, CFI and TLI > −0.01, RMSEA and SRMR < 0.015) with the exception of the CFI concerning scalar invariance (ΔCFI = −0.018) (Marsh, 1994). This means that the PHS revealed acceptable (partial metric) to strong invariance and that it is possible to compare the PHS scores between the national samples. The general hope construct measured with the PHS seemed to be conceptualized in the same way across cultures and was suitable to be examined in relationship to other constructs.

Step 1: Descriptive Statistics and Mean Value Comparisons

We continued our analysis by calculating mean values and standard deviations for perceived hope and all well-being and worldview variables (weighted by gender) and compared the values between samples. The statistics in Table 5.2 show similarities and significant differences between samples and first noteworthy findings. We firstly focused our attention on the levels of perceived hope. All values were above the center of the scale (M > 2.5) and there were significant differences between all countries except between the French Swiss and Poland. South Africa had the highest level of perceived hope, followed by Israel, the German Swiss, Germany, and finally Poland and the French speaking Swiss.

Compared to the other samples, South Africa revealed the highest levels of perceived hope, positive emotions, meaning in life, harmony in life, agency, pathways, self-control and religiosity ($p < 0.01$), the second highest in life-satisfaction, altruism, benevolence and controllability, and the lowest levels of negative emotions (together with Israel) and randomness (together with Poland) ($p < 0.01$).

On the other hand, the sample from French speaking Switzerland showed the lowest levels of perceived hope, meaning in life, altruism, pathways, benevolence, justice, luck, and religiosity and at the same time the highest level of self-worth ($p < 0.01$). This is remarkable, since according to the statistics of the World Bank,

Table 5.2 Mean values, standard deviations and analysis of variance by sample

	German Swiss		French Swiss		Germany		South Africa		Israel		Poland		Anova	
	M	SD	M	SD	M	SD	M	SD	M	SD	M	SD	F	Sig.
Perceived Hope	3.42	0.97	2.96	1.16	3.23	1.06	3.76	0.87	3.61	0.91	3.09	1.21	104.93	0.000
Subjective Well-being														
Life-satisfaction	4.94	1.36	4.14	1.50	4.63	1.42	4.90	1.31	4.83	1.21	3.90	1.38	121.21	0.000
Positive emotions	3.72	0.76	3.56	0.84	3.52	0.80	3.80	0.72	3.65	0.67	3.43	0.85	32.58	0.000
Negative emotions	2.70	0.85	2.78	0.88	2.76	0.89	2.57	0.79	2.64	0.73	2.75	0.95	8.63	0.000
Psychological Well-being														
Meaning	4.95	1.38	4.55	1.47	4.88	1.36	5.53	1.26	4.98	1.42	4.89	1.40	56.43	0.000
Helping others	4.12	0.68	3.91	0.74	4.03	0.72	4.35	0.56	4.44	0.48	4.09	0.73	98.33	0.000
Harmony in life	4.91	1.22	4.70	1.40	4.75	1.29	5.21	1.20	4.89	1.16	4.74	1.36	21.03	0.000
Goal orientation and self-confidence														
Agency	3.59	0.90	3.12	1.07	3.54	0.94	3.98	0.78	3.83	0.79	3.22	1.09	143.94	0.000
Pathways	3.76	0.85	3.33	1.07	3.71	0.90	3.99	0.80	3.74	0.82	3.81	0.91	88.13	0.000
Basic assumptions														
Benevolence	2.85	0.89	2.29	0.93	2.63	0.95	3.15	0.82	3.28	0.81	2.79	0.93	213.54	0.000
Justice	2.20	1.04	1.61	1.02	2.10	1.01	2.13	0.98	1.93	0.99	2.24	0.93	102.61	0.000
Controllability	2.42	0.94	2.18	0.98	2.46	0.96	2.51	0.96	2.20	0.88	2.73	0.94	38.75	0.000
Randomness	2.69	0.96	2.51	1.04	2.88	0.90	2.53	0.97	2.80	0.91	2.61	0.98	29.41	0.000
Self-worth	3.48	0.99	3.76	1.01	3.45	1.05	3.63	0.99	3.66	0.92	3.05	1.05	44.05	0.000
Self-control	2.68	0.78	2.97	0.86	2.86	0.78	3.49	0.71	3.43	0.73	3.06	0.86	247.06	0.000
Luck	3.24	0.98	2.22	1.20	2.93	1.02	3.16	0.99	3.59	0.86	2.75	1.04	354.82	0.000
Religiosity	1.71	0.82	1.67	0.89	1.61	0.78	2.68	0.98	1.87	0.86	2.08	0.83	196.90	0.000

Switzerland is the country in our study with the highest GDP per capita (U$S 87,100.-) and South Africa that with the lowest (U$S 5600.-). Furthermore, Switzerland has a very stable political system and social structure, while South Africa struggles with ethnic, social, and political tensions (including economic and social injustice, violence, etc.).

What additionally stands out is the fact, that despite the same national political and economic context and only little structural differences, the results of German and French Switzerland were significantly (and in some domains markedly) distinct in almost all evaluated dimensions. Notably, the French-speaking Swiss showed higher levels of self-worth and self-control and significantly worse results in all other variables, especially in luck, benevolence, and life satisfaction. Furthermore, the German-Swiss sample showed no significant difference with German participants regarding agency, pathways, negative emotions, meaning in life, controllability, and self-worth, but significantly higher levels of perceived hope, life satisfaction, positive emotions, altruism, harmony in life, benevolence, justice, luck, and religiosity ($p < 0.01$). Germans, on the other hand, had significantly higher levels of self-control and randomness.

Other interesting findings result from comparing South Africa and Israel, the two countries with the highest levels of perceived hope. No significant differences between both countries emerged in life satisfaction, negative emotions, self-worth, and self-control. Whereas South Africans had significantly higher levels of perceived hope, agency, pathways, positive feelings, meaning in life, harmony, justice, controllability, and especially religiosity, the Israeli sample expressed significantly higher levels of altruism (helping others), benevolence, randomness, and luck.

We also examined the results of the two samples with the lowest levels of hope, French Switzerland and Poland. Participants in the Polish sample had the lowest levels of life satisfaction, positive emotions, and self-worth and the second-lowest in agency and luck, and at the same time, the highest values of justice and controllability from all samples in this study. French-Swiss had even lower levels than Polish in pathways, meaning in life, altruism, benevolence, justice, controllability, luck, and religiosity but higher self-worth.

Overall, we found the largest differences between the six samples in the following domains: Luck (the highest in Israel and the lowest in French Switzerland), self-control (the highest in South Africa and Israel and the lowest in German Switzerland), benevolence (the highest in Israel and South Africa and the lowest in French Switzerland), and religiosity (the highest in South Africa and the lowest in Germany and French Switzerland).

To sum up, the results from this first step of analysis bear interesting learnings. Countries with similar economic, political, and social backgrounds like Germany and Switzerland displayed certain commonalities but also significant differences, especially regarding the level of perceived hope and basic beliefs. This is even more pronounced within Switzerland, a country with little economic inequalities (Gini-Index of 33), where people in two culturally distinct regions display huge differences in worldviews, perceived hope, and well-being. Moreover, South Africa and Poland, with lower economic income but both with higher levels of religiosity, display significant differences in hope, well-being, and some basic beliefs. On the other hand, two very dissimilar countries like Israel and South Africa, with many differences regarding their socio-cultural background and some basic beliefs but both facing social struggles and inequalities, display similar high levels of hope. In the next step, we analyzed associations between the variables in an attempt to further understand these similarities and distinctions between the six samples.

Step 2: Partial Bivariate Correlations

In this second step, we first analyzed the relationships between well-being variables, basic beliefs, and perceived hope and then investigated assessed correlations with perceived hope in each sample. The overall purpose was to identify similar and different correlates with perceived hope in the single samples. For a general overview, in Appendix 5.2 we report the partial correlation coefficients (controlled by demographics) between all variables using the entire database (N = 6548).

For our purposes, we focused our analysis on the correlation coefficients between well-being domains and basic beliefs in relation to perceived hope. Results in Table 5.3 display partial bivariate correlations for each individual sample after controlling for the demographic variables. All correlation coefficients were significant. Results in all samples displayed similar high positive correlation coefficients with perceived hope for life satisfaction, positive emotions, harmony in life, meaning in life, agency, pathways, benevolence, luck, and self-worth (slightly lower). Correlation coefficients with moderate positive associations were observed for helping others, justice, controllability, self-control, and religiosity. Negative emotions and randomness were negatively correlated with perceived hope.

A few interesting differences emerged, noteworthy to be highlighted. In the South African sample, the strength of most of the correlations was the lowest in comparison to the other samples, with the exception of helping others and religiosity. Compared to the other countries, South Africa presented significantly lower correlation coefficients of perceived hope with agency and pathways ($p < 0.01$), controllability (with the exception of Israel) ($p < 0.05$) and a higher effect with religiosity (although statistically not significant). People in French-speaking Switzerland, Israel, and Poland exhibited significantly higher correlations between hope and self-control in comparison with German-speaking Swiss and Germans ($p < 0.01$) and to a lesser extent, with South Africans (n.s.).

Regarding basic assumptions, our results suggested that variables representing a positive external locus of control such as benevolence and luck had a closer association with hope than concepts related to an internal locus of control, i.e., controllability and self-control. Furthermore, the belief in the benevolence of the world and the experience of good fortune in one's life, seemed to have similar effects as the self-oriented agency and pathways. For a more differentiated analysis, we implemented hierarchical regressions in step 3.

Table 5.3 Partial Pearson's bivariate correlation coefficients with Perceived Hope by sample

	German Swiss	French Swiss	Germany	SouthAfrica	Israel	Poland
Subjective Well-being						
Life-satisfaction	0.584**	0.605**	0.579**	0.480**	0.560**	0.590**
Positive emotions	0.597**	0.622**	0.605**	0.560**	0.561**	0.707**
Negative emotions	−0.465**	−0.468**	−0.505**	−0.395**	−0.450**	−0.556**
Psychological Well-being						
Meaning in life	0.490**	0.545**	0.463**	0.523**	0.458**	0.588**
Helping others	0.252**	0.308**	0.259**	0.389**	0.280**	0.407**
Harmony in life	0.579**	0.620**	0.592**	0.543**	0.608**	0.611**
Goal orientation and self-confidence						
Agency	0.561**	0.649**	0.555**	0.437**	0.655**	0.637**
Pathways	0.565**	0.634**	0.592**	0.451**	0.640**	0.480**
Basic assumptions						
Benevolence	0.471**	0.513**	0.520**	0.468**	0.519**	0.584**
Justice	0.303**	0.353**	0.289**	0.210**	0.353**	0.405**
Controllability	0.259**	0.300**	0.311**	0.118*	0.192**	0.387**
Randomness	−0.128**	−0.153**	−0.126**	−0.119*	−0.177**	−0.200**
Self-worth	0.401**	0.422**	0.420**	0.382**	0.497**	0.445**
Self-control	0.185**	0.333**	0.178**	0.245**	0.347**	0.327**
Luck	0.533**	0.526**	0.510**	0.317**	0.506**	0.581**
Religiosity	0.206**	0.245**	0.223**	0.326**	0.253**	0.214**

Note: **. Correlation is significant at 0.01 level; *. Correlation is significant at 0.05 level
Control variables: Gender, age, marital status, education, main activity, professional status and religion

Step 3: Hierarchical Regression Analyses

The correlation coefficients could be further explained by the results of the hierarchical regression analyses to predict perceived hope, as presented in Table 5.4. For our purpose, we entered the demographic variables in the first step, followed by the subjective well-being domains in the second step, the psychological well-being indicators in the third step, agency and pathways in the next, and all basic belief dimensions in the final step.

The first finding is that the level of perceived hope is only weakly or not at all explained by demographic characteristics. The variables in every further step contributed significantly to explaining the variance of perceived hope. Overall, the entire set of variables explains between 52% (South Africa) and 66% (Poland) of the variance of perceived hope. Remarkably, in all samples, the set of basic beliefs still has a significant effect of around 5% on perceived hope, after subjective and psychological well-being variables, agency, and pathways.

Table 5.4 Hierarchical regression analysis with Perceived Hope as dependent variable by sample

	German Swiss		French Swiss		Germany		South Africa		Israel		Poland	
	Std. β	p	Std. β	p	Std. β	p	Std. β	p	Std. β	p	Std. β	p
Step 1: Demographics												
Gender	0.037	0.003	0.025	0.187	0.047	0.058	0.009	0.797	−0.020	0.513	−0.026	0.617
Age	−0.011	0.394	0.019	0.344	−0.022	0.377	−0.063	0.244	−0.006	0.840	0.061	0.426
Marital status	0.043	0.001	0.015	0.439	0.006	0.807	0.043	0.396	−0.010	0.760	−0.021	0.698
Education	−0.016	0.198	−0.054	0.002	−0.013	0.575	0.026	0.483	−0.023	0.455	−0.084	0.101
Main activity	0.025	0.060	0.041	0.036	0.018	0.486	−0.008	0.858	0.074	0.029	0.022	0.746
Professional status	−0.019	0.113	−0.059	0.001	0.002	0.924	0.007	0.860	−0.013	0.698	−0.016	0.750
Step 2: Subjective Well-being												
Life satisfaction	0.053	0.017	0.035	0.341	0.060	0.192	−0.013	0.824	−0.073	0.143	−0.202	0.051
Positive emotions	0.139	<0.001	0.124	<0.001	0.150	<0.001	0.169	0.002	0.050	0.257	0.347	<0.001
Negative emotions	−0.087	<0.001	−0.074	0.001	−0.123	<0.001	−0.071	0.125	−0.068	0.077	−0.070	0.373
Step 3: Psychological Well-being												
Meaning	0.032	0.054	0.027	0.290	0.011	0.717	0.133	0.009	0.039	0.308	0.106	0.145
Helping others	0.075	<0.001	0.069	<0.001	0.068	0.006	0.088	0.034	−0.003	0.921	0.081	0.150
Harmony in life	0.027	0.221	0.037	0.307	0.032	0.490	0.110	0.092	0.168	<0.001	0.103	0.262
Step 4: Self-confidence												
Agency	0.096	<0.001	0.127	<0.001	0.030	0.464	−0.008	0.892	0.164	0.002	0.250	0.008
Pathways	0.200	<0.001	0.261	<0.001	0.249	<0.001	0.154	0.004	0.236	<0.001	−0.042	0.591
Step 5: Basic assumptions												
Benevolence	0.137	<0.001	0.146	<0.001	0.191	<0.001	0.166	<0.001	0.116	0.002	0.189	0.006
Justice	0.024	0.098	0.048	0.030	0.010	0.738	0.058	0.201	0.067	0.061	0.100	0.098
Control	−0.014	0.361	−0.011	0.631	0.022	0.473	−0.059	0.201	−0.016	0.631	−0.011	0.869
Randomness	−0.027	0.030	−0.045	0.014	−0.031	0.197	−0.007	0.862	−0.021	0.514	−0.038	0.507
Self-worth	0.032	0.033	−0.001	0.957	−0.015	0.629	0.024	0.606	0.080	0.042	−0.053	0.461

(continued)

Table 5.4 (continued)

	German Swiss		French Swiss		Germany		South Africa		Israel		Poland	
	Std. β	p	Std. β	p	Std. β	p	Std. β	p	Std. β	p	Std. β	p
Self-control	0.021	0.112	−0.012	0.577	0.029	0.273	0.052	0.219	−0.006	0.866	0.001	0.982
Luck	0.141	<0.001	0.134	<0.001	0.084	0.008	0.059	0.151	0.178	<0.001	0.082	0.318
Religiosity	0.095	<0.001	0.092	<0.001	0.119	<0.001	0.138	0.001	0.054	0.099	0.063	0.235
	Δ adj. R^2	Sig. Change	Δ adj. R^2	Sig. Change	Δ adj. R^2	Sig. Change	Δ adj. R^2	Sig. Change	Δ adj. R^2	Sig. Change	Δ adj. R^2	Sig. Change
Model 1 (demographics)	0.053	<0.001	0.023	<0.001	0.052	<0.001	0.027	0.067	0.043	0.002	0.048	0.168
Model 2 (demographics + SWB)	0.392	<0.001	0.430	<0.001	0.404	<0.001	0.344	<0.001	0.381	<0.001	0.484	<0.001
Model 3 (demographics + SWB + PWB)	0.035	<0.001	0.043	<0.001	0.035	<0.001	0.081	<0.001	0.072	<0.001	0.051	<0.001
Model 4 (demographics + SWB + PWB + A/P)	0.054	<0.001	0.080	<0.001	0.048	<0.001	0.018	0.001	0.093	<0.001	0.026	0.003
Model 5 (all variables)	0.044	<0.001	0.051	<0.001	0.055	<0.001	0.052	<0.001	0.049	<0.001	0.050	0.003
Total adj. R^2	0.577	<0.001	0.627	<0.001	0.595	<0.001	0.523	<0.001	0.638	<0.001	0.660	0.003

The most striking findings are related to the individual predictors of perceived hope and the patterns emerging from the single samples. In the samples from German and French Switzerland, Germany, and Israel, the highest predictor of perceived hope was pathways (i.e., the individual capacity to overcome difficulties and obstacles) followed by the belief in a benevolent world (and people), positive emotions, and luck. These patterns in contrast with results from the South African sample, where many dimensions had a significant and similar effect on perceived hope: Besides positive emotions, benevolence, and pathways, we found religiosity and meaning in life with standardized beta values above 0.1. Compared to the other countries, South Africa displayed a lower impact of agency and pathways and a stronger effect of religiosity and benevolence on perceived hope (in terms of Δ adj. R^2).

The belief in a benevolent world is the only significant predictor of perceived hope in all six samples. Pathways was significant in all countries except in Poland. The impact of positive emotions was significant in all countries but Israel and the highest in Poland. Interestingly, life satisfaction had no significant effect on perceived hope (with exception of the German-Swiss sample with a very low effect). Helping others had a small but significant effect on perceived hope in both Swiss regions, Germany, and South Africa, but not in Israel and Poland. Israel is the only country in which harmony in life had a significant effect on perceived hope and where the effect of luck was stronger than in the other countries. Interestingly, neither Israel nor Poland displayed an effect of religiosity on perceived hope but both countries showed a relatively strong effect for agency.

In sum, there seem to exist some common patterns regarding the roots and features of hope common among the country samples we examined. Hope as perceived by people indeed seems to possess a cognitive, an emotional, and a spiritual dimension as claimed by many authors (Dufault & Martocchio, 1985; Farran et al., 1995), which can be anchored in certain basic beliefs about oneself and the world. The emotional dimension of well-being seems to have a stronger effect on hope than the cognitive dimension of life satisfaction. The confidence in one's own capacity to overcome difficulties and obstacles (pathways) is more influential than one's general conviction of achieving goals (agency). The belief in the benevolence of the world and of people is a significant and recurrent predictor of hope. Furthermore, the belief in being a lucky person, religious faith, and the readiness to help other people do also have a significant impact on hope. Neither the belief in the controllability of the world nor the perception of being in control of what happens in one life have a significant effect on hope.

Despite these common features, some noteworthy differences can be identified. The South African sample stands out because of the similar effects on hope of positive emotions, meaning in life, the belief in a benevolent world, pathways, and religiosity. The predictive power of religiosity and helping others on perceived hope were the highest among all samples. South Africa also displayed the highest mean values of religiosity, meaning in life, positive emotions, pathways and perceived hope compared to all other countries. Poland, the country with the second-highest level of religiosity and the second-lowest level of hope in our study, did not reveal a significant effect of religiosity on perceived hope but a strong effect of positive emotions and agency, where it showed relatively low mean levels. In turn, Israel, the country with the second-highest level of hope and the highest levels of belief in luck and self-control, displayed stronger effects of luck, pathways, and agency on hope, besides harmony in life and benevolence.

5.4 Discussion

The purpose of this chapter is to investigate the role of basic beliefs about the world and oneself in relation to the perception of hope and to analyze similarities and possible differences between samples from several countries regarding the level and the predictors of hope. According to the definition outlined in Chap. 2, hope rests on the belief of the possibility, although not probability, that a certain desired good can be attained and the trust in the availability of personal or external resources to overcome difficulties and setbacks. Therefore, the question here is, what empowers people to believe that their hopes can become true. What kind of beliefs sustain people's general hope? Although basic beliefs are based on experiences, they are not that much anchored in facts, but rather in more generalized assumptions about the world and oneself (Janoff-Bulman, 1992). These worldviews are shaped by cultural norms and values, affect how people think, feel and act, how they look towards the future and what kind of wishes, goals and hopes they consider worthwhile to pursue (Nilsson, 2013, 2014). People in different cultures and contexts may sustain their hope from different life domains and attitudes, may hope for similar or different things and act according to their priorities and norms. Some may rely more on their own strengths, others count on the social support of family and friends and yet others may belief in luck, providence or a benevolent higher power. This means that hope could be considered a universal, complex, multifaceted and at the same time cultural and individual phenomenon.

In order to investigate the research question about the role of basic beliefs and culture specific features in the experience of perceived hope, we employed Janoff-Bulman's (1989) world assumptions about the benevolence of the external world, the meaningfulness of why things happen in life and the image people have of themselves (e.g. self-worth) and supplemented them with the belief about one's individual capacity to achieve goals (agency) and overcome difficulties (pathways) as defined by Snyder (2002) as well as with the centrality of religious faith. We evaluated whether levels of hope vary across countries and cultures and examined which experiences, attitudes and basic beliefs could be identified as possible determinants of hope. Accordingly, we employed measures to evaluate subjective and psychological well-being and investigated which basic beliefs and assumptions could have an effect on hope beside and beyond these experiences and attitudes.

First, we found that the general experience of hope as measured by the perceived hope scale seems to be conceptualized in a similar way across all investigated samples (Krafft et al., 2019). Consequently, we continued to compare levels of perceived hope and analyzed then the predictors of hope across countries.

The second main finding was that people from Switzerland, Germany, South Africa, Israel and Poland, countries with huge differences in economic wealth and ethnic, historical and social backgrounds, all demonstrated moderately high levels of hope (above the center of the scale). Interestingly, it seemed that levels of hope do not depend on the economic wealth or the social stability of the country. In our study, people in South Africa and in Israel had the highest levels of hope. In another study, South African respondents showed significantly higher perceived hope, higher harmony in life, and higher levels of positive feelings in comparison with Czech participants (Slezackova et al., 2021). Further, people with very similar economic and social conditions but different cultural contexts differed in their levels of hope and well-being, as the results of French and German-speaking Switzerland showed. Furthermore, two countries with significantly higher levels of religiosity, South Africa and Poland, displayed significant differences in hope and well-being. These findings strengthen the assumption that the level of perceived hope is strongly influenced by cultural characteristics and supports the work of Averill et al. (1990) as well as Averill and Sundararajan (2005).

Third, regarding the predictors of hope, the findings from all samples support the notion that basic beliefs have a significant effect on the level of hope, however with diverse magnitude. Across the six samples, some general patterns emerged. Recurrent and most striking predictors of hope were pathways (the belief in one's ability to overcome difficulties and find many ways to attain a goal), positive emotions, the belief in the benevolence of the world, one's own agency to achieve goals, the belief of luck in life, and to a lesser but still significant extent, the readiness to help other people as well as religiosity. These seem to be general features or sources of hope with a certain universal character across several countries and highlights the multidimensional, cognitive, emotional and volitional nature of hope as proposed by Dufault and Martocchio (1985) and many others (Farran et al., 1995; Scioli & Biller, 2009).

Beyond these more or less universal features, a number of noteworthy country-specific characteristics emerged. South Africa, the poorest and at the same time, the country with the highest level of perceived hope, stands out with many dimensions having a significant effect on perceived hope. For this South African sample, hope seemed to be very much anchored in positive emotions, social relationships and the willingness to help other people, religious faith and the connection to a higher power and the general belief in the good (see also Slezackova et al., 2021). It was remarkable that religious beliefs and the belief in the good had stronger predictive power on hope than the individualistic and self-centered beliefs in agency and pathways. This suggests that for South Africans, the social dimension and a positive external locus of control appear to be more salient than the individualist internal locus of control, which is in line with Scioli's comprehensive hope theory (Scioli, 2021) and Tennen et al.'s (2002) emphasis on trust. However, as the results of South Africa and Poland show, higher levels of religiosity on its own may not always sustain higher levels of hope, which suggests that not the magnitude, but the quality and the contents of the religious faith may be important to hope.

It is notable that religiosity predicted perceived hope in Poland before controlling for basic assumptions, which could have mediated the effect of religious faith, explaining why and how Catholic faith fosters hope. We acknowledge that some of Janoff-Bulman's values could emerge from Christian-European worldview (e.g., benevolence of the world, justice), and those values may apply to the whole contemporary Polish society regardless of religious beliefs. Religiosity of Polish people includes to a larger extent, beliefs about the benevolence and justice of the world/people, and to a lesser extent a transcendent connection with God. It is therefore not so much the connection with a Divine Being but the belief in a benevolent world that gives hope to Poles.

Furthermore, our findings could be also interpreted in the light of the historical and political role played in the past by Catholic church in Poland and macrosocial changes (see also Slezackova, Millova, & Stecz in this volume) which might have contributed to the weakening of spiritual character of religiosity and faith awareness. Religion is practiced because this is rather a national and familiar tradition rather than a deep spiritual experience that reinforces hope and helps to fulfil it (Wadowski, 2019).

The opposite is the case in Israel, the country with the second-highest level of hope. In Israel, at least in our sample, the individualistic agency and pathways were stronger predictors of hope than religious and general beliefs in the good. Furthermore, the individualistic perception of luck and self-worth were significantly related to hope. A similar pattern can be observed in French-speaking Switzerland, the sample with the lowest level of hope, where agency and pathways were stronger predictors than the belief in the good and religious faith. These findings suggest that in these countries, the individualistic, cognitive and internal locus of control are predominant for the perception of hope as maintained by Snyder (2002), but that the individualistic attitude is sometimes not sufficient to foster higher levels of hope.

In sum, the levels of hope are clearly not related to economic wealth nor to social or political stability. South Africa, the country with the lowest GDP and with social turbulences as well as Israel, a country facing violence and aggression for many decades, are those with the highest levels of hope. On the other hand, two regions in Switzerland with the same economic and political environment but with different languages and cultural backgrounds exhibited significant differences in levels of hope and other variables. People in German speaking Switzerland and Germany seem more similar regarding hope than people in two cultural distinct regions within Switzerland. Whereas in a country like South Africa higher levels of (protestant) religiosity can contribute to a higher level of hope and well-being, in the catholic Poland this is not the case. These findings, of course, should be the matter for further research. In Israel and in French speaking Switzerland the individual capacity to overcome difficulties and achieve goals is a stronger determinant of hope, with significantly higher levels in Israel and markedly lower levels in French Switzerland. All in all, the general perception of hope comprises emotional, cognitive and volitional dimensions, which are shaped by basic beliefs with diverse foci in different cultures.

5.5 Limitations

Our study has a number of limitations, which we would like to address. The cross-sectional design of our research does not allow any conclusions about causalities. Although the demographic structures of our samples are largely heterogeneous, they are not representative of the entire population of the single countries. The participants have been recruited via online platforms, which exclude population groups without or with poor internet access. There are huge differences in sample sizes and therefore in the statistical power of the samples across the countries. For this reason, with a small Polish sample size, caution must be applied for interpreting unexpected outcomes regarding the determinants of perceived hope or for making cross-country comparisons.

5.6 Conclusions

Our findings support the notion that cultural norms and basic beliefs have an important effect on hope and that countries and different cultural contexts sustain and perceive hope in different ways. At the same time, there are certain universal elements that foster hope, such as self-confidence, the belief in the good, positive experiences, religious faith, and the willingness to help other people. With regard to psychological theories of hope, our findings imply that it would be misleading to reduce the experience of general hope only to individualistic and cognitive dimensions and to ignore other experiences and elements such as the emotional, the cultural and the spiritual. Our concept of hope has the advantage to incorporate at a general level of abstraction many of these dimensions, and at the same time to address the individual, social and cultural roots and elements of hope. Further research could evaluate if similar patterns emerge in other countries and which cultural characteristics appear in other societies like the Muslim, the Hindu or in more individualistic cultures like the US. In addition, much more research is needed to fully understand specific cultural norms, practices and beliefs in relation to hope.

Appendix 5.1: Demographic Structure of the Samples

	German Swiss	French Swiss	Germany	South Africa	Israel	Poland	Total
	N/n	*N/n*	*N/n*	*N/n*	*N/n*	*N/n*	*N/n*
	%	%	%	%	%	%	%
Total	3306	1308	840	427	477	190	6548
Age (M)	44.89	45.03	50.80	38.87	36.48	44.77	44.67
Age (SD)	26.03	22.96	29.78	14.50	31.86	15.82	25.84
Gender							
Male	1458	606	480	130	73	78	2825
	44.1%	46.3%	57.1%	30.4%	15.3% a	41.1%	43.1%
Female	1848	702	360	297	404	112	3723
	55.9%	53.7%	42.9%	69.6%	84.7%	58.9%	56.9%
Marital status							
Still living with my parents	345	103	22	82	56	15	623
	10.4%	7.9%	2.6%	19.2%	11.7%	7.9%	9.5%
Single, unmarried	492	174	138	76	106	27	1013
	14.9%	13.3%	16.4%	17.8%	22.2%	14.2%	15.5%
Living in a part-nership with sepa-rate households	239	99	48	20	35	3	444
	7.2%	7.6%	5.7%	4.7%	7.3%	1.6%	6.8%
Living together in a partnership	601	254	108	40	81	26	1110
	18.2%	19.4%	12.9%	9.4%	17.0%	13.7%	17.0%
Married	1287	473	430	177	171	101	2639
	38.9%	36.2%	51.2%	41.5%	35.8%	53.2%	40.3%
Divorced/ separated	278	174	73	23	22	10	580
	8.4%	13.3%	8.7%	5.4%	4.6%	5.3%	8.9%
Widowed	64	31	21	9	6	8	139
	1.9%	2.4%	2.5%	2.1%	1.3%	4.2%	2.1%
Education							
Did not finish school	32	13	9	2	2	1	59
	1.1%	1.0%	1.1%	0.5%	0.4%	0.5%	0.9%
Primary school	182	127	31	7		7	354
	5.5%	9.5%	3.7%	1.6%		3.7%	5.4%
Secondary school	289	96	186	78	48	47	744
	8.7%	7.1%	22.1%	18.3%	10.1%	24.7%	11.3%
Professional train-ing/diploma	2188	806	444	50	2	32	3522

(continued)

	German Swiss	French Swiss	Germany	South Africa	Israel	Poland	Total
	N/n	*N/n*	*N/n*	*N/n*	*N/n*	*N/n*	*N/n*
	%	%	%	%	%	%	%
	66.2%	60.0%	52.9%	11.7%	0.4%	16.8%	53.5%
Tertiary education/ university	615	301	170	290	425	103	1904
	18.6%	22.4%	20.2%	67.9%	89.1%	54.2%	28.9%
Main activity							
In education or training	285	110	32	102	191	9	729
	8.6%	8.4%	3.8%	23.9%	40.0%	4.7%	11.1%
Household/raising children	132	59	23	11	5	6	236
	4.0%	4.5%	2.7%	2.6%	1.0%	3.2%	3.6%
Part-time job	663	260	78	29	83	9	1122
	20.1%	19.9%	9.3%	6.8%	17.4%	4.7%	17.1%
Fulltime job	1592	619	480	244	162	117	3214
	48.2%	47.3%	57.1%	57.1%	34.0%	61.6%	49.1%
Unemployed	139	80	27	16	11	12	285
	4.2%	6.1%	3.2%	3.7%	2.3%	6.3%	4.4%
Retired	495	180	200	25	25	37	962
	15.0%	13.8%	23.8%	5.9%	5.2%	19.5%	14.7%
Professional status							
No position in an organization	509	252	153	71	55	41	1081
	15.4%	19.3%	18.2%	16.6%	11.5%	21.6%	16.5%
In education/ training	236	114	31	97	160	13	651
	7.1%	8.7%	3.7%	22.7%	33.5%	6.8%	9.9%
Employee	1301	579	336	95	141	84	2536
	39.4%	44.3%	40.0%	22.2%	29.6%	44.2%	38.7%
Junior/middle management	725	159	205	76	49	34	1248
	21.9%	12.2%	24.4%	17.8%	10.3%	17.9%	19.1%
Senior management/board of directors	163	54	30	35	21	6	309
	4.9%	4.1%	3.6%	8.2%	4.4%	3.2%	4.7%
Entrepreneur/business owner	372	150	85	53	51	12	723
	11.3%	11.5%	10.1%	12.4%	10.7%	6.3%	11.1%
Religion							
Catholic	830	434	198	28	4	145	1639
	25.1%	33.2%	23.6%	6.6%	0.8%	76.3%	25.0%
Protestant	946	208	191	72	0	0	1417

(continued)

	German Swiss	French Swiss	Germany	South Africa	Israel	Poland	Total
	N/n	*N/n*	*N/n*	*N/n*	*N/n*	*N/n*	*N/n*
	%	%	%	%	%	%	%
	28.6%	15.9%	22.7%	16.9%	0.0%	0.0%	21.6%
Another Christian church	132	32	13	165	3	2	347
	4.0%	2.4%	1.5%	38.6%	0.6%	1.1%	5.3%
Muslim	65	20	4	11	7	0	107
	2.0%	1.5%	0.5%	2.6%	1.5%	0.0%	1.6%
Jewish	6	5	1	9	160	0	181
	0.2%	0.4%	0.1%	2.1%	33.5%	0.0%	2.8%
Hindu	5	2	2	7	1	0	17
	0.2%	0.2%	0.2%	1.6%	0.2%	0.0%	0.3%
Buddhist	16	2	3	2	3	0	26
	0.5%	0.2%	0.4%	0.5%	0.6%	0.0%	0.4%
I am a spiritual person outside the traditional world religions.	217	107	41	82	94	6	547
	6.6%	8.2%	4.9%	19.2%	19.7%	3.2%	8.4%
Without religion or confession	1034	466	375	31	110	32	2048
	31.3%	35.6%	44.6%	7.3%	23.1%	16.8%	31.3%
Something different	55	32	12	20	95	5	219
	1.7%	2.4%	1.4%	4.7%	19.9%	2.6%	3.3%

Appendix 5.2: Partial Pearson's Bivariate Correlation Coefficients for the Total Sample N = 6548

	Perceived Hope	Life-satisfaction	Positive emotions	Negative emotions	Meaningin Life	Helping others	Harmony in Life	Agency	Pathways	Bene-volence	Justice	Control	Random-ness	Self-worth	Self-control	Luck
Perceived Hope	1.000															
Life-satisfaction	0.597**	1.000														
Positive emotions	0.606**	0.702**	1.000													
Negative emotions	−0.472**	−0.545**	−0.601**	1.000												
Meaning in life	0.510**	0.602**	0.543**	−0.419**	1.000											
Helping others	0.289**	0.187**	0.209**	−0.060**	0.225**	1.000										
Harmony in life	0.596**	0.788**	0.718**	−0.597**	0.617**	0.217**	1.000									
Agency	0.603**	0.641**	0.551**	−0.406**	0.542**	0.209**	0.608**	1.000								
Pathways	0.597**	0.512**	0.507**	−0.379**	0.465**	0.237**	0.540**	0.742**	1.000							
Benevolence	0.509**	0.463**	0.446**	−0.356**	0.383**	0.270**	0.419**	0.371**	0.352**	1.000						
Justice	0.333**	0.339**	0.281**	−0.192**	0.250**	0.165**	0.310**	0.306**	0.275**	0.342**	1.000					
Control	0.276**	0.276**	0.235**	−0.162**	0.241**	0.113**	0.287**	0.301**	0.305**	0.219**	0.565**	1.000				
Randomness	−0.129**	−0.092**	−0.110**	0.126**	−0.173**	−00.003	−0.098**	−0.093**	−0.071**	−0.091**	−0.076**	−0.064**	1.000			
Self-worth	0.399**	0.456**	0.467**	−0.466**	0.432**	0.064**	0.519**	0.463**	0.392**	0.277**	0.078**	0.089**	−0.165**	1.000		
Self-control	0.215**	0.227**	0.211**	−0.128**	0.197**	00.020	0.272**	0.306**	0.236**	0.086**	0.256**	0.375**	0.105**	0.192**	1.000	
Luck	0.536**	0.604**	0.495**	−0.332**	0.381**	0.201**	0.492**	0.495**	0.424**	0.465**	0.368**	0.314**	0.041**	0.251**	0.216**	1.000
Religiosity	0.221**	0.088**	0.127**	−0.035**	0.223**	0.210**	0.134**	0.113**	0.107**	0.111**	0.118**	0.089**	−0.239**	00.023	0.046**	0.126**

Note: **. Correlation is significant at 0 01 level; Control variables: Gender, age, country, marital status, education, main activity, professional status and religion

References

Aerts, D., Apostel, L., De Moor, B., Hellemans, S., Maex, E., Van Belle, H., & Van der Veken, J. (1994). *Worldviews: From fragmentation to integration*. Brussels Free University, Belgium.

Allport, G. W. (1955). *Becoming: Basic considerations for a psychology of personality* (Vol. 20). Yale University Press.

Averill, J. R., Catlin, G., & Chon, K. K. (1990). *Rules of hope: Recent research in psychology*. Springer.

Averill, J. R., & Sundararajan, L. (2005). Hope as rhetoric: Cultural narratives of wishing and coping. In J. Eliott (Ed.), *Interdisciplinary perspectives on hope* (pp. 133–165). Nova Science.

Beck, A. T. (1974). The development of depression: A cognitive model. In R. Friedman & M. Katz (Eds.), *Psychology of depression: Contemporary theory and research*. Winston.

Berger, P. L., & Luckmann, T. (1966). *The social construction of reality*. Anchor/Doubleday.

Bovens, L. (1999). The value of hope. *Philosophy and Phenomenological Research, 59*(3), 667–681.

Bruininks, P., & Malle, B. (2005). Distinguishing hope from optimism and related affective states. *Motivation and Emotion, 29, no., 4*(2005), 324–352. https://doi.org/10.1007/s11031-006-9010-4

Carver, C. S., & Scheier, M. F. (2014). Dispositional optimism. *Trends in Cognitive Sciences, 18*(6), 293–299.

Chen, F. F. (2007). Sensitivity of goodness of fit indexes to lack of measurement invariance. *Structural Equation Modeling: A Multidisciplinary Journal, 14*(3), 464–504. https://doi.org/10.1080/10705510701301834

Clifton, J. D., Baker, J. D., Park, C. L., Yaden, D. B., Clifton, A. B., Terni, P., Miller, J. L., Zeng, G., Giorgi, S., Schwartz, H. A., & Seligman, M. E. (2019). Primal world beliefs. *Psychological Assessment, 31*(1), 82–99. https://doi.org/10.1037/pas0000639

Dana, R. H. (1993). *Multicultural assessment perspectives for professional psychology*. Allyn & Bacon.

Diener, E. D., Emmons, R. A., Larsen, R. J., & Griffin, S. (1985). The satisfaction with life scale. *Journal of Personality Assessment, 49*(1), 71–75. https://doi.org/10.1207/s15327752jpa4901_13

Diener, E., Wirtz, D., Tov, W., Kim-Prieto, C., Choi, D. W., Oishi, S., & Biswas-Diener, R. (2010). New Well-being measures: Short scales to assess flourishing and positive and negative feelings. *Social Indicators Research, 97*(2), 143–156. https://doi.org/10.1007/s11205-009-9493-y

Dilthey, W. (1890/1957). *Dilthey's philosophy of existence: Introduction to Weltanschauungslehre* (W. Kluback & M. Weinbaum, Trans.). Bookman Associates.

Dufault, K., & Martocchio, B. C. (1985). Hope: Its spheres and dimensions. Symposium on compassionate care and the dying experience. *The Nursing Clinics of North America, 20*(2), 379–391.

Eliott, J. A. (2005). What have we done with hope? A brief history. In J. Eliott (Ed.), *Interdisciplinary perspectives on hope* (pp. 3–45). Nova Science.

Elklit, A., Shevlin, M., Solomon, Z., & Dekel, R. (2007). Factor structure and concurrent validity of the world assumptions scale. *Journal of Traumatic Stress, 20*(3), 291–301. https://doi.org/10.1002/jts.20203

Erikson, E. H. (1998). *The life cycle completed (extended version)*. WW Norton & Company.

Farran, C. J., Herth, K. A., & Popovich, J. M. (1995). *Hope and hopelessness: Critical clinical constructs*. Sage.

Hong, Y.-Y., Morris, M. W., Chiu, C.-Y., & Benet-Martinez, V. (2000). Multicultural minds: A dynamic constructivist approach to culture and cognition. *American Psychologist, 55*, 709–720. https://doi.org/10.1037/0003-066X.55.7.709

Hu, L. T., & Bentler, P. M. (1999). Cutoff criteria for fit indexes in covariance structure analysis: Conventional criteria versus new alternatives. *Structural Equation Modeling: A Multidisciplinary Journal, 6*(1), 1–55. https://doi.org/10.1080/10705519909540118

Huber, S., & Huber, O. W. (2012). The centrality of religiosity scale (CRS). *Religions, 3*(3), 710–724. https://doi.org/10.3390/rel3030710

Ibrahim, F. A. (1984). Cross-cultural counseling and psychotherapy: An existential-psychological approach. *International Journal for the Advancement of Counselling, 7*(3), 159–169. https://doi.org/10.1007/BF00116188

Ibrahim, F. A. (1985). Effective cross-cultural counseling and psychotherapy: A framework. *The Counseling Psychologist, 13*(4), 625–638. https://doi.org/10.1177/0011000085134006

Ibrahim, F. A. (1993). Existential worldview theory: Transcultural counseling. In J. McFaddon (Ed.), *Transcultural counseling: Bilateral and international perspectives* (pp. 23–58). American Counseling Association.

Ibrahim, F. A. (2003). Existential worldview theory: From inception to applications. In F. D. Harper & J. McFadden (Eds.), *Culture and counseling: New approaches* (pp. 196–208). Pearson College Division.

Ibrahim, F. A., & Heuer, J. R. (2016). *Cultural and social justice counseling*. Springer. https://doi.org/10.1007/978-3-319-18057-1

Ibrahim, F. A., Roysircar-Sodowsky, G. R., & Ohnishi, H. (2001). Worldview: Recent developments and needed directions. In J. G. Ponterotto, M. J. Casas, L. A. Suzuki, & C. M. Alexander (Eds.), *Handbook of multicultural counseling* (p. 430). Sage Publications.

James, W. (1962). *Essays on faith and morals*. World Publishing Company.

Janoff-Bulman, R. (1989). Assumptive worlds and the stress of traumatic events: Applications of the schema construct. *Social Cognition, 7*(2), 113–136. https://doi.org/10.1521/soco.1989.7.2.113

Janoff-Bulman, R. (1992). *Shattered assumptions: Towards a new psychology of trauma*. Free Press. https://doi.org/10.1080/00029157.1994.10403078

Jaspers, K. (1919). *Psychologie der Weltanschauungen [psychology of worldviews]*. Springer.

Joseph, S., & Linley, P. A. (2005). Positive adjustment to threatening events: An organismic valuing theory of growth through adversity. *Review of General Psychology, 9*(3), 262–280. https://doi.org/10.1037/1089-2680.9.3.262

Kant, I. (1790/1987). *Critique of judgment* (W. S. Pluhar, Trans.). Hackett Publishing Co.

Kelly, G. A. (1955). *The psychology of personal constructs. Volume 1: A theory of personality*. WW Norton and Company.

Kjell, O., Daukantaitė, D., Hefferon, K., & Sikström, S. (2016). Harmony in life scale complements the satisfaction with life scale. *Social Indicators Research, 126*, 893–919. https://doi.org/10.1007/s11205-015-0903-z

Koltko-Rivera, M. E. (2004). The psychology of worldviews. *Review of General Psychology, 8*(1), 3–58. https://doi.org/10.1037/1089-2680.8.1.3

Krafft, A. M., Guse, T., & Maree, D. (2021). Distinguishing perceived Hope and dispositional optimism: Theoretical foundations and empirical findings beyond future expectancies and cognition. *Journal of Well-Being Assessment, 4*, 217–243. https://doi.org/10.1007/s41543-020-00030-4

Krafft, A. M., Martin-Krumm, C., & Fenouillet, F. (2019). Adaptation, further elaboration, and validation of a scale to measure hope as perceived by people: Discriminant value and predictive utility Vis-à-Vis dispositional hope. *Assessment, 26*(8), 1594–1609. https://doi.org/10.1177/1073191117700724

Krafft, A. M., & Walker, A. M. (2018a). Exploring the concept and experience of Hope –theoretical and methodological foundations. In A. M. Krafft, P. Perrig-Chiello, & A. M. Walker (Eds.), *Hope for a good life: Results of the Hope barometer international research program* (pp. 3–19). Springer Int. https://doi.org/10.1007/978-3-319-78470-0_1

Krafft, A. M., & Walker, A. M. (2018b). Exploring the concept and experience of Hope – Empirical findings and the virtuous circle of Hope. In A. M. Krafft, P. Perrig-Chiello, & A. M. Walker (Eds.), *Hope for a good life: Results of the Hope barometer international research program* (pp. 21–60). Springer Int.

Lerner, M. J. (1980). *The belief in a just world*. Plenum. https://doi.org/10.1007/978-1-4899-0448-5_2

Leung, K. K., Silvius, J. L., Pimlott, N., Dalziel, W., & Drummond, N. (2009). Why health expectations and hopes are different: The development of a conceptual model. *Health Expectations, 12*(4), 347–360. https://doi.org/10.1111/j.1369-7625.2009.00570.x

Lonner, W. J., & Adamopoulos, J. (1997). Culture as antecedent to behavior. In J. W. Berry, Y. H. Poortinga, & J. Panday (Eds.), *Handbook of crosscultural psychology* (Vol. 1. *Theory and method*, 2nd ed., pp. 43–83). Allyn & Bacon.

Marsh, H. W. (1994). Confirmatory factor analysis models of factorial invariance: A multifaceted approach. *Structural Equation Modeling, 1*, 5–34. https://doi.org/10.1080/10705519409539960

Meirav, A. (2009). The nature of hope. *Ratio, 22*(2), 216–233. https://doi.org/10.1111/j.1467-9329.2009.00427.x

Miceli, M., & Castelfranchi, C. (2010). Hope: The power of wish and possibility. *Theory & Psychology, 20*(2), 251–276. https://doi.org/10.1177/0959354309354393

Miller, J. G. (1999). Cultural psychology: Implications for basic psychological theory. *Psychological Science, 10*, 85–91. https://doi.org/10.1111/1467-9280.00113

Milona, M. (2019). Finding hope. *Canadian Journal of Philosophy, 49*(5), 710–729. https://doi.org/10.1080/00455091.2018.1435612

Milona, M. (2020). Philosophy of Hope. In S. van den Heuvel (Ed.), *Historical and multidisciplinary perspectives on Hope* (pp. 99–116). Springer. https://doi.org/10.1007/978-3-030-46489-9_6

Naugle, D. K. (2002). *Worldview: The history of a concept*. Eerdmans Publishing.

Nickell, G. S. (1998). *The helping attitude scale: A new measure of prosocial tendencies*. Paper presented at the American Psychological Association.

Nilsson, A. (2013). *The psychology of worldviews: Toward a non-reductive science of personality*. Lund University.

Nilsson, A. (2014). Personality psychology as the integrative study of traits and worldviews. *New Ideas in Psychology, 32*, 18–32. https://doi.org/10.1016/j.newideapsych.2013.04.008

Plante, T. G., & Boccaccini, M. T. (1997). The Santa Clara strength of religious faith questionnaire. *Pastoral Psychology, 45*(5), 375–387. https://doi.org/10.1007/BF02230993

Rokeach, M. (1968). *Beliefs, attitudes, and values: A theory of organization and change*. Jossey-Bass.

Rotter, J. B. (1966). Generalized expectancies for internal versus external control of reinforcement. *Psychological Monographs: General and Applied, 80*(1), 1–28.

Scheier, M. F., Carver, C. S., & Bridges, M. W. (2001). Optimism, pessimism, and psychological Well-being. *Optimism and Pessimism, 1*, 189–216. https://doi.org/10.1037/10385-009

Scioli, A. (2021). The psychology of Hope: A diagnostic and prescriptive account. In S. C. van den Heuvel (Ed.), *Historical and multidisciplinary perspectives on Hope* (pp. 137–163). Springer. https://doi.org/10.1007/978-3-030-46489-9_8

Scioli, A., & Biller, H. (2009). *Hope in the age of anxiety*. Oxford University Press.

Scioli, A., Chamberlin, C. M., Samor, C. M., Lapointe, A. B., Campbell, T. L., Macleod, A. R., & McLenon, J. (1997). A prospective study of hope, optimism, and health. *Psychological Reports, 81*(3), 723–733. https://doi.org/10.2466/pr0.1997.81.3.723

Slezackova, A., Guse, T., & Prosek, T. (2021). The role of perceived hope in harmony in life among Czech and south African adults. In R. Kumar Pradhan & U. Kumar (Eds.), *Emotion, Well-being, and resilience: Theoretical perspectives and practical applications*. Apple Academic Press, Taylor & Francis Group. ISBN 978-1-77188-890-5.

Snyder, C. R. (2000). Hypothesis: There is hope. In C. R. Snyder (Ed.), *Handbook of hope: Theory, measures, and applications* (pp. 3–21). Academic.

Snyder, C. R. (2002). Hope theory: Rainbows in the mind. *Psychological Inquiry, 13*(4), 249–275. https://doi.org/10.1207/S15327965PLI1304_01

Snyder, C. R., Harris, C., Anderson, J. R., Holleran, S. A., Irving, L. M., Sigmon, S. T., & Harney, P. (1991). The will and the ways: Development and validation of an individual-differences measure of hope. *Journal of Personality and Social Psychology, 60*(4), 570–585. https://doi.org/10.1037/0022-3514.60.4.570

Steger, M. F., Frazier, P., Oishi, S., & Kaler, M. (2006). The meaning in life questionnaire: Assessing the presence of and search for meaning in life. *Journal of Counseling Psychology, 53*(1), 80–93. https://doi.org/10.1037/0022-0167.53.1.80

Steiger, J. H. (1980). Tests for comparing elements of a correlation matrix. *Psychological Bulletin, 87*(2), 245–251. https://doi.org/10.1037/0033-2909.87.2.245

Storch, E. A., Roberti, J. W., Bravata, E., & Storch, J. B. (2004). Psychometric investigation of the Santa Clara strength of religious faith questionnaire - short-form. *Pastoral Psychology, 52*(6), 479–483.

Tennen, H., Affleck, G., & Tennen, R. (2002). Clipped feathers: The theory and measurement of hope. *Psychological Inquiry, 13*(4), 311–317.

Triandis, H. C. (1995). *Individualism and collectivism.* Westview Press.

Triandis, H. C. (1997). Cross-cultural perspectives on personality. In R. Hogan, J. Johnson, & S. Briggs (Eds.), *Handbook of personality psychology* (pp. 439–464). Academic.

Wadowski, D. (2019). Religion and religiosity in contemporary Poland. *Central European Journal of Contemporary Religion, 3*(1), 35–63. https://doi.org/10.14712/25704893.2019.2

Wrightsman, L. S. (1962). Philosphies of human nature. In S. W. Cook (Ed.), *Research plans in the field of religion, values, and morality* (pp. 118–122). Religious Education Assn.

Zinnbauer, B. J., & Pargament, K. I. (2005). Religiousness and spirituality. In R. F. Paloutzian & C. L. Park (Eds.), *Handbook of the psychology of religion and spirituality* (pp. 21–42). Guilford.

Andreas Krafft holds a doctoral degree in Management Sciences at the University of St. Gallen (Switzerland) with special focus on Organizational Psychology, Culture and Development. He has academic specializations in Social Psychology of Organizations, Work and Health Psychology as well as Positive Psychology from the University of Zürich. Andreas is associate researcher for Futures Studies and lecturer at the Institute of Systemic Management and Public Governance at the University of St. Gallen. Furthermore, he teaches at the University of Zürich in the field of Work and Health, at the Master of Applied Positive Psychology at the University of Lisbon, Portugal, as well as at the Master of Futures Studies from the Free University Berlin. He is co-president of swissfuture, the Swiss Society for Futures Studies, member of the executive board of SWIPPA (the Swiss Positive Psychology Association) and of the DACH-PP (German speaking Association of Positive Psychology). Since many years he leads the International Research Network of the Hope Barometer.

Dr. Tharina Guse is a counselling psychologist and obtained an MA (Counselling Psychology) degree from the Potchefstroom University (now North-West University) in 1989. She was in full-time private practice for the next 15 years providing psychotherapy for children, adolescents and adults. In 2003 she obtained her PhD (Psychology) from Potchefstroom University. She returned to academia in 2005 and joined the University of Johannesburg. Since April 2018 she is a professor and Head of the Department of Psychology at the University of Pretoria. Currently she serves on the Professional Board for Psychology of the Health Professions Council of South Africa (HPCSA). She is also President of the recently founded South African Positive Psychology Association (SAPPA). Her research focuses are on positive psychology in general and in particular on psycho-social well-being, positive psychology interventions and psychological strengths such as hope and gratitude. Closely aligned with this broad focus she also conducts research on the application of hypnosis for the promotion of mental health and well-being.

Dr hab. Elżbieta Kasprzak, psychologist, professor at the Kazimierz Wielki University in Bydgoszcz, Poland. Researcher of the determinants of careers and their consequences for the well-being of employees. An important area of her scientific interests are various aspects of positive functioning at work, job satisfaction, hope and passion at work, as well as the conditions and effects of job crafting and proactivity at work. Since 2015 she has been participating in the international research network of the Hope Barometer.

Dr. Dorit Redlich-Amirav is an occupational therapist who works in the field of hope and mental health, mainly with family members. She completed her doctoral studies in the Department of Rehabilitation Medicine at the University of Alberta, Edmonton, Canada. Hope in mothers of adult children with mental illness in an environment of socio-political conflict. She teaches in the field of hope and mental health in the school of health professions at Tel Aviv University. On the subject of hope, she teaches a 'Circle of Hope' course at Levinsky-Wingate Academic Center and at the Ono Academic Campus. In addition, she leads the Hope Index project in Israel.

Dr Patryk Stecz, a psychologist, is an assistant professor at the Institute of Psychology, University of Lodz, Poland. From 2014–2017 and 2021–2025, he was elected to the Executive Board of the Polish Suicidology Association. Dr Stecz completed his Ph.D. at the Medical University of Lodz. He published approx. 40 scientific works related to applied clinical psychology (attitudes towards suicide, positive suicidology, religious coping, well-being predictors in clinical and non-clinical populations, risk behavior in students with visual impairment, studies on hope). Dr Stecz has been serving psychological support at the Academic Counseling Centre (Technical University of Lodz) for students and employees with disabilities and special needs since 2008. Dr Stecz was aged 31 when he received the Medical University Rector's Scientific Award. Currently he is finishing a four-year post-graduate Clinical Psychology Specialization Program (Center of Postgraduate Medical Education).

Chapter 6
Trust, Social Support and Hope Resources

Andreas M. Krafft, JohnBosco Chika Chukwuorji, Rajneesh Choubisa, Stella Conte, Fabien Fenouillet, Valle Flores-Lucas, Tharina Guse, Elżbieta Kasprzak, Charles Martin-Krumm, Helena Agueda Marujo, Chitra S. Nair, Dorit Redlich-Amirav, Mark Sinclair, Alena Slezackova, Patryk Stecz, Olga Varsos, and Eduardo Wills Herrera

Abstract The current chapter is dedicated to the exploration of different sources and activities of hope across countries. In particular, we explore how these serve as expressions of trust and confidence in the availability of resources, nourishing the belief in the feasibility and supporting the realization of wished-for goods considered

---

A. M. Krafft (✉)
Institute of Systemic Management and Public Governance, University of St. Gallen, St. Gallen, Switzerland
e-mail: andreas.krafft@unisg.ch

J. C. Chukwuorji
Department of Psychology, University of Nigeria, Nsukka, Nigeria

R. Choubisa
Department of Humanities and Social Sciences, Birla Institute of Technology and Science, (BITS) Pilani, Pilani, India

S. Conte
Department of Psychology, University of Cagliari, Cagliari, Italy

F. Fenouillet
Interdisciplinary Laboratory in Neuroscience, Physiology and Psychology: Learning, Physical Activity and Health, Université Paris Nanterre, Nanterre, France

V. Flores-Lucas
Department of Psychology, University of Valladolid, Valladolid, Spain

T. Guse
Department of Psychology, University of Pretoria, Pretoria, South Africa

E. Kasprzak
Department of Work and Organisational Psychology, Institute of Psychology, Kazimierz Wielki University of Bydgoszcz, Bydgoszcz, Poland

C. Martin-Krumm
Vulnerability, Capability, and Recovery Laboratory, Ecole de Psychologues Praticiens de Paris, Paris, France

H. A. Marujo
Instituto Superior de Ciências Sociais e Politicas, University of Lisbon, Lisbon, Portugal

A. M. Krafft et al. (eds.), *Hope across cultures*, Cross-Cultural Advancements in Positive Psychology 14, https://doi.org/10.1007/978-3-031-24412-4_6

to be possible, although not necessarily probable. Following an interdisciplinary approach, we integrated perspectives from the disciplines of Positive Psychology, Risk Management, and the Philosophy of Hope to elucidate the difference between trust and confidence. We further differentiate between perceived hope, on the one hand, and dispositional hope and optimism, on the other, backed in this interdisciplinary approach. Using data from the Hope Barometer in 2018 and 2019 we investigated the role of internal and external sources and activities of hope in two studies. Study 1 comprised 12 countries ($N = 10{,}193$) and aimed to analyze several personal and external hope sources with a specific focus on social support, religiosity and the feeling of luck in relation to hope. Study 2 was performed with 8 samples from 7 countries ($N = 6245$), centering on the assessment of several hope activities and their effects on perceived hope. Our findings highlight the importance of social, religious and other external factors of hope, demonstrate the differential nature of perceived and dispositional hope, and show significant differences between countries regarding the role of trust in individual capabilities, in emotional and instrumental support as well as in religious/spiritual experiences and practices.

6.1 Introduction

In previous chapters, hope was defined as a wish or desire related to the attainment of an important future good of which the realization is considered to be possible (although not necessarily probable) and trust in the availability of personal and other resources to overcome obstacles and setbacks. Averill and his colleagues (Averill et al., 1990; Averill & Sundararajan, 2005) reported that people in diverse

C. S. Nair
K. N. M. Government Arts and Science College Kanjiramkulam, University of Kerala, Thiruvananthapuram, India

D. Redlich-Amirav
Sackler Faculty of Medicine, Tel Aviv University, Tel Aviv, Israel

M. Sinclair
Mentor Education, Melbourne, VIC, Australia

A. Slezackova
Department of Medical Psychology and Psychosomatics, Faculty of Medicine, Masaryk University, Brno, Czech Republic

P. Stecz
Department of Clinical Psychology and Psychopathology, Institute of Psychology, University of Łódź, Łódź, Poland

O. Varsos
Centre for Positive Change, Melbourne, VIC, Australia

E. W. Herrera
Interdisciplinary Center for Development Studies (CIDER), School of Management, University of los Andes, Bogotá, Colombia

cultures differ not only in relation to the targets they hope for, but also regarding the actions performed to achieve their hopes and the sources which support their hopes in difficult situations. On the one hand, activities and sources of hope can be based on one's own resources and capabilities (e.g., working harder, assessing the situation more accurately, being more creative etc.). On the other hand, hope can be nurtured by activities entailing social support as well as spiritual, religious and other sources of faith (e.g., praying and meditating). Trust, faith and social support are particularly important when people feel they can do little to get their hopes fulfilled, either because they encounter their own limitations (e.g., a lack of knowledge or experience) or because their hopes are directed towards other people or to external events out of their control (e.g., the well-being of a family member or the weather) (Bruininks & Malle, 2005; Tennen et al., 2002; Tong et al., 2010).

In this chapter we aim to contribute to the knowledge of hope in two ways: Firstly, by theoretically investigating the concepts of trust and confidence in relation to hope. For this purpose, we adopted an interdisciplinary approach integrating psychological and philosophical perspectives with the discipline of Risk Management (e.g., Earle & Siegrist, 2006). Secondly, we explore and evaluate several sources and activities of hope across countries with a particular emphasis on trust and social support. How people hope and whom they generally trust can be better understood by assessing what people do to get their hopes fulfilled and which sources they connect with in order to remain hopeful, especially in times of struggle and disillusionment. In doing so, we address the third element in the proposed hope model, which is the trust in the availability of personal and other external resources as demonstrated in concrete activities and sources of hope.

6.2 Theoretical Background

6.2.1 Hope and Trust

Over the last decades, psychological theories and research on hope have evolved in two different directions. On the one hand, theories which emphasize the cognitive and individual dimensions, and on the other hand, psychological and philosophical works which highlight the emotional, social, and spiritual roots of hope. In the first category, hope has been conceptualized and investigated within a cognitive framework of self-regulation and goal-setting (Snyder, 2000; Stotland, 1969). One of the most prominent cognitive hope theories is that of Snyder (2000), which focuses on individual goals, together with the personal determination (will-power) and ability (way-power) to achieve these goals. According to Snyder (2002, p. 249): "Hope is defined as the perceived capability to derive pathways to desired goals, and motivate oneself via agency thinking to use those pathways." Agency, is basically the conviction that "I can do this" and pathways involve the self-confidence that "I'll find a way to get this done!" (Snyder, 2002, p. 251). This conceptualization of hope is fundamentally based on cognition, personal control and achievement and makes no distinction regarding different types of hoped-for ends.

Several authors in psychology and other disciplines have consistently argued and empirically demonstrated that hope is much more than a goal-setting process along with the personal will-power and capability to achieve individual goals (Averill et al., 1990; Bruininks & Malle, 2005; Farran et al., 1995; Scioli & Biller, 2009; Tennen et al., 2002). For Scioli and his colleagues (Scioli et al., 2016) fundamental hope is not only about personal mastery and individual goals, but likewise and principally about attachment, interpersonal trust, connection to other people as well as to a spiritual higher power. These psychologists have encouraged researchers to recognize the relevance of social relationships and to incorporate other elements such as trust in the conceptualization and investigation of hope. According to these authors, hope is to a large extent, emotional in nature and comprises a sense of trust that can be manifested in many different forms: trust in others (e.g., friends, therapists, and teachers), trust in the meaningfulness of things, trust in the benevolence of the world, trust in a higher power etc. From this point of view, trust is a constitutive and fundamental feature of hope (Tennen et al., 2002).

Erikson (1950) was one of the first psychologists to emphasize the role of a basic sense of trust in the formation of the fundamental virtue of hope. In his developmental theory, hope is the phenomenon emerging from the positive resolution of the existential conflict between fear and trust, which leaves a lasting tendency in the child to believe in the fulfilment of his/her existential needs despite the distress and the anger associated with them. Hope is the first human virtue that grows in the context of reliable and predictable bonds to caregivers in the form of primal trust, and becomes an essential part of one's own biography and character strength. This basic trust and hope become part of human identity, a basic sense of communion with other people, and of order and consistency between past, present and future, which is maintained throughout life. In this sense, fundamental hope and trust are the conditions for human life and human development par excellence. The initial basic trust in the caregivers expands in subsequent phases of life to trust in institutions of the social environment, which is why hope is fundamentally a dynamic and socio-psychological phenomenon in Erikson's work. Since hope in the future is based on a general and superior sense of belonging and togetherness, it can be sustained even in the face of specific threats and frustrations.

6.2.2 *Distinguishing Trust and Confidence*

In order to understand the phenomenon of trust in the context of hope, we turn to the Risk Management Model of Earle and Siegrist (2006), together with the work of other authors that have conceptually and empirically distinguished between the experiences of trust and confidence (for an overview, see Adams, 2005; Luhmann, 1988; Perry, 2011; White, 2009). Based on previous works of Rousseau et al. (1998), Rempel et al. (1985), Deutsch (1973), and Rotter (1980) among others,

Earle and Siegrist developed the TCC model (Trust, Confidence and Cooperation). Rousseau et al. (1998) proposed that there are three basic forms of trust, which correspond to different psychological processes: calculative, relational and institutional trust. Calculative trust is based on rational behavioral calculations, institutional trust relies on institutional controls and relational trust is rooted in social relationships.

Referring to the work of Luhmann (1988) and based on their own empirical studies, Earle and Siegrist (2006) made a clear conceptual distinction between confidence (calculative and institutional) and trust (relational) as two different psychological states. Whereas trust is defined "as the willingness to make oneself vulnerable to another based on a judgement of similarity of intentions or values", confidence, in contrast, "is the belief, based on experience or evidence (e.g., past performance), that certain future events will occur as expected." (Earle, 2009, p. 786). For the purpose of our study, we will explain these two concepts more in detail and relate them to the concepts of perceived hope (Krafft et al., 2017), dispositional optimism (Scheier & Carver, 1987) and dispositional hope (Snyder, 2000, 2002).

6.2.2.1 General Confidence and Self-Confidence

According to authors in the discipline of risk management, confidence is basically an intellectual, cognitive, analytical, and rational phenomenon rooted in judgements of past performance, objective facts, and personal or institutional control (Earle, 2001; Keller et al., 2011). Confidence arises as a result of specific knowledge and is built on reason and facts (Shaw, 1997). At the personal level, the antecedents of confidence are ability, competence and past performance. Furthermore, we rely on people that have already proved to be capable of performing a certain task and to generate the expected results. From an institutional point of view, confidence is related to regulations, social norms and institutions (political, economic etc.), that constrain future outcomes and make them foreseeable (Earle et al., 2001). Confidence is therefore linked to stability, consistency of past behaviors, objective facts, and all sorts of rules and routines (Earle, 2001). While trust relates to people, confidence is put in material objects like a bridge, an impersonal social system (e.g., a regulatory body) or in people treated like performance factors (Earle & Siegrist, 2006; Ullmann-Margalit, 2004). Whereas the scope of trust is cooperation and solidarity, the scope of confidence is accuracy and capabilities.

Confidence emerges in situations where the level of control and the ascribed probability of a certain outcome seem to be high and uncertainty is perceived as low (Adams, 2005). General confidence is therefore "the belief that things in general are under control, uncertainty is low, and events will occur as expected" (Earle, 2001, p. 32). In a broader sense, general confidence is the positive expectation that society can cope with future challenges and that everything is under control (Keller et al., 2011). In psychological terms, general confidence in the proper functioning of other people and the efficacy of social institutions is like a buffer which reduces tension and anxiety and conveys a feeling of security. Similar to unrealistic optimism (Weinstein, 1980), these beliefs can sometimes be positive illusions that help people cope with difficult life events with the often unconscious expectation of not being harmed or disappointed (Luhmann, 1988). Although confidence is an expectation about the future, its function is to reduce complexity and increase the sense of certainty and controllability either through extrapolation of knowledge from the past or by imposing constraints on the future (Earle, 2010).

A special type of confidence is the notion of self-confidence, which comprises beliefs in personal success, achievements, persistence, courage and self-awareness (White, 2009). Self-confidence is the confidence in oneself and in one's powers and abilities supporting the belief of one's competence to successfully complete a task (Lundberg, 2008; Perry, 2011). To feel self-confident, one firstly assesses his or her knowledge, abilities and skills in relation to a certain task or challenge. Based on this assessment, one develops a belief about how successful one will be (Koriat et al., 1980). How close the conceptualization of self-confidence is to Snyder's concept of dispositional hope is demonstrated by the following features: A recurrent characteristic in the definition of self-confidence is the personal belief that in a certain situation one can attain a positive outcome (Gesell, 2007; Mellalieu et al., 2006). The opposite of self-confidence is self-doubt and the fear of failure when confronted with upcoming tasks (Oleson et al., 2000). Another feature of self-confidence is persistence in the face of obstacles toward the accomplishment of personal goals (Hutchinson & Mercier, 2004). A third element is self-awareness and self-esteem in relation to an internal locus of control (Schunk & Pajares, 2005). The elements of self-confidence are in sum: goal-orientation, knowledge, personal skills, experience, autonomy, individual expectations, certainty, self-esteem, persistence and success, almost identical to the characteristics Snyder (2002) attributed to agency and pathways.

6.2.2.2 Interpersonal and General Trust

Trust is defined "as the willingness to make oneself vulnerable to another based on a judgement of similarity of intentions and values" (Earle & Siegrist, 2006, p. 386). Unlike confidence, which is based on evidence, performance and norms, trust is related to social interactions and therefore primarily intuitive and emotional (Siegrist, 2010). This social, intuitive and emotional trust is particularly relevant in absence of knowledge and when facing uncertainty (Siegrist et al., 2005). Social trust develops when feeling oneself part of a community (such as the family and friends) with shared values related to benevolence, integrity, fairness, and caring (Earle, 2001). Whereas confidence is backed in the observation of past performance, trust appears in the emotional and moral assessment of future intentions. We trust people whom we consider to have good intentions, support our values and would help us in case of necessity. In this sense, social trust is the first condition for solidarity, mutual cooperation and support.

According to Luhmann (1988), trust emerges only in the presence of risk and is associated with uncertainty and vulnerability (Adams, 2005; Mayer et al., 1995). Trust is the recognition of our mutual dependency. We all depend on the positive intentions of other people in one way or another. General trust is hence the sort of trust we maintain in connection to the larger society, based on the perception of common social values and purposes (Rotter, 1980). In a broader sense, trust is based on faith beyond reason and available evidence (Shaw, 1997). A generalized interpersonal trust rests on the belief that most people are good and can be trusted (Siegrist et al., 2005). A community or society which is only kept together on the basis of rules and constraints will be much more fragile and less resilient than a society where people trust each other because affective bonds and common values tie them together. In a community where people share common interests and values, they will be ready and willing to work together in order to pursue their visions and aspirations (Earle, 2009). Consequently, whereas confidence is a future expectation anchored in the past, trust is future oriented in that it entails taking risks and being open to uncertainty (Earle, 2001). That is why trust usually is concerned with affect laden promotion-oriented ideals while confidence is connected to prevention-oriented goals (Earle, 2010).

6.2.2.3 The Practical Dominance of Trust Over Confidence

Trust based on information about values and intentions seems to be more robust and dominant than confidence founded on rules, control, and performance information (De Bruin & Van Lange, 1999, 2000). At least with regard to trust and cooperation, values are more important than performance (Wojciszke et al., 1998). As long as one appreciates the values and intentions of another person, the failure of this person to perform and attain certain results will not affect the trust deposited in her/him. In other words, performance is interpreted in the light of morality and intentions (Earle et al., 2001). It is usually more relevant to know that the intentions of another person towards oneself or a common cause are good, than to know if the person is capable to perform (Earle, 2010). Whereas confidence is focused on concrete facts and rules constraining behavior, the nature of trust is to open up oneself to recognize the freedom of the other person. Consequently, hope and trust tend to expand the range of alternatives, while in the case of confidence the focus is on a few predefined possibilities (Luhmann, 1988). Conversely, of course, doubts about the good intentions of another person automatically affect trust and cooperation (Earle & Siegrist, 2006).

Table 6.1 summarizes the antecedents and fundamental elements of trust and (self-) confidence as discussed in the literature.

Table 6.1 Distinguishing trust and confidence

Trust	Confidence
Emotional and intuitive	Cognitive and rational
Relational, attachment-based	Rule-based, calculative, regulatory
Faith	Reason
Intentions	Abilities
Freedom	Control
Morality and values	Performance
Future oriented	Past oriented
Promotion oriented	Prevention oriented
Risk taking	Risk avoiding
Change	Constancy
Broadening future alternatives	Constraining future alternatives
Motivation	Reliance
Resilient	Fragile
Vulnerability and dependence	Capabilities and independence
Solidarity	Accuracy
Subjective	Objective
Cooperation	Individualism
Human relations	Technical processes
Uncertainty	Knowledge, evidence and facts

6.2.3 *Hope and Optimism*

6.2.3.1 Confident Optimism and Trustful Hope

The core features and characteristics of trust and confidence can be related to the main differences between hope and optimism (see also Milona, 2020b). Scheier and Carver (1987) conceptualized dispositional optimism as a positive future expectation assuming that "everything will go well" despite existing barriers and difficulties (Scheier et al., 2001). Originally, the concept of dispositional optimism emerged from the broader cognitive theory of self-regulation, which assumes that a person's behavior is oriented towards the achievement of certain goals (Carver & Scheier, 1981). Based on positive past experiences, individuals with an optimistic attitude have particularly positive expectations about the achievement of personal goals and, even when obstacles arise, they persist in their plans. Positive expectations are characterized as assessments of confidence about the feasibility of achieving a valuable goal. How close the notion of confidence is to the concept of optimism was shown in the exemplary work of de Jonge and his colleagues (de Jonge et al., 2007, 2008), who conceptualized consumer confidence in the safety of food as basically consisting of the dimensions optimism and pessimism.

Gray (1959, p. 225) considered the virtue of hope to be "that quality of character which is directed toward the future in trust rather than in confidence". Bruininks and Malle (2005) have investigated the differences between hope and optimism from the point of view of the layperson. Unlike optimism, people hope for things that are particularly relevant to them, but which are perceived to be less likely and less under their control (see also Averill et al., 1990). Hope is perceived as a fundamental emotion that enables people not to give up or despair when they feel unable to reach something they desire (Bruininks & Malle, 2005). This means that hope is particularly relevant when people face setbacks and difficulties. Optimism and dispositional hope, on the other hand, have been characterized as cognitions with a higher degree of personal control (Scheier & Carver, 1987; Snyder, 2000). People feel optimistic when things go smoothly. Furthermore, whereas hope is more connected to relational and altruistic goals (many times we hope for other people instead of for ourselves), optimism (and dispositional hope) seems to be especially related to personal achievement related targets.

To summarize: While dispositional optimism and dispositional hope have been conceptualized as cognitive states and traits, perceived hope, in a broader sense, is mainly an emotion with cognitive elements (Staats & Stassen, 1985). Whereas cognitive theories of dispositional optimism and hope are grounded in evidence, as well as in rational estimates about the likelihood of a desired outcome and confidence in personal efficacy, broader perceived hope is rooted in interpersonal trust and influenced by social attachment and support (Scioli et al., 1997). Basically, hope is particularly relevant and salient when people are confronted with uncertainty, adversity, and existential threats in which they cannot be optimistic anymore (Pruyser, 1986).

This is the reason why "hope dies last". As long as we are confident about the future, we can remain optimistic (Bury et al., 2016; Milona, 2020b). In these cases, trust and hope play a secondary role. Once we cannot rely on past experiences anymore and have lost control over future events, we have to face uncertainty, recognize our vulnerability and place our trust and hope in others. This suggests that hope and trust (and therefore values and positive emotions) would be more resilient and of a more fundamental value than confidence and optimism (based on facts and figures). In order to be able to retrieve our optimism in threatening times we must preserve hope and trust through the affection and assistance of others.

6.2.3.2 Exploring Trustful Hope

In this section we further explore the concept of trustful hope, integrating philosophical and psychological writings and highlighting the main features of personal and interpersonal hope based on trust. Meirav (2009) proposed that hope needs something more than a wish or desire and the belief in its possibility. To be able to hope, people must trust in the benevolence and support of some external factor (such as other people, luck, fate, God), which works in favor of the hoped-for good. As we have seen in a previous section, Erikson (1950) anchors the phenomenon of hope and trust in the quality of care in early childhood, which in later age can be extended to loving friends and family as well as to a caring community and a higher power (Marcel, 1962; Vaillant, 1993). The experience of hope and trust in the communion with other people is based on shared beliefs, values and concerns for something larger than oneself. This means that hope is grounded not only in the self but in a community of people (Martin, 2019).

McGeer (2008) elaborated on the concepts of substantial trust and substantial hope and explained their strong interdependence. Substantial trust involves a positive affective judgement about the goodwill of others that goes beyond the available evidence. We can trust people who in the past have not always demonstrated to be reliable. In such cases we place our hope and trust in the person not because the person has proved to be trustworthy, but just because we like, esteem or love her. By doing so, we are neither confident nor optimistic but believe in the good intentions of the other person and his/her potential to improve and grow. Therefore, substantial hope starts by accepting our limitations and those of others, but without surrendering to them. With this kind of hope we believe and trust ourselves and the others will continue to focus our attention on the desired good and, when possible, engage ourselves for its attainment. This indicates again that a hopeful trust goes beyond mere confidence. Moreover, it empowers people to develop their agency and willpower as well as their capabilities and possibilities transcending current limitations, caring and supporting each other in a process of mutual growth.

This is what McGeer (2004) referred to as "the art of good hope". She distinguished between a wishful, a willful, and a responsive kind of hope. Whereas a wishful hope involves an overreliance on external factors (too much confidence) and willful hope fearfully neglects one's own limitations (too much self-confidence), the good responsive and scaffolding hope emphasizes mutual dependency, trust and care. "Well-balanced hopers understand the need for relying on and developing their own powers of agency in formulating and pursuing their hopes, but such hopers also understand how others can significantly affect their powers, enhancing or inhibiting them depending on the quality of their various interactions. Hence, hoping well has an interpersonal dimension as well: it depends on finding—or making—a community in which individual hopers can experience the benefits of peer scaffolding" (McGeer, 2004, p. 123). McGeer (2004) defined peer scaffolding as "a particular mode of engagement in which individuals are supported in their capacity to hope, not primarily by way of material aid but rather by way of psychological aid" (p. 118).

6.2.4 *Integrating Both Worlds: Hope Sources and Activities*

To conclude the theoretical part of this chapter, we integrate the emotional and the cognitive dimensions of hope, as well as trust and (self-)confidence, focusing on the concrete sources and activities people relate to and perform in order to sustain their hopes and see their hopes fulfilled. People differ not only with regard to what they hope for but also in the way they hope. Walker (2006) recognized a motivational force incorporating different forms of attention, expression and behavior in hope. Martin's (2013) "Incorporation Theory of Hope" argued that the key to hope is to combine the value of what we hope for with the belief in the possibility of its fulfillment as a license to engage in different hope activities. A meaningful hope emerges when the value of what we hope for is expressed by engaging in meaningful and intrinsically valuable actions in order to make it happen (Bovens, 1999; McGeer, 2004; Milona, 2020a). This means that hope is fundamentally associated with action. Alternately, people cease to engage in hopeful activities either because they no longer believe in the possibility of their hopes and therefore give up or because their hopes are not considered desirable anymore (Blöser & Stahl, 2017).

Hope activities can be as varied as situations encountered and have been classified as cognitive, achievement, social and spiritual oriented activities (Averill et al., 1990; Scioli & Biller, 2009). The first two activities emphasize self-reliance on one's own possibilities, while the latter two activities emphasize trust in others and faith (Averill & Sundararajan, 2005). Cognitive activities are rooted in the intellectual human capacity of mental imaging, fantasizing, gathering information and planning (Bovens, 1999; Martin, 2011). Achievement and coping oriented activities such as working harder are related to active problem solving, personal effort, ambition and will (Snyder, 2002). Social oriented activities, as we have seen, are based on the availability of a valued person and can be differentiated as emotional and instrumental support (Shakespeare-Finch & Obst, 2011). To trust is an activity reflecting openness, disclosure, intimacy and the appreciation of the helpfulness of other people (Scioli & Biller, 2003). Even having faith and trust in a benevolent higher power by praying, meditating or going to church is an active engagement to remain hopeful in seemingly hopeless situations such as in case of an illness (Scioli et al., 2016). Furthermore, what people hope-for and how people hope seem to be influenced by the culture in which they live. Whereas in individualistic cultures people seem to be more self-confident and believe primarily in themselves, in more collectivistic cultures people tend to connect to other people and value external sources of hope (Averill & Sundararajan, 2005).

Beyond concrete actions to foster the realization of specific hopes, people can draw on several resources in order to remain hopeful and to nurture their hopefulness, even when there is little they can practically do to fulfill their desires. Shade (2001) characterized hope by its implicit resourcefulness in terms of finding and developing resources to support, direct and expand the ability to nurture one's general hopefulness and to foster the realization of one's particular hopes. In order to be hopeful, people must basically trust in the availability of resources to make their hopes happen, especially when confronting difficulties and obstacles (Scioli & Biller, 2003). Snyder et al. (1991) argued that hope is the belief that personal goals can be attained by one's own resources. However, especially in times of adversity, people can make use of numerous sources of hope in order to promote their hope. When personal resources are depleted, people can remain hopeful when they trust that external resources are available and can contribute to realizing their hopes (Tong et al., 2010).

Scioli and Biller (2003) distinguished several potential sources of trust and hope: Besides the self, they recognized external factors such as culture and tradition, diversity and equality, the economic system, nature, other people, science and a Higher Power. Whereas personal hope sources are grounded in the self, in one's own talents, experiences and abilities, which include imagination and creativity, external resources come into play in situations in which people perceive little control over their hoped-for targets. External resources can be the perceived emotional and instrumental support awaited from family members, friends and others (such as teachers, therapists, lawyers. etc.) but also the faith in a benevolent transcendent Higher Power or energy such as God, nature or simply luck (Shade, 2001).

Both internal and external sources of hope require an attitude of readiness and engagement on the part of the hoping person. According to Shade (2001), one important resource of hope is the ability to request and accept the support of others. This presupposes personal strengths such as the humility and courage to recognize one's own limitations and appreciate the abilities of others, the patience to wait for the right moment and the openness to accept new ideas. In a community of hope, the connection with others and the faith in a higher power are not only sources of hope but also valuable resources to maintain and expand one's own agency and abilities (McGeer, 2004, 2008). Social and spiritual resources can contribute to the empowerment, expansion and development of one's agency, which is especially of value in times of adversity (Lear, 2006). As soon as trust in another person or a higher power comes into play, hoping may well become a mutual activity (Stitzlein, 2019). Hopeful people accept external support when they need it and give support to others when they are able to do so.

6.3 Our Studies

6.3.1 Main Aim

Conceptualizing hope as a wish or desire for a valuable good which is considered to be possible (however not necessarily probable), together with trust in the availability of individual, social or spiritual resources to overcome difficulties and obstacles, the aim of our empirical studies reported in this chapter was to explore the sources and activities of hope relevant for maintaining hope and making one's hopes happen across several countries. Specifically, we focused on trust and social support. In the following sections we present two studies based on data collected through the Hope Barometer in 2018 and 2019. Study 1 examined the role of several sources of hope, with a specific focus on social support and further external hope resources such as religiosity and luck. We also explored their relationship with perceived and dispositional hope. Study 2 extended the findings of study 1 by centering on concrete activities people perform in order to get their hopes fulfilled and by evaluating their possible impact on hope.

6.3.2 *Study 1: Hope Sources, Social Support, Religiosity, and Luck*

6.3.2.1 Objectives

Study 1 examined several sources of hope across 12 countries as well as the relationship of these sources of hope with levels of perceived and dispositional (individualistic-cognitive) hope. Furthermore, we investigated the different aspects of social support (giving and receiving emotional and instrumental support) as indicators of social trust, together with the trust in a higher power and in an unspecific benevolent force experienced as "luck" in relation to hope.

We predicted that levels of perceived hope will be more strongly positively associated with social and spiritual sources than dispositional hope. We also expected that in more collectivist countries (e.g., Portugal, Nigeria, Colombia, India and South Africa), hope will be more related to social and spiritual sources than in more individualistic countries (Australia, Czechia, Italy, Israel, Poland, Spain, and Switzerland). Assuming the relevance of emotions and the role of peer scaffolding to maintain hope as suggested by McGeer (2004), we assumed that receiving and giving emotional support will be more important than receiving and giving instrumental support. Furthermore, we explored the impact of several external factors (social support, religiousness and luck) in different countries to predict hope.

6.3.2.2 Procedure and Participant Samples

Data was collected as part of the Hope Barometer in November 2019 through announcements in online newspapers, social media and e-mails. No incentives were offered. For this study we selected 12 countries each displaying a robust database of at least 200 participants. People younger than 18 were excluded from the analysis. A total of 10,287 participants completed the questionnaire, of 94 were removed due to a high number of missing values and obvious erroneous answers (e.g., always 0 or 1).

Participants were recruited in Australia ($N = 474$), Colombia ($N = 311$), the Czech Republic ($N = 469$), India ($N = 1092$), Israel ($N = 884$), Italy ($N = 272$), Nigeria ($N = 665$), Poland ($N = 481$), Portugal ($N = 507$), South Africa ($N = 574$), Spain ($N = 529$) and Switzerland ($N = 3935$). The questionnaire was delivered in English (Australia, Northern and Southern India, Nigeria and South Africa), Spanish (Colombia and Spain), Czech (Czech Republic), Hebrew (Israel), Italian (Italy and Switzerland), Polish (Poland), Portuguese (Portugal), Malayalam (Southern India) as well as French and German (Switzerland).

The demographic structure of the samples is exhibited in Appendix 6.1. Gender distribution is quite balanced in Australia, Colombia, India, South Africa and Switzerland. In the Czech Republic, Israel, Italy, Poland, Portugal and Spain, more women than men (about 70/30) and in Nigeria more men than women took part to the survey. The mean age varied, with the youngest sample being from Colombia ($M = 26.29$, $SD = 8.63$) and the oldest in Australia ($M = 47.53$, $SD = 13.05$) and Switzerland ($M = 46.82$, $SD = 15.67$). Regarding marital status and education, the samples were diverse. However, the Australian and Israeli samples included a large number of married people, the Colombian sample contained many people still living with their parents, and the Nigerian sample included a large number of single individuals. Many participants had a full- or part-time job, especially in Australia, Israel and Poland. In Colombia, Czechia, India and Spain, the samples included a larger number of people still in education or training.

6.3.2.3 Measures

Hope Sources

Krafft and Walker (2018) developed a list of 18 items describing different sources of hope fitting into 7 categories: (1) Religious ("I have experienced God's support"), (2) social-relational ("the support of family and friends"), (3) coping ("I have recovered well from illness"), (4) hedonic ("I have experienced great concerts and parties"), (5) personal mastery ("I have solved difficult problems"), (6) material-financial ("I have earned a lot of money"), and (7) altruistic ("Doing good for a meaningful cause"). The items could be rated on a scale from 0 (not at all) to 3 (very much).

Perceived Hope Scale

The general level of personal hope was assessed with the Perceived Hope Scale (PHS) (Krafft et al., 2017, 2021; Marujo et al., 2021; Slezackova et al., 2020). The PHS consists of six items to measure the level of hope as perceived by people in a direct manner and free from any preconceptions regarding the nature and quality of hope. The PHS is especially suitable to assess the level of general hope in different cultures since it avoids any bias regarding potential sources, roots, dimensions and elements of hope. The items of the PHS evaluate the degree of hope in general ("I feel hopeful"), in one's life ("I am hopeful with regard to my life") and in difficult situations. Further items assess the belief in the possibility of fulfillment of one's hopes and the intensity of general hope vis-à-vis the feeling of anxiety ("In my life hope outweighs anxiety"). The six positively worded items were rated on a 6-point Likert scale from 0 (strongly disagree) to 5 (strongly agree). In the current study the six items achieved a high internal consistency in all samples with Cronbach alpha values between $\alpha = 0.79$ and $\alpha = 0.90$.

Dispositional Hope Scale

To assess the individualistic-cognitive concept of hope we applied Snyder's Adult Dispositional Hope Scale (Snyder et al., 1991). The scale consists of four items to assess the motivational dimension of agency (will-power, e.g. "I energetically pursue my goals") and four items to assess the cognitive dimension of pathways (way-power, e.g. "I can think of many ways to get the things in life that are most important to me"). The eight items were scored on a 6-point scale ranging from 0 (strongly disagree) to 5 (strongly agree) and attained high internal consistency with values between $\alpha = 0.84$ and $\alpha = 0.91$.

Receiving and Giving Social Support

In order to measure the reciprocal nature of social support and trust we administered the 2-Way Social Support Scale (Shakespeare-Finch & Obst, 2011). The scale consists of 21 items designed to assess receiving emotional support (7 items, e.g. "There is at least one person that I feel I can trust"), receiving instrumental support (4 items, e.g. "There is someone who can help me fulfil my responsibilities when I am unable"), giving emotional support (5 items, e.g. "People confide in me when they have problems"), and giving instrumental support (5 items, e.g. "I am a person others turn to for help with tasks"). Participants were asked to indicate the degree to which each statement was true for them on a 6-point Likert scale ranging from 0 (not at all) to 5 (always). Reliability coefficients ranged between $\alpha = 0.91$ and $\alpha = 0.96$ for receiving emotional support, between $\alpha = 0.81$ and $\alpha = 0.90$ for receiving instrumental support, between $\alpha = 0.84$ and $\alpha = 0.91$ for giving emotional support and between $\alpha = 0.71$ and $\alpha = 0.83$ for giving instrumental support.

6.3.2.4 Data Analysis

All statistical analyses were performed with IBM SPSS and AMOS version 27.0. We first determined mean values of the sources of hope and compared them between countries. Thereafter, we calculated partial bivariate Pearson correlations controlling for demographic variables between the sources of hope and both constructs to assess perceived and dispositional hope.

Further analyses established levels of receiving and giving emotional and instrumental support as well as of religiosity and luck in all countries. By means of hierarchical regression analyses we then estimated the predictive power of different constructs representing several external factors of hope. After starting with demographic variables in step 1, we entered the two variables which measured receiving emotional and instrumental support in step 2, after which we included the two factors for giving emotional and instrumental support in step 3. This was followed by a composite variable to determine the level of religiousness in step 4, and finally the item "I have been always lucky" in step 5. To assess religiousness we combined two items describing religious sources of hope ("My prayers have been answered" and "I have experienced God's support") with an item describing a religious wish ("More religious and spiritual experiences"). The Cronbach Alpha indices for religiousness yielded high levels of reliability, between $\alpha = 0.82$ and $\alpha = 0.90$.

Group invariance across the 12 samples for the Perceived Hope Scale was already tested in Chap. 4, and the results indicated that we can assume that the PHS demonstrated satisfactory invariance across the investigated countries and that the individual scores can be compared. This would indicate that perceived hope has been conceptualized in a similar form across countries and that correlation analyses with other constructs are possible.

6.3.2.5 Results

Hope Sources: Descriptive Statistics

Table 6.2 displays the mean values and standard deviations of the 18 hope sources. We commence with an overview of the most general results which emerged as common patterns in most countries. The principal hope sources highly valued by most people were the social support of family and friends and the experience of doing good for a meaningful cause. Further important social oriented resources were the support of other people in difficult times as well as the gratitude of people one has helped. Cognitive and achievement-oriented experiences (success in education, in the job and solving difficult problems) were as important as the social sources. Less relevant in almost all countries were financial and technological resources, hedonic experiences (such as parties) and political engagement. The item "I have been always lucky" usually ranked at the center of the list. Furthermore, religious resources were of little importance for most people, but there were pronounced differences between countries.

Considering specific items, significant differences between countries emerged. Some Latin countries such as Spain, Colombia and Portugal stand out regarding both, social as well as achievement-oriented sources of hope. Experiencing support of family and friends, the helpfulness of other people in difficult times as well as the gratitude of people they have helped were significantly stronger for participants in these countries than those in Switzerland and Italy. Likewise, the achievement-oriented sources of hope such as successful education or studies, professional accomplishments and having been able to solve difficult problems in the past were scored higher in Colombia and Portugal than for example in Switzerland.

Memories of a happy childhood were experienced as a hope source most often in India, Spain, Colombia and South Africa, and the least in Poland and Czechia. Having earned a lot of money was significantly more relevant, although at a lower level, in Poland, Australia, India, Colombia, Nigeria and South Africa than in Spain, Italy, Switzerland, Israel, Portugal and Czechia. On the other hand, participants in Switzerland, Czechia and India especially benefited from pleasant experiences in nature, significantly more so than people in Nigeria, Italy, Spain, Israel and Poland.

Table 6.2 Hope sources—mean values, standard deviations and analysis of variance

	Australia		Colombia		Czech Rep.		India		Israel		Italy		Nigeria	
	M	*SD*	*M*	*SD*	*M*	*SD*	*M*	*SD*	*M*	*SD*	*M*	*SD*	*M*	*SD*
The support of family and friends	2.36	0.78	2.62	0.59	2.40	0.78	2.43	0.79	2.50	0.69	2.32	0.79	2.18	0.84
Doing good for a meaningful cause	2.17	0.86	2.36	0.77	2.29	0.81	2.31	0.81	2.45	0.71	2.16	0.86	2.43	0.66
Pleasant experiences in the free nature	1.99	0.90	2.00	0.95	2.09	0.87	2.09	0.90	1.84	0.90	1.75	1.03	1.69	0.80
Successful education or studies	1.91	0.92	2.42	0.77	1.97	0.89	2.25	0.88	2.01	0.86	1.93	0.98	2.26	0.77
I have solved difficult problems	2.03	0.83	2.25	0.75	1.94	0.93	1.98	0.87	1.87	0.86	2.01	0.82	2.03	0.78
The gratitude of those people I have helped	1.92	0.89	2.24	0.87	1.87	0.93	2.00	0.93	2.09	0.82	1.73	0.94	1.85	0.88
My professional successes and achievements	1.98	0.85	2.41	0.74	1.62	0.92	1.94	0.95	2.20	0.75	1.80	0.94	1.89	0.86
Other people have helped me in difficult times	1.82	0.90	2.29	0.81	2.00	0.92	1.98	0.92	1.81	0.87	1.75	0.89	1.87	0.87
Memories of a happy childhood	1.59	1.01	1.98	0.95	1.50	0.99	2.16	0.91	1.76	0.94	1.60	1.05	1.59	0.87
I have recovered well from illness	1.61	1.02	1.78	1.11	1.60	1.07	2.07	0.91	1.18	1.10	1.16	1.09	2.15	0.89
I have been always lucky	1.19	0.88	1.54	0.93	1.28	0.91	1.75	1.00	1.44	0.89	1.55	1.00	1.84	0.83
I have experienced great parties and concerts	1.45	1.04	1.43	1.07	1.17	1.01	1.51	1.09	1.26	0.96	1.35	1.02	1.12	0.89
I have experienced God's support	1.16	1.15	1.76	1.19	0.99	1.18	2.09	1.06	1.12	1.16	1.15	1.16	2.71	0.60
I have profited from technological progress	1.23	0.94	1.77	0.93	0.78	0.78	1.54	1.03	1.13	0.96	1.20	0.90	1.53	0.89
My prayers have been answered	1.11	1.11	1.46	1.18	1.06	1.15	2.09	1.01	1.36	1.11	1.12	1.01	2.32	0.76
I have earned a lot of money	1.24	0.87	1.17	0.88	0.88	0.86	1.20	1.09	0.87	0.84	0.57	0.74	1.08	0.82
Successful political involvement	0.62	0.86	0.73	0.92	0.31	0.61	0.88	1.07	0.52	0.78	0.28	0.61	0.64	0.85
Participation at political events	0.44	0.73	0.61	0.80	0.49	0.74	0.77	1.01	0.42	0.68	0.38	0.75	0.62	0.75

(continued)

Table 6.2 (continued)

	Poland		Portugal		South Africa		Spain		Switzerland		ANOVA		
	M	*SD*	*M*	*SD*	*M*	*SD*	*M*	*SD*	*M*	*SD*	*F*	Sig.	η^2
The support of family and friends	2.37	0.80	2.56	0.66	2.42	0.82	2.63	0.58	2.20	0.87	31.44	<0.001	0.033
Doing good for a meaningful cause	2.06	0.83	2.43	0.72	2.37	0.78	2.33	0.69	1.81	0.92	95.27	<0.001	0.093
Pleasant experiences in the free nature	1.85	0.93	1.97	0.90	2.05	0.92	1.80	0.91	2.13	0.92	23.15	<0.001	0.024
Successful education or studies	1.80	0.94	2.31	0.73	2.11	0.90	2.16	0.82	1.78	0.94	51.61	<0.001	0.053
I have solved difficult problems	2.27	0.77	2.13	0.82	2.10	0.84	1.93	0.77	1.83	0.87	22.92	<0.001	0.024
The gratitude of those people I have helped	1.89	0.90	2.08	0.87	2.16	0.85	2.27	0.79	1.75	0.92	34.47	<0.001	0.036
My professional successes and achievements	2.01	0.85	2.29	0.76	1.95	0.95	2.01	0.82	1.72	0.90	50.36	<0.001	0.052
Other people have helped me in difficult times	2.10	0.89	2.12	0.84	2.04	0.90	2.16	0.79	1.68	0.96	38.15	<0.001	0.040
Memories of a happy childhood	1.50	1.01	1.86	0.96	1.94	0.94	2.08	0.93	1.60	1.01	44.24	<0.001	0.046
I have recovered well from illness	1.86	1.00	1.53	1.16	1.83	1.03	1.43	1.10	1.46	1.09	66.58	<0.001	0.067
I have been always lucky	1.17	0.95	1.34	0.94	1.33	0.95	1.19	0.81	1.39	0.94	36.70	<0.001	0.038
I have experienced great parties and concerts	1.14	0.96	1.20	0.98	1.37	1.07	1.36	1.04	1.44	1.06	13.16	<0.001	0.014
I have experienced God's support	1.21	1.15	1.30	1.20	2.16	1.04	0.71	0.95	0.84	1.06	289.72	<0.001	0.238
I have profited from technological progress	1.36	0.88	1.39	0.90	1.38	0.99	1.31	0.90	1.23	0.92	37.17	<0.001	0.039
My prayers have been answered	1.13	1.14	1.33	1.14	1.99	1.04	0.72	0.91	0.86	1.02	225.66	<0.001	0.196
I have earned a lot of money	1.51	0.89	.088	0.87	1.06	0.89	0.49	0.70	0.83	0.85	60.73	<0.001	0.062
Successful political involvement	0.45	0.71	.072	0.90	0.77	0.96	0.42	0.71	0.32	0.67	51.61	<0.001	0.062
Participation at political events	0.46	0.69	0.59	0.79	0.52	0.83	0.38	0.69	0.35	0.68	30.25	<0.001	0.032

In Nigeria and India, the experience of having recovered well from an illness was an important hope source in contrast to people in Italy and Israel.

The most remarkable difference emerged with regard to the religious and spiritual sources of hope. People in Nigeria, India and South Africa have felt God's support and that their prayers have been answered more intensely than people in all other countries, especially those in Switzerland, Czechia and Spain, who displayed the lowest scores. Furthermore, people in Nigeria and India remarked they have been always lucky, a feeling that was significantly lower in Australia, Spain and Poland.

Hope Sources as Correlates of Perceived and Dispositional Hope

The next step was dedicated to analyzing levels of hope across all samples (see Table 6.3). Perceived and dispositional hope scores were moderately high (clearly above the center of the scale) in all countries. Furthermore, mean values of dispositional hope (expressing self-confidence) were slightly but statistically significantly higher than perceived hope (expressing trust) in almost all countries with exception of Nigeria and Czechia, where they were similar. Participants in Nigeria, Australia, India, South Africa and Israel exhibited the highest levels of perceived hope, and people in Switzerland, Poland, Spain, Czechia and Italy the lowest. Regarding dispositional hope, scores were the highest in Nigeria, Colombia, Australia, Italy and South Africa and the lowest in Czechia, Switzerland, Spain and Poland.

In the next step partial bivariate correlations were calculated between the 18 hope sources, on the one hand, and the general levels of perceived and dispositional hope, on the other (see Table 6.4). The analyses of the results were focused on three main questions: 1. Which sources of hope are the most strongly related to the general level of hope? 2. Which similarities and differences emerge regarding the coefficients

Table 6.3 Perceived and dispositional hope—mean values and standard deviations

	Perceived hope		Dispositional hope	
	M	*SD*	*M*	*SD*
Australia	3.71	0.88	3.89	0.78
Colombia	3.55	0.86	3.90	0.69
Czech Rep.	3.41	0.97	3.41	0.82
India	3.69	0.82	3.74	0.79
Israel	3.60	0.94	3.73	0.77
Italy	3.43	1.11	3.82	0.74
Nigeria	4.21	0.61	4.17	0.65
Poland	3.26	0.99	3.57	0.85
Portugal	3.50	1.00	3.75	0.69
South Africa	3.65	0.98	3.78	0.86
Spain	3.28	0.95	3.54	0.71
Switzerland	3.24	1.08	3.48	0.92
F/Sig.	70.21	<0.001	54.59	<0.001
eta2	0.07		0.06	

Table 6.4 Sources of hope—partial bivariate Pearson correlations with perceived and dispositional hope

	Australia		Colombia		Czech Rep.		India		Israel		Italy	
	PHS	DHS	PHS	DHS	PHS	DHS	PHS	DHS	PHS	DHS	PHS	DHS
Correlation PHS/DHS	0.706**		0.641**		0.552**		0.569**		0.680**		0.611**	
The support of family and friends	0.239**	0.189**	0.242**	0.180**	0.261**	0.187**	0.274**	0.200**	0.236**	0.208**	0.266**	0.187**
Doing good for a meaningful cause	0.287**	0.263**	0.203**	0.200**	0.278**	0.305**	0.276**	0.251**	0.287**	0.284**	0.264**	0.278**
Pleasant experiences in the free nature	0.211**	0.217**	0.131*	0.161**	0.167**	0.103*	0.148**	0.166**	0.264**	0.247**	0.211**	0.143*
Successful education or studies	0.208**	0.297**	0.107	0.149**	0.137**	0.216**	0.153**	0.182**	0.158**	0.132**	0.159**	0.348**
I have solved difficult problems	0.262**	0.396**	0.284**	0.324**	0.104*	0.180**	0.200**	0.285**	0.260**	0.330**	0.249**	0.440**
The gratitude of those people I have helped	0.182**	0.160**	0.105	0.108	0.191**	0.198**	0.210**	0.245**	0.182**	0.175**	0.226**	0.222**
My professional successes and achievements	0.392**	0.492**	0.319**	0.425**	0.168**	0.330**	0.169**	0.191**	0.258**	0.387**	0.240**	0.445**
Other people have helped me in difficult times	0.251**	0.215**	0.223**	0.181**	0.284**	0.202**	0.118**	0.093**	0.230**	0.191**	0.209**	0.142*
Memories of a happy childhood	0.247**	0.222**	0.268**	0.214**	0.214**	0.131**	0.202**	0.246**	0.287**	0.232**	0.286**	0.222**
I have recovered well from illness	0.178**	0.120**	0.103	0.184**	0.116*	0.155**	0.219**	0.240**	0.139**	0.098**	0.158**	0.138*
I have been always lucky	0.374**	0.317**	0.317**	0.234**	0.223**	0.208**	0.229**	0.203**	0.398**	0.327**	0.394**	0.248**
I have experienced great parties and concerts	0.171**	0.178**	0.232**	0.226**	0.061	0.095*	0.085**	0.058	0.176**	0.178**	0.148*	0.201**
I have experienced God's support	0.313**	0.164**	0.325**	0.208**	0.205**	0.045	0.203**	0.211**	0.278**	0.129**	0.403**	0.252**
I have profited from technological progress	0.218**	0.225**	0.206**	0.268**	0.016	0.132**	0.135**	0.149**	0.214**	0.239**	0.144*	0.178**
My prayers have been answered	0.314**	0.185**	0.296**	0.189**	0.209**	0.052	0.324**	0.264**	0.242**	0.142**	0.460**	0.340**
I have earned a lot of money	0.253**	0.263**	0.122*	0.154**	−0.073	0.121**	0.091**	0.096**	0.149**	0.139**	0.180**	0.194**
Successful political involvement	0.083	0.060	0.068	0.110	−0.046	0.026	0.143**	0.044	0.110**	0.101**	0.078	0.038
Participation at political events	0.007	0.042	0.085	0.077	0.032	0.066	0.139**	0.011	0.084*	0.099**	0.092	0.047

	Nigeria		Poland		Portugal		South Africa		Spain		Switzerland	
	PHS	DHS	PHS	DHS	PHS	DHS	PHS	DHS	PHS	DHS	PHS	DHS
Correlation PHS/DHS	0.582**		0.559**		0.577**		0.654**		0.653**		0.684**	
The support of family and friends	0.221**	0.207**	0.314**	0.215**	0.172**	0.167**	0.353**	0.255**	0.232**	0.165**	0.311**	0.252**
Doing good for a meaningful cause	0.300**	0.364**	0.281**	0.243**	0.204**	0.275**	0.385**	0.323**	0.216**	0.202**	0.333**	0.274**
Pleasant experiences in the free nature	0.268**	0.313**	0.135**	0.128**	0.221**	0.213**	0.250**	0.317**	0.200**	0.218**	0.299**	0.325**
Successful education or studies	0.225**	0.308**	0.117*	0.203**	0.214**	0.257**	0.209**	0.280**	0.188**	0.191**	0.225**	0.273**
I have solved difficult problems	0.285**	0.422**	0.277**	0.335**	0.253**	0.275**	0.369**	0.461**	0.255**	0.392**	0.352**	0.478**
The gratitude of those people I have helped	0.193**	0.230**	0.223**	0.167**	0.255**	0.230**	0.266**	0.254**	0.150**	0.132**	0.222**	0.177**
My professional successes and achievements	0.259**	0.385**	0.263**	0.367**	0.209**	0.254**	0.287**	0.426**	0.228**	0.347**	0.349**	0.448**
Other people have helped me in difficult times	0.254**	0.248**	0.265**	0.181**	0.154**	0.214**	0.310**	0.201**	0.215**	0.191**	0.262**	0.175**
Memories of a happy childhood	0.188**	0.255**	0.250**	0.095*	0.271**	0.198**	0.281**	0.203**	0.280**	0.179**	0.250**	0.174**
I have recovered well from illness	0.109**	0.152**	0.165**	0.099*	0.143**	0.084	0.215**	0.229**	0.096*	0.157**	0.263**	0.261**
I have been always lucky	0.303**	0.381**	0.299**	0.261**	0.229**	0.204**	0.276**	0.334**	0.358**	0.319**	0.403**	0.349**
I have experienced great parties and concerts	0.123**	0.189**	0.100*	0.103*	0.145**	0.091*	0.170**	0.234**	0.156**	0.104*	0.200**	0.193**
I have experienced God's support	0.295**	0.240**	0.356**	0.109*	0.266**	0.147**	0.375**	0.266**	0.203**	0.212**	0.249**	0.160**
I have profited from technological progress	0.175**	0.313**	0.152**	0.260**	0.156**	0.109*	0.196**	0.252**	0.180**	0.205**	0.229**	0.250**
My prayers have been answered	0.374**	0.309**	0.366**	0.101*	0.253**	0.073	0.390**	0.253**	0.195**	0.192**	0.272**	0.175**
I have earned a lot of money	0.192**	0.305**	0.115*	0.145**	0.061	−0.001	0.176**	0.264**	0.117**	0.149**	0.235**	0.305**
Successful political involvement	0.074	0.173**	0.029	0.034	0.065	0.166**	0.200**	0.209**	0.053	0.053	0.128**	0.114**
Participation at political events	0.048	0.126**	0.051	0.056	0.092*	0.141**	0.198**	0.235**	0.092*	0.086*	0.160**	0.127**

Note: **. Correlation is significant at 0.01 level, *. Correlation is significant at 0.05 level, *PHS* Perceived Hope Scale, *DHS* Dispositional Hope Scale, control variables: Gender, age, marital status, education, main activity, professional status related to both constructs of hope? 3. Which similarities and differences can be detected between countries?

The first noteworthy results were the high correlation coefficients between perceived and dispositional hope (between $r = 0.55$ and $r = 0.70$) and that most of the hope sources correlate significantly with both hope constructs (with exception of the two items portraying political activities) but with notable differences in effect sizes within and between samples. Achievement oriented sources such as "I have solved difficult problems" and "my professional successes and achievements" were moderately associated with hope but clearly stronger with dispositional hope than with perceived hope. On the other hand, religious and social related sources as well as the experience of luck in one's life were also moderately related to hope, but more markedly with perceived hope.

In several countries such as Australia, Colombia, Italy, Nigeria, Poland and South Africa, the religious and spiritual sources of hope especially displayed moderately high correlation coefficients with perceived hope, while the achievement-oriented items also showed moderately high effects with dispositional hope. In Portugal, India and the Czech Republic the correlation effects between the achievement-oriented hope sources (having solved difficult problems in the past and professional successes) and dispositional hope are notably weaker. Whereas in the Italian and the South African samples the correlation coefficients between perceived hope and the religious items were the highest among all countries, the Czech and Spanish samples displayed the lowest. The correlation coefficients between luck and perceived hope were the strongest in Switzerland, Israel and Italy.

In the South African sample, the association of the social sources of hope (family, friends, and other people) as well as "doing good for a meaningful cause" in relation to perceived hope were especially strong. Interestingly, in South Africa, the religious items and "doing good…" were not only the strongest correlators with perceived hope, but did also display moderate correlation effects with dispositional hope. Remarkably, "luck" exhibited a stronger association with dispositional hope than with perceived hope, which could indicate that one's will- and way-power not only results from the appreciation of one's own capabilities but also from a benevolent external factor. Even more pronounced was a similar effect in Nigeria and in Italy, where dispositional hope correlated moderately high with achievement-oriented sources, but also with doing good and having luck as well as with the faith related to prayers. This could mean that people in Nigeria, Italy and South Africa are able to connect and integrate personal, religious and other external sources of hope in a very natural manner.

Having earned a lot of money displayed low effects on both hope types, with the highest coefficients emerging in Switzerland and Nigeria. In Switzerland (and with lower effects also in Israel) both hope constructs were similarly related to achievement experiences, to social sources as well as to the external factor of luck, while the effects of the religious resources were less pronounced. Furthermore, the item "doing good…", which unites accomplishment and social values displayed a moderate effect on perceived and dispositional hope too.

Consequently, it can be concluded that social and religious hope sources anchored in trust experiences with other people and a higher power are moderately associated with perceived hope. Achievement and mastery-oriented hope sources are more likely associated with dispositional hope, emphasizing the closeness of dispositional hope to the concept of self-confidence. Whereas self-centered hope sources were more pronounced in countries such as Switzerland, Spain, Israel and Czechia, social and religious hope sources were more salient in countries such as Nigeria, South Africa, India, and Italy. Furthermore, it can be assumed that people in certain countries like South Africa, Italy and Nigeria could integrate social, religious and achievement-oriented hope sources more smoothly. In other countries such as Switzerland and Israel, the religious sources seem to be replaced by the experience of luck and nature, underscoring the importance of some external factor in countries with low levels of religiosity.

Social Support, Religiosity, and Luck: Descriptive Statistics

We started our next analyses calculating mean values and standard deviations for the four social support dimensions as well as for religiosity and luck (see Table 6.5). Mean scores of receiving emotional and instrumental support were relatively high (above the scale center of 2.5) but with significant differences between countries. Interestingly, in almost all countries (with exception of India) the degrees of receiving emotional support were significantly higher than receiving instrumental support. Likewise, mean values of giving emotional and instrumental support to others were also above the center of the scale in all countries, but giving emotional support was significantly more pronounced than giving instrumental support.

Receiving emotional support was especially evident in Spain, Colombia, Portugal and Israel and the least in Nigeria, South Africa, India and Switzerland. Similarly, mean scores of receiving instrumental support were the highest in Spain, Colombia, Poland and Israel and the lowest in Nigeria, Switzerland, South Africa, Czechia and India. Giving emotional support was more pronounced in Portugal, Poland, Spain and Colombia and less evident in India, Switzerland, Nigeria and South Africa. Furthermore, giving instrumental support achieved the highest scores in Portugal, Nigeria, Australia, South Africa, and Poland and the lowest in Italy, Switzerland, Czechia, Israel, and Colombia.

We also determined mean values for two further external hope sources, religiosity and luck, which displayed significant differences between countries. People in Nigeria, South Africa, and India presented mean values of religiosity and luck clearly above the center of the scale. In Colombia Portugal, Israel and Poland religiosity scores were moderate and in Spain, Switzerland and Czechia especially low. The experience of luck was particularly strong in Nigeria and India, moderate in Italy, Colombia, Israel, Switzerland, Portugal and South Africa, and rather low in Poland, Spain, Australia and Czechia. The relationship between religiosity and luck was also of interest. Whereas in Nigeria, South Africa and India religiosity scores were higher than luck, in Switzerland, Spain, Italy, Czechia and Israel the experience

Table 6.5 Social support, religiosity and luck—mean values, standard deviations and analysis of variance

	Australia		Colombia		Czech Rep.		India		Israel		Italy		Nigeria	
	M	*SD*	*M*	*SD*	*M*	*SD*	*M*	*SD*	*M*	*SD*	*M*	*SD*	*M*	*SD*
Receiving Emotional Support	3.97	1.20	4.32	0.83	4.01	1.12	3.74	1.21	4.21	0.96	4.09	0.97	3.65	1.14
Receiving Instrumental Support	3.73	1.28	3.99	0.98	3.56	1.11	3.68	1.15	3.92	1.06	3.73	1.05	3.21	1.24
Giving Emotional Support	4.05	0.85	4.14	0.72	4.13	0.70	3.89	0.92	4.11	0.69	4.10	0.72	4.03	0.77
Giving Instrumental Support	3.80	0.85	3.61	0.86	3.46	0.89	3.64	0.99	3.57	0.84	3.29	0.82	3.83	0.79
Religiosity	1.16	0.99	1.58	1.05	1.03	1.02	1.99	0.82	1.22	0.96	1.16	0.93	2.48	0.55
Luck	1.19	0.88	1.54	0.93	1.28	0.91	1.75	1.00	1.44	0.89	1.55	1.00	1.84	0.83

	Poland		Portugal		South Africa		Spain		Switzerland		ANOVA		
	M	*SD*	*M*	*SD*	*M*	*SD*	*M*	*SD*	*M*	*SD*	*F*	Sig.	η^2
Receiving Emotional Support	4.17	1.06	4.30	0.95	3.76	1.30	4.39	0.76	3.96	1.22	31.31	<.001	0.03
Receiving Instrumental Support	3.95	1.09	3.83	1.07	3.54	1.37	4.12	0.89	3.48	1.38	32.08	<.001	0.03
Giving Emotional Support	4.21	0.71	4.34	0.62	4.06	0.90	4.21	0.63	3.97	0.89	17.82	<.001	0.02
Giving Instrumental Support	3.75	0.80	3.88	0.78	3.80	0.93	3.68	0.69	3.45	0.97	31.01	<.001	0.03
Religiosity	1.21	1.03	1.30	1.03	2.07	0.91	0.70	0.79	0.81	0.89	333.26	<.001	0.27
Luck	1.17	0.95	1.34	0.94	1.33	0.95	1.19	0.81	1.39	0.94	36.70	<.001	0.04

of luck had primacy over religiosity. In Colombia, Portugal, Poland and Australia both constructs scored at a similar level.

Regression Analyses Predicting Perceived Hope

Before presenting the results of the regression analyses, a first look at the partial bivariate correlations for the entire data including all countries presented in Table 6.6 reveal moderate positive associations of perceived hope with receiving emotional and instrumental support, religiosity and luck, and low effects with giving emotional and instrumental support (after controlling for samples and demographic variables). Furthermore, the correlation coefficients between all four dimensions of social support and religiosity and luck were rather low.

Turning to the results of the regression analyses predicting perceived hope reported in Table 6.7, some common and some individual results came forward. In general terms, receiving social support had a greater impact on hope (between 6.7% and 20.3% of the explained variance) than giving social support (between 0 and 8.5% of hope's variance). Moreover, the predictive effect of receiving emotional support was more salient than the effect of receiving instrumental support in almost all countries except Poland. Receiving instrumental support displayed a positive impact on hope only in Israel, Poland, Spain and Switzerland, but not in the other country samples. With regards to giving support to others, the patterns were less uniform. Whereas giving emotional support had a positive association with hope in the Israeli, Nigerian, Spanish and Swiss samples, giving instrumental support displayed a positive predictive effect in India, Nigeria, Poland, and Portugal.

Religiosity revealed a positive impact on hope in all countries (explained variance from 2.5% in Spain to 15.8% in Italy), with the highest coefficients arising in South Africa, Poland, Italy and Nigeria. The unspecific external factor of luck had an additional predictive effect on hope, between 1.6% in Nigeria and 5.4% in Spain. Whereas in Switzerland, Spain and Israel the effect of luck on hope is visibly higher than the effect of religiosity, in South Africa, Poland and Italy the contribution of religiosity is clearly stronger than the effect of luck. In Australia and Colombia, the impact of religiosity and luck on hope are almost at the same level (in terms of adjusted beta).

6.3.2.6 Summary of Findings

The general objective of this study was to assess a variety of hope sources and the expression of trust, social support and other external factors on hope across several countries. We assumed that social and spiritual sources would be associated with perceived hope more strongly than with dispositional hope and that they would be more pronounced in collectivistic than in individualistic countries. The results of Study 1 reveal four major findings: (1) the importance and role of different hope sources; (2) the distinct characteristics of perceived and dispositional hope; (3) the

Table 6.6 Perceived hope, social support, religiosity and luck—partial bivariate Pearson correlations

	Perceived Hope	Receiving Emotional Support	Receiving Instrumental Support	Giving Emotional Support	Giving Instrumental Support	Religiosity
Perceived Hope	1					
Receiving Emotional Support	0.337**	1				
Receiving Instrumental Support	0.345**	0.791**	1			
Giving Emotional Support	0.250**	0.403**	0.363**	1		
Giving Instrumental Support	0.266**	0.301**	0.329**	0.622**	1	
Religiosity	0.382**	0.032**	0.064**	0.085**	0.167**	1
Luck	0.363**	0.195**	0.233**	0.101**	0.128**	0.285**

Note: **. Correlation is significant at 0.01 level; control variables: Country, gender, age, marital status, education, main activity, professional status

Table 6.7 Hierarchical regression analyses predicting perceived hope

	Australia		Colombia		Czech Republic		India		Israel		Italy	
	Std. β	Sig.	Std. β	Sig.	Std. β	Sig.	Std. β	Sig.	Std. β	Sig.	Std. β	Sig.
Step 1: Demographics							Std. β					
Gender	−0.112	0.006	−0.054	0.301	0.030	0.458	0.016	0.571	−0.022	0.448	0.062	0.259
Age	0.017	0.705	0.167	0.027	0.153	0.057	0.072	0.159	0.052	0.155	0.116	0.103
Family Status	0.097	0.022	−0.033	0.616	0.055	0.372	−0.042	0.381	0.032	0.339	−0.096	0.123
Education	0.096	0.013	−0.025	0.640	0.001	0.988	0.085	0.003	−0.014	0.646	−0.041	0.434
Main activity	0.024	0.544	−0.160	0.033	−0.004	0.957	−0.063	0.103	0.031	0.340	−0.003	0.967
Professional Status	0.072	0.070	0.110	0.085	0.037	0.437	0.156	<0.001	0.051	0.092	0.093	0.098
Step 2: Receiving Social Support												
Receiving Emotional Support	0.225	0.002	0.273	0.001	0.268	<0.001	0.129	0.001	0.215	<0.001	0.153	0.058
Receiving Instrumental Support	0.024	0.745	0.027	0.743	0.080	0.233	0.031	0.425	0.132	0.005	0.109	0.145
Step 3: Giving Social Support												
Giving Emotional Support	0.094	0.142	−0.011	0.859	0.079	0.148	0.002	0.957	0.085	0.013	0.057	0.379
Giving Instrumental Support	0.079	0.200	0.097	0.122	0.026	0.631	0.176	<0.001	0.046	0.165	−0.022	0.730
Step 4: Religiosity	0.231	<0.001	0.226	<0.001	0.158	<0.001	0.224	<0.001	0.195	<0.001	0.340	<0.001
Step 5: Luck	0.223	<0.001	0.222	<0.001	0.131	0.002	0.103	<0.001	0.240	<0.001	0.190	0.001
											Adj. R^2	
	Adj R^2	Sig.	Adj. R^2	Sig.	Adj. R^2	Sig.	Adj. R^2	Sig.	Adj. R^2	Sig.	Adj. R^2	Sig.
Model 1: Step 1	0.040	<0.001	0.034	0.011	0.056	<0.001	0.062	<0.001	0.045	<0.001	0.015	0.123
Model 2: Steps 1–2	0.180	<0.001	0.170	<0.001	0.233	<0.001	0.139	<0.001	0.226	<0.001	0.137	<0.001
Model 3: Steps 1–3	0.211	<0.001	0.185	<0.001	0.238	<0.001	0.173	<0.001	0.246	<0.001	0.132	<0.001
Model 4: Steps 1–4	0.290	<0.001	0.238	<0.001	0.264	<0.001	0.228	<0.001	0.312	<0.001	0.290	<0.001
Model 5: Steps 1–5	0.333	<0.001	0.283	<0.001	0.278	<0.001	0.236	<0.001	0.358	<0.001	0.317	<0.001
Δ Step 2	0.141	<0.001	0.136	<0.001	0.177	<0.001	0.077	<0.001	0.181	<0.001	0.122	<0.001
Δ Step 3	0.030	<0.001	0.015	0.024	0.005	0.075	0.034	<0.001	0.019	<0.001	−0.005	0.808
Δ Step 4	0.080	<0.001	0.053	<0.001	0.026	<0.001	0.055	<0.001	0.066	<0.001	0.158	<0.001
Δ Step 5	0.042	<0.001	0.045	<0.001	0.014	0.002	0.008	<0.001	0.046	<0.001	0.027	0.001

(continued)

Table 6.7 (continued)

	Nigeria		Poland		Portugal		South Africa		Spain		Switzerland	
	Std. β	Sig.	Std. β	Sig.	Std. β	Sig.	Std. β	Sig.	Std. β	Sig.	Std. β	Sig.
Step 1: Demographics												
Gender	−0.031	0.363	−0.048	0.250	−0.070	0.061	−0.040	0.273	−0.018	0.638	0.018	0.199
Age	0.082	0.071	0.046	0.368	0.172	0.005	0.000	0.996	0.164	0.018	0.120	<0.001
Family Status	−0.019	0.658	0.096	0.047	0.081	0.142	0.026	0.562	−0.121	0.045	−0.014	0.340
Education	−0.012	0.734	−0.052	0.251	−0.011	0.772	−0.022	0.554	0.018	0.627	0.088	<0.001
Main activity	−0.057	0.108	−0.087	0.125	0.122	0.028	0.053	0.182	0.126	0.049	0.016	0.311
Professional Status	0.032	0.360	0.084	0.056	0.038	0.372	0.049	0.185	0.056	0.188	0.082	<0.001
Step 2: Receiving Social Support												
Receiving Emotional Support	0.108	0.034	0.063	0.370	0.232	<0.001	0.154	0.023	0.193	0.002	0.193	<0.001
Receiving Instrumental Support	0.011	0.822	0.173	0.016	0.011	0.849	0.039	0.549	0.161	0.009	0.164	<0.001
Step 3: Giving Social Support												
Giving Emotional Support	0.139	0.003	0.038	0.479	−0.007	0.889	0.029	0.750	0.117	0.020	0.097	<0.001
Giving Instrumental Support	0.120	0.010	0.124	0.019	0.128	0.007	0.112	0.233	0.009	0.846	0.001	0.939
Step 4: Religiosity	0.289	<0.001	0.302	<0.001	0.199	<0.001	0.325	<0.001	0.120	0.002	0.167	<0.001
Step 5: Luck	0.140	<0.001	0.159	<0.001	0.128	0.001	0.169	<0.001	0.251	<0.001	0.221	<0.001
	Adj. R^2	Sig.	Adj. R^2	Sig.	Adj. R^2	Sig.	Adj. R^2	Sig.	Adj. R^2	Sig.	Adj. R^2	Sig.
Model 1: Step 1	0.008	0.078	0.053	<0.001	0.204	<0.001	0.014	0.031	0.042	<0.001	0.072	<0.001
Model 2: Steps 1–2	0.075	<0.001	0.180	<0.001	0.284	<0.001	0.126	<0.001	0.221	<0.001	0.275	<0.001
Model 3: Steps 1–3	0.160	<0.001	0.200	<0.001	0.300	<0.001	0.158	<0.001	0.232	<0.001	0.283	<0.001
Model 4: Steps 1–4	0.254	<0.001	0.298	<0.001	0.348	<0.001	0.266	<0.001	0.257	<0.001	0.324	<0.001
Model 5: Steps 1–5	0.270	<0.001	0.320	<0.001	0.362	<0.001	0.291	<0.001	0.310	<0.001	0.365	<0.001
Δ Step 2	0.067	<0.001	0.127	<0.001	0.080	<0.001	0.113	<0.001	0.179	<0.001	0.203	<0.001
Δ Step 3	0.085	<0.001	0.020	0.001	0.016	0.001	0.032	<0.001	0.011	0.010	0.008	<0.001
Δ Step 4	0.094	<0.001	0.098	<0.001	0.048	<0.001	0.108	<0.001	0.025	<0.001	0.041	<0.001
Δ Step 5	0.016	<0.001	0.022	<0.001	0.014	0.001	0.025	<0.001	0.054	<0.001	0.041	<0.001

relevance of several dimensions of social support and other external factors such as religiosity and luck for hope; as well as (4) the distinctive nature of diverse hope sources across people in different countries.

In general terms and across all samples, social sources of hope such as the support of family and friends, doing good for a meaningful cause, and the gratitude of people one has helped, are at least as important as self-centered, performance and mastery-oriented sources such as a successful education or job and having solved difficult problems. Of lesser significance in most countries were financial and technical resources, political events as well as (however not in all countries) religious experiences. The factor "luck" was of moderate importance in most of the samples.

Social, religious, and achievement-oriented sources displayed moderate correlation coefficients with perceived and dispositional hope but with major differences between samples. Overall, as expected, whereas achievement and mastery-oriented hope sources were more strongly related to dispositional hope, social and religious oriented hope sources displayed a greater association with perceived hope. Despite the huge economic and social differences between the 12 countries under study, the levels of perceived and dispositional hope were of a moderately high magnitude in all samples. Moreover, participants in Nigeria, India, South Africa, Australia, and Israel displayed significantly higher levels of perceived and dispositional hope than those in Switzerland, Spain, Czechia, and Poland (with Italy in between).

Hope sources related to social support were of special importance in some Latin countries such as Spain, Colombia, and Portugal and of lesser importance in Switzerland and Italy. However, social sources of hope were moderately associated with perceived hope in all countries and especially in South Africa. In line with the emotional nature of hope, to receive and give emotional support is, as assumed, for most people much more significant in terms of hope than receiving and giving instrumental support, especially for people in Latin countries (Spain, Portugal and Colombia). Surprisingly, participants in Nigeria, South Africa and India, together with those in Switzerland expressed lower levels of receiving and giving emotional support. Alternately, the samples from Nigeria, South Africa and India reported to give more instrumental support as well as having higher levels of religiosity and luck. For people in non-European countries the hope supporting factor of earning money was significantly more important than for people in European countries.

Religious and spiritual hope sources paired with the experience of luck were mainly relevant for people in Nigeria, India and South Africa and to a much lower extent in Switzerland, Czechia and Spain. On the other hand, people in Switzerland and Czechia nurtured their hope through inspiring experiences in nature, which could also be considered as a significant external factor fostering hope. In South Africa, Nigeria and Italy, the experiences of doing good, luck and faith in God were highly associated with both perceived and dispositional hope. Religious sources were the least related to perceived hope in the Czech, Spanish and Swiss samples. Luck, instead, was more related to hope in Switzerland, Israel and Italy. The relevance of religiosity and the perception of being lucky was furthermore substantiated by the regression analyses.

Concluding, the results of this study revealed the general importance of trust, social support, religiosity and the perception of luck, as well as other external factors of hope like stimulating experiences in nature, as significant sources of hope. However, they also disclosed significant differences and notable results across countries. Specifically, people with higher levels of hope located in Nigeria, South Africa and India were those with the highest levels of religiosity and luck along with the strongest predictive effects of these factors on perceived hope. To the contrary, people in Switzerland, Czechia and Spain expressed both the lowest levels of hope and the lowest levels of religiosity. Furthermore, people in some Latin countries such as Spain, Portugal and Colombia drew hope the most from social sources, especially from receiving and giving emotional support, which for people in Switzerland, Nigeria, South Africa and India seemed to be less relevant.

Beyond these practical findings, our results could also reveal an important insight regarding the association between religiosity and luck as external factors of hope. For example, for people in Italy, a country with deep Catholic roots and where the Church enjoys a high reputation, trusting God and considering oneself lucky both exhibited a strong correlation with hope (see Table 6.4). In the regression analysis, however, religiosity accounted for the largest proportion of explained variance, absorbing most of the effect of luck. This could imply, that the perception of luck has its roots in religious faith. However, in Spain, where resentment against the Catholic Church is still strong, the predominant external factor was not religiosity but the experience of luck, with beta scores and variance explained of hope exceeding those in Italy, indicating that the perception of luck is either related to an unspecific benevolent external force, which people probably cannot describe or even be aware of, or to one's own efforts. In this sense, we could go one step further and assume that whereas the nature of religiosity is clearly relational (one's communion with God), the nature of "luck" might be either rooted in an external (religious, spiritual or metaphysical) force, or otherwise be the expression of a self-centered attitude ("I'm the lucky one" or even more extreme "I'm the creator of my own luck"). However, in any case, we still assume that both factors, religiosity and luck, by and large, should be considered external sources of hope.

6.3.3 Study 2: Hope Activities

6.3.3.1 Objectives

Departing from the notion of hope as a disposition to act (Martin, 2013), the aim of study 2 was to investigate several cognitive, social, spiritual and other activities people perform in order to see their hopes fulfilled. We assessed common patterns and differences between countries regarding the intensity of such activities and evaluated to what extent these hope activities were associated with the general level of perceived hope. We expected that participants in more individualistic countries such as Switzerland, Italy and Australia, would prefer cognitive activities and that these activities would show a stronger impact on hope than social and spiritual activities, while in more collectivistic countries such as Nigeria, South Africa, Colombia and India it would be the other way around.

6.3.3.2 Procedure and Participant Samples

Data was collected with the Hope Barometer survey in November 2018, announcing it in online newspapers, social media and e-mails. No incentives were offered. For this study we selected eight samples from German ($N = 3049$) and French ($N = 1109$) speaking Switzerland, France ($N = 135$), Spain ($N = 528$), Portugal ($N = 808$), Czechia ($N = 338$), Poland ($N = 169$) and South Africa ($N = 109$). People younger than 18 were excluded from the analysis. A total of 6548 people completed the questionnaire, from which 303 were removed due to a high number of missing values, obvious erroneous answers (e.g., always 0 or 1) and multivariate outliers.

The demographic structure of the samples is exhibited in Appendix 6.2. Gender distribution was quite balanced in the two Swiss samples (around 40% male and 60% female). In the other samples, we have considerably more female than male participants. Regarding age, Swiss and South African participants were on average the oldest and Czech were the youngest. The distribution of the marital status was quite comparable across countries, however with significantly more married people being part of the South African and Polish samples, and more single people belonging to the Portuguese group. As in the previous studies, the education level was difficult to compare due to different education systems. Most of the (older) South African participants held a university degree, which is clearly not representative for the general population in this country. Overall, most of the participants had a full-time or a part-time job as employees or in management positions.

6.3.3.3 Measures

Hope Activities

Participants could assess a list of 13 activities people perform in order to fulfil their hopes (Krafft & Walker, 2018). The 13 items belong to four dimensions: (1) The cognitive-rational dimension (e.g., "I think a lot and analyze circumstances"), (2) the social-relational dimension (e.g., "I talk about my hopes with my spouse/partner"), (3) the spiritual-religious dimension (e.g., "I pray, meditate"), and (4) the engagement dimension (e.g., "I take responsibility and engage myself"). The items were rated on a scale from 0 (not at all) to 3 (very often).

Perceived Hope Scale

As in Study 1, the general level of personal hope was assessed with the six items of the Perceived Hope Scale (PHS) (Krafft et al., 2017, 2021; Marujo et al., 2021; Slezackova et al., 2020). In the current study the six items achieved a high internal consistency in all samples with Cronbach alpha values between $\alpha = 0.89$ and $\alpha = 0.92$.

6.3.3.4 Data Analysis

Statistical analyses were performed with IBM SPSS and AMOS version 27.0. The first step was to calculate the mean values of the hope activities, analyze the rank order within the samples and compare the scores of the single activities across samples. The next step was dedicated to determining partial bivariate correlation coefficients between the 13 hope activities and the general level of perceived hope (controlling for demographic variables).

In order to demonstrate measurement invariance of the Perceived Hope Scale across the eight investigated samples a multi-group Confirmatory Factor Analysis (MGCFA) was performed. The fit of the general model by means of maximum likelihood estimation was evaluated using the following indices: Comparative fit index (CFI) and Tucker-Lewis index (TLI) (study criterion $\geq$0.95 as ideal and $\geq$ 0.90 as the minimum acceptable level), root mean square error of approximation (RMSEA) (study criterion $\leq$0.08) and the standardized root mean residual SRMR (study criterion $\leq$0.08) (Hu & Bentler, 1999). The test for measurement invariance was performed in four steps, from configurational invariance (equal form), to metric invariance (equal loadings), to scalar invariance (equal intercepts), and finally to strict invariance (equal residuals). The recommended criteria to demonstrate invariance are changes in CFI and TLI between comparison and nested models of $\geq -$ 0.010, a change in RMSEA of $\leq$0.015 and a variation in SRMR of $\leq$0.030 (for loading invariance) and $\leq$ 0.010 (for intercept invariance) (Chen, 2007).

6.3.3.5 Results

Hope Activities: Descriptive Statistics

Table 6.8 displays the mean values, standard deviations and variance analyses of the 13 hope activities. The most highly endorsed hope activities in all countries were of a cognitive and self-centered nature: "I think a lot and analyze circumstances" as well as taking personal responsibility and committing oneself. These were followed by social activities related to friends and families or talking about one's hopes with a partner. Religious and spiritual activities of trusting God, praying, meditating and going to church received much lower scores especially in Switzerland, France, Spain

Table 6.8 Hope activities—mean values, standard deviations and analysis of variance

	German Swiss		French Swiss		France		Spain		Portugal		Czech Rep.		Poland		South Africa		ANOVA		
	M	*SD*	*M*	*SD*	*M*	*SD*	*M*	*SD*	*M*	*SD*	*M*	*SD*	*M*	*SD*	*M*	*SD*	*F*	Sig.	η^2
I think a lot and analyze circumstances.	2.24	0.73	2.24	0.63	2.35	0.66	2.56	0.59	2.62	0.54	2.30	0.70	2.62	0.53	2.61	0.56	48.82	<0.001	0.052
I inform myself (read widely, use internet, etc.).	1.34	1.03	1.52	1.00	1.93	0.92	2.44	0.70	2.58	0.60	2.03	0.77	2.65	0.59	2.64	0.63	277.51	<0.001	0.237
I take responsibility and commit myself.	2.16	0.73	2.22	0.65	2.30	0.57	2.57	0.57	2.70	0.50	2.03	0.68	2.61	0.57	2.83	0.43	99.09	<0.001	0.100
I engage myself entrepreneurially.	1.51	1.00	1.66	0.93	1.64	0.88	2.16	0.74	2.44	0.65	0.89	0.96	2.12	0.92	1.94	0.83	156.29	<0.001	0.149
I have a job that allows me to fulfil my hopes.	1.48	1.13	1.65	1.05	1.96	0.87	1.73	1.06	1.79	0.95	1.78	0.94	2.35	0.77	2.13	0.92	29.63	<0.001	0.032
I talk about my hopes with my spouse/partner.	1.65	1.17	1.79	1.13	2.07	0.99	1.91	1.12	2.12	1.05	1.57	1.07	2.13	1.10	2.43	0.93	27.32	<0.001	0.030
I motivate my family.	1.90	0.86	1.91	0.86	1.99	0.82	2.35	0.73	2.48	0.71	1.67	0.88	2.21	0.78	2.46	0.73	74.03	<0.001	0.077
I motivate my friends.	2.00	0.77	1.89	0.82	1.99	0.77	2.35	0.71	2.56	0.62	1.81	0.79	2.25	0.78	2.37	0.69	79.64	<0.001	0.082
I trust in God.	1.14	1.17	0.79	1.06	0.67	0.96	1.10	1.16	1.76	1.24	1.22	1.22	1.68	1.27	2.31	1.10	70.60	<0.001	0.073
I pray, meditate.	0.93	1.03	0.89	0.99	0.95	1.02	1.09	1.00	1.57	1.11	1.00	1.01	1.41	1.16	2.16	1.05	59.66	<0.001	0.063
I go to church/other place of worship.	0.64	0.89	0.46	0.77	0.58	0.88	0.63	0.92	1.14	1.13	0.66	0.92	1.10	1.14	1.45	1.26	54.55	<0.001	0.058
I save money.	1.43	0.99	1.66	0.98	1.75	0.81	2.03	0.89	2.05	0.80	1.66	0.89	1.92	0.94	2.07	0.92	62.22	<0.001	0.065
I donate money to the object of my hopes.	0.80	0.87	1.02	0.92	1.19	0.89	1.33	0.99	1.20	0.97	1.36	0.92	2.09	0.81	1.77	0.91	91.20	<0.001	0.093

and Czechia. In South Africa, trusting God and praying/meditating were situated clearly above the center of the scale, and in Portugal and Poland around the center.

Beyond these general findings, some further noteworthy differences between countries emerged. Participants in Portugal and Spain seemed to engage themselves in entrepreneurial activities, which was rarely the case in Czechia, Switzerland and France. To inform oneself through widely reading newspapers or consulting the internet was less chosen in Switzerland. Polish participants endorsed cognitive activities and were more likely to endorse religious activities than participants in most other countries. In South Africa and Portugal, participants placed special emphasis on social activities involving a partner, family members and friends. In South Africa, to trust God had nearly the same value as connecting with family and friends.

Group Invariance of the Perceived Hope Scale

In order to compare mean values of the PHS and relate them to other variables, we tested invariance using all eight investigated samples. Table 6.9 exhibits the results of the MGCFA including the fit indices for the general sample followed by the four models to test different types of invariance. The overall fit indices for the total sample revealed that the one-factor model achieved good model fit (CFI and TLI > 0.95, RMSEA and SRMR < 0.08) (Hu & Bentler, 1999). Furthermore, the model fit of the individual samples revealed adequate results too. The equal form used as baseline model provided a good fit to the data, suggesting reasonable support for configurational invariance across the groups. Likewise, all indices comparing the further models with the baseline model were under the threshold values recommended by the literature (Chen, 2007, CFI and TLI > -0.01, RMSEA and SRMR < 0.015). This means that the PHS revealed a strong measurement invariance and that it is possible to compare the PHS scores between the national samples. The general hope construct measured with the PHS seemed to be conceptualized in a

Table 6.9 Multigroup confirmatory factor analysis and group invariance for the perceived hope scale

	X^2	df	CFI	TLI	RMSEA	SRMR
Total sample (N = 6245)	282.14	9	0.987	0.979	0.070	0.019
Country/sample invariance						
Configurational Invariance (equal form)	1815.19	180	0.922	0.948	0.038	0.028
Metric Invariance (equal loadings)	1849.86	185	0.921	0.949	0.038	0.028
Scalar Invariance (equal intercepts)	1916.95	191	0.918	0.948	0.038	0.028
Full uniqueness (measurement residuals)	1954.58	198	0.916	0.949	0.038	0.027

Note: *CFA* Confirmatory factor analysis, *CFI* Comparative fit index, *TLI* Tucker-Lewis index, *RMSEA* Root mean square error of approximation, *SRMR* Standardized root mean residual

similar way across cultures and was suitable to be examined in relationship to other constructs.

Hope Activities as Correlates of Perceived Hope

Regarding the level of perceived hope, people in South Africa ($M = 3.62$, $SD = 0.99$), Poland ($M = 3.61$, $SD = 0.99$), Portugal ($M = 3.59$, $SD = 0.95$), and Czechia ($M = 3.59$, $SD = 0.95$) showed significantly higher levels in comparison to people in France ($M = 3.37$, $SD = 1.03$), Spain ($M = 3.42$, $SD = 0.93$) and German speaking Switzerland ($M = 3.40$, $SD = 1.02$) ($p < 0.05$), but the differences were small. Significant and markedly lower levels of hope were expressed by people in the French Swiss sample ($M = 2.93$, $SD = 1.15$) ($p < 0.01$). We correlated the hope activities with the general level of perceived hope with noteworthy results (see Table 6.10). The highly appreciated cognitive activities of thinking a lot and informing oneself barely correlated with hope in most of the countries, with the exception of France and French speaking Switzerland. In all countries, the social activities of engaging one's family and friends or talking with one's partner displayed higher correlation coefficients than the cognitive activities. Furthermore, religious activities of praying, trusting God and going to church showed stronger correlations with hope than the cognitive activities. Religious activities has the lowest correlation with hope in Spain and Switzerland. In the South African, Polish and Portuguese samples social and religious activities correlated moderately high with perceived hope. Beyond this, in all samples the activities of taking responsibility and engaging oneself as well as having a good job exhibited moderate correlation coefficients with perceived hope.

6.3.3.6 Summary of Findings

The most striking finding in Study 2 was the fact that whilst people in most countries expressed a strong engagement in cognitive behaviors along with social actions and to a much lesser extent in religious practices to fulfill their hopes, the statistical impact on hope was mostly related to social and religious activities rather than to cognitive accomplishments.

In line with the results of study 1, participants from Switzerland, Spain and Czechia were the least likely to perform religious practices, whereas those in South Africa, Portugal and Poland displayed higher levels of religiosity and social activities, which also showed the strongest associations with perceived hope. Moreover, similar findings as in study 1 were found regarding lower levels of religiosity and also of perceived hope in Switzerland and Spain, and higher levels of both dimensions for participants in South Africa and to a lesser extent also in Portugal and Poland. Findings for people in Czechia were slightly different, with participants

Table 6.10 Hope activities—partial bivariate Pearson correlations with perceived hope

	Swiss German	Swiss French	France	Spain	Portugal	Czech Rep.	Poland	South Africa
I think a lot and analyze circumstances.	0.107**	0.296**	0.301**	0.067	0.021	0.031	0.064	0.059
I inform myself (read widely, use internet, etc.).	0.158**	0.204**	0.357**	0.152**	0.077*	0.177**	0.076	0.117
I take responsibility and commit myself.	0.294**	0.331**	0.250**	0.234**	0.193**	0.273**	0.222**	0.272**
I engage myself entrepreneurially.	0.174**	0.268**	0.421**	0.258**	0.251**	0.178**	0.086	0.067
I have a job that allows me to fulfil my hopes.	0.196**	0.293**	0.325**	0.348**	0.294**	0.236**	0.218**	0.231*
I talk about my hopes with my spouse/partner.	0.244**	0.258**	0.198*	0.330**	0.211**	0.359**	0.317**	0.282**
I motivate my family.	0.318**	0.349**	0.406**	0.323**	0.312**	0.292**	0.342**	0.113
I motivate my friends.	0.285**	0.286**	0.407**	0.239**	0.272**	0.137*	0.147	0.109
I trust in God.	0.227**	0.212**	0.191*	0.150**	0.239**	0.230**	0.356**	0.235*
I pray, meditate.	0.188**	0.193**	0.298**	0.172**	0.279**	0.246**	0.389**	0.321**
I go to church/other place of worship.	0.191**	0.145**	0.189*	0.139**	0.195**	0.234**	0.339**	0.294**
I save money.	0.203**	0.252**	0.215*	0.088*	0.078*	0.136*	0.121	0.179
I donate money to the object of my hopes.	0.216**	0.237**	0.258**	.228**	0.229**	0.163**	0.159*	0.173

Note: **. Correlation is significant at 0.01 level; *. Correlation is significant at 0.05 level; control variables: Gender, age, marital status, education, main activity, professional status

reporting low levels of religiosity in both studies, but in this study expressed slightly higher levels of perceived hope.

Similar to the findings in study 1, people in South Africa (and now also in Portugal and Poland) demonstrated that taking personal responsibility and engaging oneself, is not in contradiction to the belief in a higher power and to prayers or meditation. Rather, it seems that these activities can be smoothly complemented and integrated in order to foster a higher sense of hopefulness.

6.3.4 General Findings and Discussion

In the theoretical part of this chapter we maintained that trust in others, e.g., family members, friends, the wider community, a spiritual higher power or a benevolent external factor such as luck or nature, is a constitutive element of hope (Scioli et al., 2016). Trust especially comes into play when people hope for a desired good, when they also believe in the possibility but not necessarily in a high probability of its realization, and therefore have to remain hopeful even in dire situations characterized by little personal control (Bruininks & Malle, 2005; Tennen et al., 2002). Based on the TCC risk management model (Earle, 2001; Earle & Siegrist, 2006; Siegrist, 2010) we explained the distinctive characteristics between confidence and trust and argued that whereas the self-centered concepts of dispositional hope and optimism are grounded in (self-) confidence (performance oriented and evidence based), a much broader concept of (perceived) hope would be eminently rooted in trust (based in relationships and value oriented). Moreover, it was argued that trustful hope is characterized by three interrelated aspects, a disposition to act (Martin, 2013), mutual social care and support (McGeer, 2004, 2008), as well as trust in further external resources (Bovens, 1999; Shade, 2001). Finally, it was assumed that people in different cultures might cultivate hope backed in diverse individual, social and religious hope sources and would likewise perform different activities in order to get their hopes fulfilled (Averill et al., 1990; Averill & Sundararajan, 2005).

The overall purpose of the two empirical studies in this chapter was to explore the sources and activities of hope relevant to maintaining hope and making one's hopes happen, with special focus on trust, social support and further external factors such as religiosity and luck in several countries. Study 1 was focused on the importance of several hope sources for people in 12 countries and analyzed the role of social support and other external hope resources on perceived and dispositional hope. Study 2 broadened the findings of study 1 by centering on concrete activities people use to perform in order to get their hopes fulfilled and by evaluating their possible impact on perceived hope among different countries.

As suggested by several authors (Averill & Sundararajan, 2005; Scioli et al., 2016; Tennen et al., 2002), the general findings of our studies support the importance of external hope sources and activities such as social support, luck, nature as well as religious experiences and practices along with self-centered, performance and mastery-oriented sources and activities but with distinct emphases in different countries. Based on the results of our studies we identified three groups of countries which differed with regard to the importance assigned to several hope sources and activities as well as the level of general hope. Social resources and activities such as supporting each other emotionally and talking with family and friends were especially important for people in some Latin countries (Spain, Portugal, and Colombia). People in African countries (Nigeria and South Africa) and India received and nurtured hope especially from religious sources and practices (trusting God, praying, meditating, etc.). Finally, people in more individualistic countries like Switzerland and Czechia relied the most on self-centered, performance and mastery-oriented sources and activities, but also acknowledged the importance of external factors such as social support, luck and inspiring experiences in nature.

Remarkably, people in countries in which religious sources and practices were especially valued and could also be combined with individual capabilities, expressed the highest levels of perceived and dispositional hope and vice-versa, people in countries with the lowest levels and effects of religious sources and practices displayed the lowest levels of hope. Conceptually, the broader notion of perceived hope was related to several individual, social, religious and further factors (such as luck and nature) in a more balanced way than dispositional hope (more centered on individual mastery and performance) (Krafft et al., 2017). Moreover, people in countries like South Africa, Nigeria and India seem to be able to integrate the reliance in one's own personal capabilities with the trust in a higher religious or spiritual power. When focusing on social support, our studies exposed that in most countries emotional support had a greater effect on perceived hope than instrumental support. Moreover, cognitive practices such as reading and analyzing, although highly endorsed, demonstrated lower effects on hope than social activities supporting the eminently emotional character of hope as suggested by several authors (Fredrickson, 2013; Scioli & Biller, 2009; Tong et al., 2010).

6.3.5 Limitations

Our studies contain a number of limitations necessary to acknowledge. As in the previous chapters, the design of our research is cross-sectional, impeding us to infer any kind of causality. We assume that the relationship between hope and trust is largely reciprocal: Hopeful people are able to trust others and vise-versa, trusting others will foster one's hope. A recurring limitation already addressed in other chapters is the very unequal sample sizes, the dissimilar demographic structures and the lack of representativeness across countries. Results of countries with rather a small number of participants should be interpreted with caution and dealt with as possible hints to motivate more exhaustive research in the future. Furthermore, the online survey makes the participation of socio-economic groups with limited or no internet access, especially in developing countries, difficult or even impossible.

6.4 Conclusions

In this chapter we aimed to contribute to the knowledge of hope by highlighting and exploring the nature and role of trust expressed in several individual, social and religious/spiritual sources and activities held and performed by people in different countries. Trustful hope comes into play especially in dire situations when people cease to be optimistic and cannot rely on a positive outcome anymore, but at the same time don't want to give up their hopes and despite all difficulties still decide to believe in the possibility of their realization. In these cases, the central role of external resources related to mutual care and support, to a Divine Higher Power or to a benevolent metaphysical force such as luck or nature becomes apparent, not only to nurture hopefulness but also to encourage and develop confidence in one's own capabilities and agency. People in different countries and cultures differ in the way they hope and in the activities they perform in order to see their hopes become true. Future research should be sensitive to such differences, choose a broader conceptualization of hope and integrate a variety of theoretical frameworks and empirical measures in order to do justice to such diverse phenomena.

Appendix 6.1: Demographic Structure of the Samples Study 1

Number of Participants, Mean Age and Standard Deviation and GDP Per Capita

	Australia	Colombia	Czech Rep.	India	Israel	Italy	Nigeria	Poland	Portugal	South Africa	Spain	Switzerland
N	474	311	469	1092	884	272	665	481	507	574	529	3935
%	4.7%	3.1%	4.6%	10.7%	8.7%	2.7%	6.5%	4.7%	5.0%	5.6%	5.2%	38.6%
M_{age}	47.53	26.19	32.75	31.15	41.65	41.86	32.26	31.58	36.45	39.27	35.19	15.22
SD_{age}	13.05	8.63	15.54	12.60	14.98	13.78	8.47	10.82	14.74	14.85	46.82	15.67
GDP per capita in U$S	51,693	5335	22,932	1928	44,169	31,714	2097	15,721	22,176	5656	27,063	87,097

Gender

		Australia	Colombia	Czech Rep.	India	Israel	Italy	Nigeria	Poland	Portugal	South Africa	Spain	Switzerland
Male	n	232	151	132	529	262	75	434	140	124	*252*	116	1797
	%	48.9%	48.6%	28.1%	48.4%	29.6%	27.6%	65.3%	29.1%	24.5%	*43.9%*	21.9%	45.7%
Female	n	242	160	337	563	622	197	231	341	383	*322*	413	2138
	%	51.1%	51.4%	71.9%	51.6%	70.4%	72.4%	34.7%	70.9%	75.5%	*56.1%*	78.1%	54.3%

Marital Status

		Australia	Colombia	Czech Rep.	India	Israel	Italy	Nigeria	Poland	Portugal	South Africa	Spain	Switzerland
Still living with my parents	n	20	182	136	469	92	45	112	85	142	106	206	231
	%	4.2%	58.5%	29.0%	42.9%	10.4%	16.5%	16.8%	17.7%	28.0%	18.5%	38.9%	5.9%
Single, unmarried	n	41	63	67	140	108	36	295	71	84	82	67	589
	%	8.6%	20.3%	14.3%	12.8%	12.2%	13.2%	44.4%	14.8%	16.6%	14.3%	12.7%	15.0%

(continued)

		Australia	Colombia	Czech Rep.	India	Israel	Italy	Nigeria	Poland	Portugal	South Africa	Spain	Switzerland
Living in a partnership but in separate households	n	16	10	44	9	46	33	11	43	17	14	26	314
	%	3.4%	3.2%	9.4%	0.8%	5.2%	12.1%	1.7%	8.9%	3.4%	2.4%	4.9%	8.0%
Living together in a partnership	n	54	17	70	18	82	60	4	101	65	92	58	719
	%	11.4%	5.5%	14.9%	1.6%	9.3%	22.1%	0.6%	21.0%	12.8%	16.0%	11.0%	18.3%
Married	n	298	35	117	428	500	79	228	166	150	224	150	1531
	%	62.9%	11.3%	24.9%	39.2%	56.6%	29.0%	34.3%	34.5%	29.6%	39.0%	28.4%	38.9%
Divorced/separated	n	42	4	27	16	45	16	11	14	46	43	21	459
	%	8.9%	1.3%	5.8%	1.5%	5.1%	5.9%	1.7%	2.9%	9.1%	7.5%	4.0%	11.7%
Widowed	n	3	0	8	12	11	3	4	1	3	13	1	92
	%	0.6%	0.0%	1.7%	1.1%	1.2%	1.1%	0.6%	0.2%	0.6%	2.3%	0.2%	2.3%

Education

		Australia	Colombia	Czech Rep.	India	Israel	Italia	Nigeria	Poland	Portugal	South Africa	Spain	Switzerland
Did not finish school	n	4	0	0	4	5	0	1	0	0	6	12	41
	%	0.8%	0.0%	0.0%	0.4%	0.6%	0.0%	0.2%	0.0%	0.0%	1.0%	1.1%	1.0%
Primary school	n	0	0	16	36	1	18	0	4	1	4	61	190
	%	0.0%	0.0%	3.4%	3.3%	0.1%	6.6%	0.0%	0.8%	0.2%	0.7%	5.9%	4.8%
Secondary school	n	54	67	287	214	96	54	23	185	147	211	361	1111
	%	11.4%	21.5%	61.2%	19.6%	10.9%	19.9%	3.5%	38.5%	29.0%	32.1%	34.5%	28.2%
Professional training/ Diploma	n	126	14	0	526	110	69	22	64	226	140	271	2146
	%	40.0%	4.5%	0.0%	48.2%	12.4%	52.7%	3.3%	13.3%	44.6%	24.4%	25.9%	54.5%
Tertiary education/ University	n	131	230	166	312	672	131	619	228	124	212	349	447
	%	41.6%	74.0%	35.4%	28.6%	76.0%	48.2%	93.1%	47.4%	24.5%	37.1%	66.0%	11.4%

Main Activity

		Australia	Colombia	Czech Rep.	India	Israel	Italy	Nigeria	Poland	Portugal	South Africa	Spain	Switzerland
In education or training (student)	n	23	178	236	504	150	62	171	144	171	83	216	197
	%	4.9%	57.2%	50.3%	46.2%	17.0%	22.8%	25.7%	29.9%	33.7%	14.5%	40.8%	5.0%
Household/raising children	n	16	2	15	118	17	13	7	18	2	16	12	181
	%	3.4%	0.6%	3.2%	10.8%	1.9%	4.8%	1.1%	3.7%	0.4%	2.8%	2.3%	4.6%
Part-time job	n	77	13	33	57	143	41	102	33	45	73	62	830
	%	16.2%	4.2%	7.0%	5.2%	16.2%	15.1%	15.3%	6.9%	8.9%	12.7%	11.7%	21.1%
Fulltime job	n	312	113	155	352	492	126	276	269	260	293	202	1777
	%	65.8%	36.3%	33.0%	32.2%	55.7%	46.3%	41.5%	55.9%	51.3%	51.0%	38.2%	45.2%
Unemployed	n	22	5	0	46	28	16	103	7	17	68	13	212
	%	4.6%	1.6%	0.0%	4.2%	3.2%	5.9%	15.5%	1.5%	3.4%	11.8%	2.5%	5.4%
Retired	n	24	0	30	15	54	14	6	10	12	41	24	738
	%	5.1%	0.0%	6.4%	1.4%	6.1%	5.1%	0.9%	2.1%	2.4%	7.1%	4.5%	18.8%

Professional Status

		Australia	Colombia	Czech Rep.	India	Israel	Italy	Nigeria	Poland	Portugal	South Africa	Spain	Switzerland
No position in an organization (eg. at school, housekeeping, unemployed, retired)	n	47	63	154	224	101	69	101	32	111	127	136	657
	%	9.9%	20.3%	32.8%	20.5%	11.4%	25.4%	15.2%	6.7%	21.9%	22.1%	25.7%	16.7%
In education/training	n	23	101	91	499	110	34	159	147	68	90	98	168
	%	4.9%	32.5%	19.4%	45.7%	12.4%	12.5%	23.9%	30.6%	13.4%	15.7%	18.5%	4.3%
Employee	n	150	58	155	242	319	55	162	195	199	138	196	1705
	%	31.6%	18.6%	33.0%	22.2%	36.1%	20.2%	24.4%	40.5%	39.3%	24.0%	37.1%	43.3%

(continued)

		Australia	Colombia	Czech Rep.	India	Israel	Italy	Nigeria	Poland	Portugal	South Africa	Spain	Switzerland
Junior/Middle management	n	64	53	32	70	151	16	79	49	71	102	42	729
	%	13.5%	17.0%	6.8%	6.4%	17.1%	5.9%	11.9%	10.2%	14.0%	17.8%	7.9%	18.5%
Senior management/ Board of directors	n	49	24	6	18	95	21	47	9	22	37	37	275
	%	10.3%	7.7%	1.3%	1.6%	10.7%	7.7%	7.1%	1.9%	4.3%	6.4%	7.0%	7.0%
Entrepreneur/Business owner	n	141	12	31	39	108	77	117	49	36	80	20	401
	%	29.7%	3.9%	6.6%	3.6%	12.2%	28.3%	17.6%	10.2%	7.1%	13.9%	3.8%	10.2%

Religion

		Australia	Colombia	Czech Rep.	India	Israel	Italy	Nigeria	Poland	Portugal	South Africa	Spain	Switzerland
Catholic	n	80	163	101	224	8	130	326	308	244	41	288	1100
	%	16.9%	52.4%	21.5%	20.5%	0.9%	47.8%	49.0%	64.0%	48.1%	7.1%	54.4%	28.0%
Protestant	n	43	8	11	14	4	0	131	4	10	69	2	796
	%	9.1%	2.6%	2.3%	1.3%	0.5%	0.0%	19.7%	0.8%	2.0%	12.0%	0.4%	20.2%
Another Christian church or community	n	66	8	26	25	0	2	155	11	5	265	1	138
	%	13.9%	2.6%	5.5%	2.3%	0.0%	0.7%	23.3%	2.3%	1.0%	46..2%	0.2%	3.5%
Muslim	n	5	0	0	215	9	1	14	0	2	16	2	71
	%	1.1%	0.0%	0.0%	19.7%	1.0%	0.4%	2.1%	0.0%	0.4%	2.8%	0.4%	1.8%
Jewish	n	17	0	1	0	496	1	0	0	0	5	0	11
	%	3.6%	0.0%	0.2%	0.0%	56.1%	0.4%	0.0%	0.0%	0.0%	0.9%	0.0%	0.3%
Hindu	n	14	0	0	533	3	1	0	0	0	8	0	1
	%	3.0%	0.0%	0.0%	48.8%	0.3%	0.4%	0.0%	0.0%	0.0%	1.4%	0.0%	0.0%
Buddhist	n	9	0	5	0	3	9	0	2	3	1	0	27
	%	1.9%	0.0%	1.1%	0.0%	0.3%	3.3%	0.0%	0.4%	0.6%	0.2%	0.0%	0.7%
	n	95	60	156	37	138	32	28	50	96	92	35	340

(continued)

		Australia	Colombia	Czech Rep.	India	Israel	Italy	Nigeria	Poland	Portugal	South Africa	Spain	Switzerland
I am a spiritual person outside the traditional world religions	%	20.0%	19.3%	33.3%	3.4%	15.6%	11.8%	4.2%	10.4%	18.9%	16.0%	6.6%	8.6%
Without religion or confession	n	121	56	137	24	132	86	4	96	120	48	170	1352
	%	25.5%	18.0%	29.2%	2.2%	14.9%	31.6%	0.6%	20.0%	23.7%	8.4%	32.1%	34.4%
Something different	n	24	16	32	20	91	10	7	10	27	29	31	99
	%	5.1%	5.1%	6.8%	1.8%	10.3%	3.7%	1.1%	2.1%	5.3%	5.1%	5.9%	2.5%

Appendix 6.2: Demographic Structure of the Samples Study 2

		German Swiss	French Swiss	France	Spain	Portugal	Czech Rep.	Poland	South Africa
Total	*N*	3049	1109	135	528	808	338	169	109
Age (M)		43.71	44.16	39.09	37.79	37.49	30.92	37.59	42.63
Age (SD)		15.92	14.15	15.78	14.78	15.53	11.90	15.54	13.85
Gender									
Male	n	1255	472	32	134	153	117	31	21
	%	41.2%	42.6%	23.7%	25.4%	18.9%	34.6%	18.3%	19.3%
Female	n	1794	637	103	394	655	221	138	88
	%	58.8%	57.4%	76.3%	74.6%	81.1%	65.4%	81.7%	80.7%
Marital Status									
Still living with my parents	n	234	69	13	139	222	56	19	6
	%	7.7%	6.2%	9.6%	26.3%	27.5%	16.6%	11.2%	5.5%

(continued)

		German Swiss	French Swiss	France	Spain	Portugal	Czech Rep.	Poland	South Africa
Single, unmarried	n	526	160	16	76	149	62	16	14
	%	17.3%	14.4%	11.9%	14.4%	18.4%	18.3%	9.5%	12.8%
Living in a partnership with separate households	n	263	93	23	20	25	42	14	10
	%	8.6%	8.4%	17.0%	3.8%	3.1%	12.4%	8.3%	9.2%
Living together in a partnership	n	592	226	32	69	99	75	20	9
	%	19.4%	20.4%	23.7%	13.1%	12.3%	22.2%	11.8%	8.3%
Married	n	1111	395	38	186	236	86	84	60
	%	36.4%	35.6%	28.1%	35.2%	29.2%	25.4%	49.7%	55.0%
Divorced/separated	n	267	143	10	34	68	13	14	7
	%	8.8%	12.9%	7.4%	6.4%	8.4%	3.8%	8.3%	6.4%
Widowed	n	56	23	3	4	9	4	2	3
	%	1.8%	2.1%	2.2%	0.8%	1.1%	1.2%	1.2%	2.8%
Education									
Did not finish school	n	9	5	0	1	0	0	0	1
	%	0.3%	0.5%	0.0%	0.2%	0.0%	0.0%	0.0%	0.9%
Primary school	n	105	71	1	12	1	9	0	0
	%	3.4%	6.4%	0.7%	2.3%	0.1%	2.7%	0.0%	0.0%
Secondary school	n	255	68	16	87	227	157	29	13
	%	8.4%	6.1%	11.8%	16.5%	28.1%	46.4%	17.2%	11.9%
Professional training/Diploma	n	2050	687	32	68	6	28	23	13
	%	67.2%	61.9%	23.7%	12.9%	0.7%	8.3%	13.6%	11.9%
Tertiary education/University	n	630	278	86	360	574	144	117	82
	%	20.7%	25.1%	63.7%	68.2%	71.0%	42.6%	69.2%	75.2%
Main activity									
In education or training	n	202	68	38	159	283	131	29	18
	%	6.6%	6.1%	28.1%	30.1%	35.0%	38.8%	17.2%	16.5%

(continued)

		German Swiss	French Swiss	France	Spain	Portugal	Czech Rep.	Poland	South Africa
Household/raising children	n	123	56	1	18	6	15	7	4
	%	4.0%	5.0%	0.7%	3.4%	0.7%	4.4%	4.1%	3.7%
Part-time job	n	617	230	17	46	70	19	9	12
	%	20.2%	20.7%	12.6%	8.7%	8.7%	5.6%	5.3%	11.0%
Fulltime job	n	1580	562	57	269	404	162	115	69
	%	51.8%	50.7%	42.2%	50.9%	50.0%	47.9%	68.0%	63.3%
Unemployed	n	109	62	10	17	17	5	6	0
	%	3.6%	5.6%	7.4%	3.2%	2.1%	1.5%	3.6%	0.0%
Retired	n	418	131	12	19	28	6	3	6
	%	13.7%	11.8%	8.9%	3.6%	3.5%	1.8%	1.8%	5.5%
Professional Status									
No position in an organization	n	407	208	25	95	173	71	8	12
	%	13.3%	18.8%	18.5%	18.0%	21.4%	21.0%	4.7%	11.0%
In education/training	n	170	69	33	106	140	58	38	23
	%	5.6%	6.2%	24.4%	20.1%	17.3%	17.2%	22.5%	21.1%
Employee	n	1248	519	23	181	313	146	51	28
	%	40.9%	46.8%	17.0%	34.3%	38.7%	43.2%	30.2%	25.7%
Junior/Middle management	n	729	143	16	65	79	31	30	12
	%	23.9%	12.9%	11.9%	12.3%	9.8%	9.2%	17.8%	11.0%
Senior management/Board of directors	n	147	70	11	42	29	7	13	11
	%	4.8%	6.3%	20.0%	8.0%	3.6%	2.1%	7.7%	10.1%
Entrepreneur/Business owner	n	348	100	27	39	74	25	29	23
	%	11.4%	9.0%	5.9%	7.4%	9.2%	7.4%	17.2%	21.1%
Religion									
Catholic	n	770	330	51	277	405	91	109	4
	%	25.3%	29.8%	37.8%	52.5%	50.1%	26.9%	64.5%	3.7%

(continued)

		German Swiss	French Swiss	France	Spain	Portugal	Czech Rep.	Poland	South Africa
Protestant	n	822	203	0	4	21	9	1	23
	%	27.0%	18.3%	0.0%	0.8%	2.6%	2.7%	0.6%	21.1%
Another Christian church	n	141	24	1	1	7	4	3	38
	%	4.6%	2.2%	0.7%	0.2%	0.9%	1.2%	1.8%	34.9%
Muslim	n	43	13	1	2	2	1	1	0
	%	1.4%	1.2%	0.7%	0.4%	0.2%	0.3%	0.6%	0.0%
Jewish	n	6	3	1	0	0	0	0	3
	%	0.2%	0.3%	0.7%	0.0%	0.0%	0.0%	0.0%	2.8%
Hindu	n	4	0	0	0	1	0	0	0
	%	0.1%	0.0%	0.0%	0.0%	0.1%	0.0%	0.0%	0.0%
Buddhist	n	22	6	1	1	6	1	1	2
	%	0.7%	0.5%	0.7%	0.2%	0.7%	0.3%	0.6%	1.8%
I am a spiritual person outside the traditional world religions.	n	204	130	23	55	160	109	22	25
	%	6.7%	11.7%	17.0%	10.4%	19.8%	32.2%	13.0%	22.9%
Without religion or confession	n	989	382	57	164	174	103	27	9
	%	32.4%	34.4%	42.2%	31.1%	21.5%	30.5%	16.0%	8.3%
Something different	n	48	18	0	24	32	20	5	5
	%	1.6%	1.6%	0.0%	4.5%	4.0%	5.9%	3.0%	4.6%

References

Adams, B. D. (2005). *Trust vs. confidence*. Humansystems.

Averill, J. R., Catlin, G., & Chon, K. K. (1990). *Rules of hope: Recent research in psychology*. Springer.

Averill, J. R., & Sundararajan, L. (2005). Hope as rhetoric: Cultural narratives of wishing and coping. In J. Eliott (Ed.), *Interdisciplinary perspectives on hope* (pp. 133–165). Nova Science.

Blöser, C., & Stahl, T. (2017). Fundamental Hope and Practical Identity. *Philosophical Papers, 46*(3), 345–371. https://doi.org/10.1080/05568641.2017.1400918

Bovens, L. (1999). The value of hope. *Philosophy and Phenomenological Research, 59*(3), 667–681.

Bruininks, P., & Malle, B. F. (2005). Distinguishing hope from optimism and related affective states. *Motivation and Emotion, 29*(4), 324–352. https://doi.org/10.1007/s11031-006-9010-4

Bury, S. M., Wenzel, M., & Woodyatt, L. (2016). Giving hope a sporting chance: Hope as distinct from optimism when events are possible but not probable. *Motivation and Emotion, 40*(4), 588–601. https://doi.org/10.1007/s11031-016-9560-z

Carver, C., & Scheier, M. F. (1981). *Attention and self-regulation: A control-theory approach to human behavior*. Springer.

Chen, F. F. (2007). Sensitivity of goodness of fit indexes to lack of measurement invariance. *Structural Equation Modeling: A Multidisciplinary Journal, 14*(3), 464–504. https://doi.org/10.1080/10705510701301834

De Bruin, E. N. M., & Van Lange, P. A. M. (1999). Impression formation and cooperative behavior. *European Journal of Social Psychology, 29*, 305–328. https://doi.org/10.1002/(SICI)1099-0992(199903/05)29:2/3<305::AID-EJSP929>3.0.CO;2-R

De Bruin, E. N. M., & Van Lange, P. A. M. (2000). What people look for in others: Influences of the perceiver and the perceived on information selection. *Personality and Social Psychology Bulletin, 26*, 206–219. https://doi.org/10.1177/0146167200264007

De Jonge, J., Van Trijp, H., Renes, R. J., & Frewer, L. (2007). Understanding consumer confidence in the safety of food: Its two-dimensional structure and determinants. *Risk Analysis, 27*, 729–740. https://doi.org/10.1111/j.1539-6924.2007.00917.x

De Jonge, J., Van Trijp, J. C. M., Van Der Lans, I. A., Renes, R. J., & Frewer, L. (2008). How trust in institutions and organizations builds general consumer confidence in the safety of food: A decomposition of effects. *Appetite, 51*, 311–317. https://doi.org/10.1016/j.appet.2008.03.008

Deutsch, M. (1973). *The resolution of conflict: Constructive and destructive processes*. Yale University Press.

Earle, T. C. (2001). From risk perception to social trust: an outline of recent contributions of psychology to risk management. In OECD NEA (ed.) *Better integration of radiation protection in modern society*, Workshop Proceedings, Villingen, 27–33.

Earle, T. C. (2009). Trust, confidence, and the 2008 global financial crisis. *Risk Analysis: An International Journal, 29*(6), 785–792. https://doi.org/10.1111/j.1539-6924.2009.01230.x

Earle, T. C. (2010). Trust in risk management: A model-based review of empirical research. *Risk Analysis: An International Journal, 30*(4), 541–574. https://doi.org/10.1111/j.1539-6924.2010.01398.x

Earle, T. C., & Siegrist, M. (2006). Morality information, performance information, and the distinction between trust and confidence. *First Journal of Applied Social Psychology, 36*(2), 383–416. https://doi.org/10.1111/j.0021-9029.2006.00012.x

Earle, T. C., Siegrist, M., & Gutscher, H. (2001). The influence of trust and confidence on perceived risks and cooperation. *Perception, 2*, 353–362.

Erikson, E. (1950). *Childhood and society*. Norton.

Farran, C. J., Herth, K. A., & Popovich, J. M. (1995). *Hope and hopelessness: Critical clinical constructs*. Sage.

Fredrickson, B. L. (2013). Positive emotions broaden and build. *Advances in Experimental Social Psychology, 47*(1), 1–53. https://doi.org/10.1016/B978-0-12-407236-7.00001-2

Gesell, I. (2007). Am I talking to me? The power of internal dialogue to help or hinder our success. *Journal for Quality & Participation, 30*(2), 20–21.

Gray, J. G. (1959). *The warriors: Reflections on men in battle*. Harcourt Brace.

Hu, L. T., & Bentler, P. M. (1999). Cutoff criteria for fit indexes in covariance structure analysis: Conventional criteria versus new alternatives. *Structural Equation Modeling: A Multidisciplinary Journal, 6*(1), 1–55. https://doi.org/10.1080/10705519909540118

Hutchinson, G. E., & Mercier, R. (2004). Using social psychological concepts to help students. *Journal of Physical Education. Recreation & Dance, 75*(7), 22–26. https://doi.org/10.1080/07303084.2004.10607269

Keller, C., Siegrist, M., Earle, T. C., & Gutscher, H. (2011). The general confidence scale: coping with environmental uncertainty and threat. *Journal of Applied Social Psychology, 41*(9), 2200–2229. https://doi.org/10.1111/j.1559-1816.2011.00811.x

Koriat, A., Lichtenstein, S., & Fischoff, B. (1980). Reasons for confidence. *Journal of Experimental Psychology: Human Learning and Memory, 6*(2), 107–118. https://doi.org/10.1037/0278-7393.6.2.107

Krafft, A. M., Guse, T., & Maree, D. (2021). Distinguishing Perceived Hope and Dispositional Optimism: Theoretical Foundations and Empirical Findings beyond Future Expectancies and Cognition. *Journal of Well-Being Assessment, 4*(7), 1–27. https://doi.org/10.1007/s41543-020-00030-4

Krafft, A. M., Martin-Krumm, C., & Fenouillet, F. (2017). Adaptation, further elaboration, and validation of a scale to measure hope as perceived by people: Discriminant Value and Predictive Utility Vis-à-Vis Dispositional Hope. *Assessment, 26*(8), 1594–1609. https://doi.org/10.1177/1073191117700724

Krafft, A. M., & Walker, A. M. (2018). Exploring the concept and experience of Hope – Empirical findings and the virtuous circle of Hope. In A. M. Krafft, P. Perrig-Chiello, & A. M. Walker (Eds.), *Hope for a good life: Results of the Hope Barometer International Research Program* (pp. 21–60). Springer. https://doi.org/10.1007/978-3-319-78470-0_2

Lear, J. (2006). *Radical hope: Ethics in the face of cultural devastation*. Harvard University Press.

Luhmann, N. (1988). Familiarity, Confidence, Trust: Problems and Alternatives. In D. Gambetta (Ed.), *Trust: Making and Breaking Cooperative Relations* (pp. 94–107). Department of Sociology; University of Oxford.

Lundberg, K. M. (2008). Promoting self-confidence in clinical nursing students. *Nurse Educator, 33*(2), 86–89. https://doi.org/10.1097/01.NNE.0000299512.78270.d0

Marcel, G. (1962). *Homo viator: Introduction to a metaphysic of hope* (Crauford. E. Trans.). New York: Harper and Row (Original work published 1944).

Martin, A. (2011). Hopes and dreams. *Philosophy and Phenomenological Research, 83*(1), 148–173. https://doi.org/10.1111/j.1933-1592.2010.00422.x

Martin, A. (2013). How we hope. *Princeton University Press*. https://doi.org/10.1515/9781400848706

Martin, A. (2019). Interpersonal hope. In C. Blöser & T. Stahl (Eds.), *The moral psychology of hope* (pp. 229–248). Rowman & Littlefield International.

Marujo, H. Á., Velez, M. J., Gonçalves, S. P., Neto, L. M., Krafft, A. M., & Casais, M. (2021). The value of hope: Validation of the perceived hope scale in the Portuguese population. *Current Psychology, 1-9*. https://doi.org/10.1007/s12144-021-02115-6

Mayer, R. C., Davis, J. H., & Schoorman, F. D. (1995). An integrative model of organizational trust. *Academy of Management Review, 20*(3), 709–734. https://doi.org/10.5465/amr.1995.9508080335

McGeer, V. (2004). The art of good hope. *The Annals of the American Academy of Political and Social Science, 592*(1), 100–127. https://doi.org/10.1177/0002716203261781

McGeer, V. (2008). Trust, hope and empowerment. *Australasian Journal of Philosophy, 86*(2), 237–254. https://doi.org/10.1080/00048400801886413

Meirav, A. (2009). The nature of hope. *Ratio, 22*(2), 216–233. https://doi.org/10.1111/j.1467-9329.2009.00427.x

Mellalieu, S. D., Neil, R., & Hanton, S. (2006). Self-confidence as a mediator of the relationship between competitive anxiety intensity and interpretation. *Research Quarterly for Exercise and Sport, 77*, 263–227.

Milona, M. (2020a). Philosophy of Hope. In S. Van den Heuvel (Ed.), *Historical and multidisciplinary perspectives on Hope* (pp. 99–116). Springer. https://doi.org/10.1007/978-3-030-46489-9_6

Milona, M. (2020b). *Hope and Optimism*. John Templeton Foundation.

Oleson, K. C., Poehlmann, K. M., Yost, J. H., Lynch, M. E., & Arkin, R. M. (2000). Subjective overachievement: Individual differences in self-doubt and concern with performance. *Journal of Personality, 68*, 491–524. https://doi.org/10.1111/1467-6494.00104

Perry, P. (2011). Concept analysis: Confidence/self-confidence. *Nursing Forum, 46*(4), 218–223., Malden, USA: Blackwell Publishing Inc. https://doi.org/10.1111/j.1744-6198.2011.00230.x

Pruyser, P. W. (1986). Maintaining hope in adversity. *Pastoral Psychology, 35*(2), 120–131.

Rempel, J. K., Holmes, J. G., & Zanna, M. P. (1985). Trust in close relationships. *Journal of Personality and Social Psychology, 49*, 95–117.

Rotter, J. B. (1980). Interpersonal trust, trustworthiness, and gullibility. *American Psychologist, 35*, 1–7. https://doi.org/10.1037/0003-066X.35.1.1

Rousseau, D. M., Sitkin, S. B., Burt, R. S., & Camerer, C. (1998). Not so different after all: A cross-discipline view of trust. *Academy of Management Review, 23*, 393–404. https://doi.org/10.5465/amr.1998.926617

Scheier, M. E., & Carver, C. S. (1987). Dispositional optimism and physical well-being: The influence of generalized outcome expectancies on health. *Journal of Personality, 55*(2), 169–121. https://doi.org/10.1111/j.1467-6494.1987.tb00434.x

Scheier, M. F., Carver, C. S., & Bridges, M. W. (2001). Optimism, pessimism, and psychological well-being. *Optimism and Pessimism, 1*, 189–216. https://doi.org/10.1037/10385-009

Schunk, D. H., & Pajares, F. (2005). Competence perceptions and academic functioning. In A. J. Elliot & C. S. Dweck (Eds.), *Handbook of competence and motivation* (pp. 85–104). Guilford Press.

Scioli, A., & Biller, H. (2003). Hope, attachment and love. Published Conference Proceedings. *Works of Love: Scientific and Religious Perspectives on Altruism. An international, interfaith and interdisciplinary conference* sponsored by the Metanexus Institute on Religion & Science and the Institute for Unlimited Love, Philadelphia, PA.

Scioli, A., & Biller, H. (2009). *Hope in the age of anxiety*. Oxford University Press.

Scioli, A., Chamberlin, C. M., Samor, C. M., Lapointe, A. B., Campbell, T. L., Macleod, A. R., & McLenon, J. (1997). A prospective study of hope, optimism, and health. *Psychological Reports, 81*(3), 723–733. https://doi.org/10.2466/pr0.1997.81.3.723

Scioli, A., Scioli-Salter, E. R., Sykes, K., Anderson, C., & Fedele, M. (2016). The positive contributions of hope to maintaining and restoring health: An integrative, mixed-method approach. *The Journal of Positive Psychology, 11*(2), 135–148. https://doi.org/10.1080/17439760.2015.1037858

Shade, P. (2001). *Habits of hope - A pragmatic theory*. Vanderbilt University Press.

Shakespeare-Finch, J., & Obst, P. L. (2011). The Development of the 2-Way Social Support Scale: A Measure of Giving and Receiving Emotional and Instrumental Support. *Journal of Personality Assessment., 93*(5), 483–449. https://doi.org/10.1080/00223891.2011.594124

Shaw, R. (1997). *Trust in the balance*. John Wiley.

Siegrist, M. (2010). Trust and confidence: The difficulties in distinguishing the two concepts in research. *Risk Analysis: An International Journal, 30*(7), 1022–1024.

Siegrist, M., Gutscher, H., & Earle, T. C. (2005). Perception of risk: The influence of general trust and general confidence. *Journal of Risk Research, 8*, 145–156. https://doi.org/10.1080/1366987032000105315

Slezackova, A., Prošek, T., Malatincová, T., & Krafft, A. M. (2020). Psychometrické vlastnosti české verze Škály prožívané naděje: faktorová struktura a vnitřní konzistence [Psychometric

characteristics of the Czech version of The Perceived Hope Scale: Factor structure and internal consistency]. *Československá psychologie/Czechoslovak Psychology, 64*(3), 288–305.
Snyder, C. R. (2000). Hypothesis: There is hope. In C. R. Snyder (Ed.), *Handbook of hope: Theory, measures, and applications* (pp. 3–21). Academic Press.
Snyder, C. R. (2002). Hope theory: Rainbows in the mind. *Psychological Inquiry, 13*(4), 249–275. https://doi.org/10.1207/S15327965PLI1304_01
Snyder, C. R., Harris, C., Anderson, J. R., Holleran, S. A., Irving, L. M., Sigmon, S. T., & Harney, P. (1991). The will and the ways: Development and validation of an individual-differences measure of hope. *Journal of Personality and Social Psychology, 60*(4), 570–585. https://doi.org/10.1037/0022-3514.60.4.570
Staats, S. R., & Stassen, M. A. (1985). Hope: An affective cognition. *Social Indicators Research, 17*(3), 235–242. https://doi.org/10.1007/BF00319312
Stitzlein, S. (2019). Pragmatist Hope. In C. Blöser & T. Stahl (Eds.), *2019* (pp. 93–112). The Moral Psychology of Hope.
Stotland, E. (1969). *The psychology of hope*. Jossey-Bass.
Tennen, H., Affleck, G., & Tennen, R. (2002). Clipped feathers: The theory and measurement of hope. *Psychological Inquiry, 13*(4), 311–317.
Tong, E. M., Fredrickson, B. L., Chang, W., & Lim, Z. X. (2010). Re-examining hope: The roles of agency thinking and pathways thinking. *Cognition and Emotion, 24*(7), 1207–1215. https://doi.org/10.1080/02699930903138865
Ullmann-Margalit, E. M. (2004). Trust, distrust and in between. In R. Hardin (Ed.), *Distrust* (pp. 60–82). Russell Sage Foundation.
Vaillant, G. (1993). *The wisdom of the ego*. Harvard University Press.
Walker, M. U. (2006). *Moral Repair: Reconstructing Moral Relations after Wrongdoing*. Cambridge University Press.
Weinstein, N. D. (1980). Unrealistic optimism about future life events. *Journal of Personality and Social Psychology, 39*(5), 806–820. https://doi.org/10.1037/0022-3514.39.5.806
White, K. A. (2009). Self-confidence: A concept analysis. *Nursing Forum, 44*(2), 103–114. https://doi.org/10.1111/j.1744-6198.2009.00133.x
Wojciszke, B., Bazinska, R., & Jaworski, M. (1998). On the dominance of moral categories in impression formation. *Personality and Social Psychology Bulletin, 24*, 1251–1263. https://doi.org/10.1177/01461672982412001

Andreas Krafft holds a doctoral degree in Management Sciences at the University of St. Gallen (Switzerland) with special focus on Organizational Psychology, Culture and Development. He has academic specializations in Social Psychology of Organizations, Work and Health Psychology as well as Positive Psychology from the University of Zürich. Andreas is associate researcher for Futures Studies and lecturer at the Institute of Systemic Management and Public Governance at the University of St. Gallen. Furthermore, he teaches at the University of Zürich in the field of Work and Health, at the Master of Applied Positive Psychology at the University of Lisbon, Portugal, as well as at the Master of Futures Studies from the Free University Berlin. He is co-president of swissfuture, the Swiss Society for Futures Studies, member of the executive board of SWIPPA (the Swiss Positive Psychology Association) and of the DACH-PP (German speaking Association of Positive Psychology). Since many years he leads the International Research Network of the Hope Barometer.

JohnBosco Chika Chukwuorji is a Senior Lecturer at the Department of Psychology, University of Nigeria, Nsukka. He was a Fulbright scholar and visiting researcher at Cleveland State University Cleveland, Ohio USA (2019–2020). He holds a PhD in clinical psychology obtained from the University of Nigeria Nsukka. As a research fellow in the Center for Translational and Implementation Research (CTAIR), University of Nigeria Nsukka, he is a core team member in the use of implementation science to enhance the effectiveness and quality of healthcare services in Nigeria.

His research is focused on finding innovative approaches to provide quality mental healthcare for people living with challenging health conditions, forcibly displaced persons, justice-involved individuals, underserved communities and the general population. In addition to being the Editor of Nigerian Journal of Psychological Research, he is associate editor of three Journals (Fulbright Chronicles, Nigerian Journal of Psychology, Journal of International Politics & Development Studies) and editorial board member of four journals (BMC Psychology, Journal of Child & Adolescent Trauma, CPQ Women and Child Health, Journal of Psychology and Allied Disciplines).

Rajneesh Choubisa is Associate Professor of Psychology in the Department of Humanities and Social Sciences at Birla Institute of Technology and Science, (BITS) Pilani, Pilani Campus, India. He is a behavioral scientist by training and specializes in Positive Psychology from IIT Delhi. He has carried out meaningful research in the area of positive psychological measurement, positive organizational psychology and well-being promotion. He has rendered his expertise for reviewing projects at the European Commission's Institute of Advance Studies, among others. He is actively providing his expertise in the capacity of reviewer and academic editor for many top quality journals in the field. As an Indian collaborator of the Hope Barometer project, he has keen interest in exploring positive psychological variables theoretically, and also testing the practicability of these variables through customized, theory-driven, tailor-made programs and interventions.

Stella Conte is professor at the University of Cagliari, Italy. She is a member of the Italian Association of Psychology (A.I.P., Experimental Session) and of the Italian Association of Ethology. She is a referee for "Psychological Research" and "International Journal of Psychology". Her main research interest focuses on the following areas: the methodological issues of research on cognitive activity in human and animal: Vigilance and Attention, Language, Perception and Memory, as well as Cooperative Learning, Ethological studies of gulls, BFC and changes after treatment in children and adults and Theater therapy in adults and children. She has been the Scientific Responsible of a number of research projects: 2020 Creation of Help Desk for the Prevention of New Technology Addictions Foundation. She is the author of 180 scientific works, including monographies, chapters of books, scientific papers and proceedings published in national and international Journals.

Fabien Fenouillet is a professor of positive psychology of learning at the University of Paris Nanterre (UPN) and deputy director of the Interdisciplinary Laboratory in Neuroscience, Physiology and Psychology: Learning, Physical Activity and Health (LINP2-2APS). He is a specialist in motivation, particularly when this concept is applied to school, university or adult learning. He has written several books on this topic and published numerous scientific articles on the relationship between motivation and cognitive processes related to intelligence, memory, or in connection with technologies. He is committed to the optimal functioning of the human being. His research and publications apply more globally to consider different aspects of learning such as those related to well-being, interests, values but also anxiety.

Valle Flores-Lucas is Associate Professor at Valladolid University, in the psychology department. She led the Postgraduate course on Positive Psychology and Humour sense at Valladolid University. Her research work has been centred on two main research lines: developmental language and communication disorders. In the last years, she started another research line in the field of Positive Psychology mainly in the study of hope and its relations with other positive strengths and its applications on education. She is member of the Spanish Positive Psychology Society.

Tharina Guse is a counselling psychologist and obtained an MA (Counselling Psychology) degree from the Potchefstroom University (now North-West University) in 1989. She was in full-time private practice for the next 15 years providing psychotherapy for children, adolescents and adults. In 2003 she obtained her PhD (Psychology) from Potchefstroom University. She returned to academia in 2005 and joined the University of Johannesburg. Since April 2018 she is a professor and Head of the Department of Psychology at the University of Pretoria. Currently she serves on the Professional Board for Psychology of the Health Professions Council of South Africa (HPCSA). She is also President of the recently founded South African Positive Psychology Association (SAPPA). Her research focuses are on positive psychology in general and in particular on psycho-social well-being, positive psychology interventions and psychological strengths such as hope and gratitude. Closely aligned with this broad focus she also conducts research on the application of hypnosis for the promotion of mental health and well-being.

Elżbieta Kasprzak, psychologist, professor at the Kazimierz Wielki University in Bydgoszcz, Poland. Researcher of the determinants of careers and their consequences for the well-being of employees. An important area of her scientific interests are various aspects of positive functioning at work, job satisfaction, hope and passion at work, as well as the conditions and effects of job crafting and proactivity at work. Since 2015 she has been participating in the international research network of the Hope Barometer.

Charles Martin-Krumm is full Professor at the Ecole de Psychologues Praticiens de Paris (EPP). He is the director of the Vulnerability, Capability, and Recovery Laboratory at EPP. He is researcher at APEMAC UR 4360 UDL in Metz and associate at the Institut de Recherche Biomédicale des Armées (IRBA), in Brétigny. He is received the Fellow Award of the International Positive Psychology Association. Author of ten books and more than a hundred scientific publications, his research themes are related to quality of life and education in the fields of school, physical activity and sports, health and organizations.

Helena Agueda Marujo has a PhD in Psychology. She is Associate Professor at the Instituto Superior de Ciências Sociais e Politicas of the University of Lisbon, where she holds the positions of Executive Coordinator of Masters and PhDs programs in Development Human Resources Policies; of Scientific Coordinator of the Postgraduate Degree in Applied Positive Psychology; of researcher at the Centre for Administration and Public Policy (CAPP); and of member of the Ethics Committee. She is the Coordinator of the UNESCO Chair in Education for Global Peace Sustainability at the University of Lisbon. Helena is a member of the Advisory Board of the International Positive Psychology Association and of the Board of Directors of the European Positive Psychology Network.

Chitra S. Nair started her career as Assistant Professor of Sociology at Government K.N.M. College, Thiruvananthapuram under University of Kerala in 2015. Her ongoing research focuses on positive psychology, improving quality of life and happiness of the marginalized, social exclusion and human rights issues, life course of centenarians and understanding the indigenous approaches to "Healthy Ageing". Her social engagements include advocacy for aged and women through local self-governments, NGOs, student level interventions, industrial partners and academic institutions. Her ongoing engagements include the Major Research Project from National Commission for Women, India to conduct research study titled 'Reproductive Rights and Choices of Fisher Women in Coastal Kerala—an Ethnographic Enquiry' and the Minor Research Project from Indian Council for Social Science Research for the research study on Intimate Partner Violence.

Dorit Redlich-Amirav is an occupational therapist who works in the field of hope and mental health, mainly with family members. She completed her doctoral studies in the Department of Rehabilitation Medicine at the University of Alberta, Edmonton, Canada. Hope in mothers of adult children with mental illness in an environment of socio-political conflict. She teaches in the field of hope and mental health in the school of health professions at Tel Aviv University. On the subject of hope, she teaches a 'Circle of Hope' course at Levinsky-Wingate Academic Center and at the Ono Academic Campus. In addition, she leads the Hope Index project in Israel.

Mark Sinclair is an experienced educator, governance and technology professional. Dr Sinclair's career spans multi-sector education; corporate advisory at KPMG and AT Kearney and IT strategy (banking & public sectors). Dr. Sinclair has advised senior executives at over 100 organizations in a broad range of industries throughout Australia, Southeast Asia and the Middle East, helped establish a successful technology start-up and, over the last 20 years, overseen the development of an Education College that has provided education to 100,000 students.

Alena Slezackova, Ph.D., is an Associate Professor of Psychology and a Vice Head of the Dept. of Psychology and Psychosomatics, Faculty of Medicine, Masaryk University, in Brno, Czech Republic. Her scientific interests include mainly hope, mental health, and well-being. She also has a special interest in the research and practice of mindfulness. Alena is a founder and director of the Czech Positive Psychology Centre (CPPC), a member of the Advisory Council of the International Positive Psychology Association (IPPA), and a member of the Executive Board of the European Network for Positive Psychology (ENPP). She has been a member of several international research projects, and she serves on the editorial boards of five academic psychological journals. Alena is the author of the first comprehensive monograph on positive psychology in the Czech language and dozens of scientific publications in positive psychology and health psychology.

Patryk Stecz, a psychologist, is an assistant professor at the Institute of Psychology, University of Lodz, Poland. From 2014–2017 and 2021–2025, he was elected to the Executive Board of the Polish Suicidology Association. Dr Stecz completed his Ph.D. at the Medical University of Lodz. He published approx. 40 scientific works related to applied clinical psychology (attitudes towards suicide, positive suicidology, religious coping, well-being predictors in clinical and non-clinical populations, risk behavior in students with visual impairment, studies on hope). Dr Stecz has been serving psychological support at the Academic Counseling Centre (Technical University of Lodz) for students and employees with disabilities and special needs since 2008. Dr Stecz was aged 31 when he received the Medical University Rector's Scientific Award. Currently he is finishing a four-year post-graduate Clinical Psychology Specialization Program (Center of Postgraduate Medical Education).

Olga Varsos is the co-Author of the POWER Coaching and the GOAL Models, with extensive experience in executive, adult, homeless and at-risk youth coaching. These leading programs are used extensively in Australia and internationally in the not-for-profit, education, community, and indigenous youth sectors, focusing on instilling hope to establish goals to help ensure positive lasting change. Olga started her career as a social worker, firstly in the health sector before moving to project managing service delivery in the community sector. Olga has post graduate degrees in Social Work, Human Resources and is an accredited EQ Practitioner.

Eduardo Wills Herrera is an organizational and well-being scholar and has developed his academic career at Universidad de Los Andes in Bogotá Colombia where he has been Director and full professor at the Interdisciplinary Center for Development Studies (CIDER) and full professor at the Management School where he was Director of the Ph.D. program. He earned a Ph.D. in Organizational behavior from Tulane University, New Orleans, and a Master's in Development Studies from the Institute of Social Studies ISS at The Hague. His research is related to exploring Subjective Well-being as an indicator of development and quality of life in countries and as an indicator of the flourishing of people in organizations. He contributed as the director of Plan Nacional de Rehabilitación, PNR, and was Director of the Mission for State Moralization and efficiency at the Presidency of the Republic of Colombia.

Chapter 7
Hope and Mental Health Among Czech and Polish Adults in a Macrosocial Perspective and Religiosity Context

Alena Slezackova, Patryk Stecz, and Katarina Millova

Abstract Czechia and Poland underwent a significant sociopolitical change following the fall of communism in the 1980s. Despite having a lot in common (i.e., culture, language), the two significantly differ in other areas, such as religiosity. Therefore, this study aimed to examine the role of hope in the context of depression and anxiety, positive mental health, and loneliness and to explore age- and religion-related differences between their citizens.

The sample consisted of 526 Czech and 481 Polish adults. The 2019 Hope Barometer questionnaire included measures of satisfaction with the past year and expectations for the upcoming year, perceived and dispositional hope, anxiety and depression, positive mental health, and loneliness.

All respondents were most satisfied with their personal lives and shared a generally low level of optimism about their national politics. However, significant differences were observed in positive and negative indicators of mental health, where Czechs obtained generally higher positive indicators than Poles. Compared to both older generations, the youngest respondents in both countries reported lower levels of perceived hope, positive mental health, and satisfaction with the climate and environment, and greater loneliness, anxiety, and depression; they also reported more pessimistic expectations for the national economy. However, regardless of cultural background, religious participants showed higher levels of perceived hope. Both samples demonstrated similar patterns in predictors of positive mental health, as found by regression analysis. Perceived hope and dispositional hope positively

A. Slezackova (✉)
Department of Medical Psychology and Psychosomatics, Faculty of Medicine, Masaryk University, Brno, Czech Republic
e mail: alena.slezackova@med.muni.cz

P. Stecz
Department of Clinical Psychology and Psychopathology, Institute of Psychology, University of Łódź, Łódź, Poland

K. Millova
Institute of Psychology, University of Ostrava, Ostrava, Czech Republic

A. M. Krafft et al. (eds.), *Hope across cultures*, Cross-Cultural Advancements in Positive Psychology 14, https://doi.org/10.1007/978-3-031-24412-4_7

predicted mental health, while negative emotivity and loneliness predicted mental health negatively.

These results are discussed within a broader framework of life experiences on the micro- and macrolevel in the context of Central European countries that recently underwent macrosocial transitions.

7.1 Introduction

Czechia and Poland are two West Slavic countries located in the heart of Europe. The two share a similar modern history, including being separated from Western Europe by the Iron Curtain and undergoing a post-communist transformation in the early 1990s. In this chapter, we originate from several life course and lifespan models that deal with human functioning in the context of macrosocial (or sociohistorical) changes and highlight the interaction between microlevel related to an individual and macrolevel, such as economy, politics, and other structures of a specific society. We propose that theoretical and empirical studies focused on understanding hope, its nature and experience, should account for the degree of embeddedness of an individual in a particular culture and its sets of beliefs. The inclusion of a sociocultural context not only allows the general concept of hope and its dimensions to be broadened but also helps identify its unique elements and sources. People across cultures face specific challenges in their life trajectories, which are related to the number of cultivated traditions and the macrosocial changes they experience, both in their countries and globally. Little is currently known about whether people from the same geographic regions and similar historical backgrounds share the same or similar hopes and wishes. Furthermore, we found it interesting to explore whether these two countries differ in their levels of mental health characteristics, particularly perceived and dispositional hope, and whether these characteristics are influenced by age.

7.1.1 Macrosocial Changes

The countries of Central and Eastern Europe have undergone substantial macrosocial changes in the past few decades as they have transitioned from totalitarian to democratic societies. These changes took place both on the level of social institutions (political, social, cultural, or educational systems) and in a broader sociocultural context. These institutions create certain societal structures that also provide a more general view of human development across the lifespan, since any social change, to a greater or lesser degree, is reflected in the individual level (Elder Jr., 1998). For example, according to Bronfenbrenner's bioecological model, personal development is influenced by several ecological systems acting at different distances to the individual (Bronfenbrenner & Morris, 1998). The nearest (proximal) system includes microsystems such as family, peers, school, or workplace, while the furthermost (distal) system includes cultural and societal macrosystems, which incorporate social norms and opinions, historical events, and cultural values. The elements of the proximal system change much more rapidly than social values and attitudes, which transform very slowly and gradually in stable societies (Bronfenbrenner, 2005).

Macrosocial factors significantly influence both the psychological and social aspects of human development. Psychological functioning is substantially shaped substantially by norms and worldviews approved and appreciated by society. Schwartz (2012) viewed values as central constituents of the personality and self; these play an essential role in the motivation of behavior and attitudes and can be used for describing individuals, societies, and cultural groups. Pursuing 'healthy' values (e.g., benevolence, self-direction, achievement, and universalism) can contribute to higher subjective well-being, while pursuing 'unhealthy' values (e.g., conformity, power, tradition, and security) can reduce it (Sagiv & Schwartz, 2000). Personal desired goals, and their stability and change, are also very good indicators of the macrosocial and historical events occurring in a certain society and moderate their influence on the individuals therein (Hnilica, 2007). Major macrosocial changes can often provoke a significant generational gap in worldview; however, intergenerational similarities and differences can also be influenced by other factors such as family norms, membership in specific social groups, or sociocultural background (Knafo & Schwartz, 2012; Ranieri & Barni, 2012).

Social functioning, on the other hand, is more closely connected to social norms and requirements, both of which are affected by fundamental macrosocial transitions. Societies in transition show several unique attributes that differentiate them from stable societies. One of these is considerably lower intergenerational stability in areas like education level or social status, as well as in personal worldviews in general. In contrast to stable societies, which are characterized by high intergenerational stability, societies in transition often undergo major changes in institutional structures, such as transformations in educational or economic systems. This leads to the emergence of key differences between the individual experiences of the younger generation and those of their parents (Silbereisen & Tomasik, 2008; Titma & Tuma, 2005).

The influence of macrosocial changes on individual successful development is also moderated by age. The most extensive losses usually occur in elderly people (Hofäcker et al., 2010). This was the case in post-communist countries, where those older than 50 when the macrosocial transition occurred felt the strongest negative impact. They lost many sources of security that were previously ensured by the state and were often unable to compete with younger generations in new economic conditions. In contrast, young people in their 20s or 30s could use the new social situation to improve their lives: they were at the start of their careers; it was much easier for them to change career direction, start their own businesses, or work abroad (Titma & Tuma, 2005).

7.1.1.1 Macrosocial Changes in Czechia

The macrosocial changes that took place during the second half of the twentieth century have affected the lives of several consecutive generations differently. In societies that went through major macrosocial changes throughout the past decades (see Silbereisen & Chen, 2010), such as Czechia, where the downfall of communism, the so-called Velvet Revolution in 1989, and the subsequent dissolution of the former Czechoslovakia in 1993, was followed by an economic and technological boom and globalization beginning in the 1990s (Švejnar, 1999); these changes resulted in profound intergenerational differences in multiple interdependent domains of functioning. One such difference can be found in the domains of education and career: Career lines, which used to be highly uniform and stable in Czech society before the 1990s, became diversified by the introduction of phenomena like unemployment, free choice of study, career flexibility, and free travel abroad (Klicperová et al., 1997; Millová et al., 2015). The percentage of adults with university education has also grown substantially, especially compared to western countries (Eurostat, 2018). During the totalitarian regime, Czech society also exhibited uniformity in the domain of family and romantic relationships. After the downfall of communism at the end of the 1980s, romantic and family relationship structures have become substantially diversified (Chaloupková, 2006), and the age at first marriage increased sharply (OECD, 2018), as did the age of parenthood (Eurostat, 2015). Taken together, it could be argued that changes such as these are likely to cause profound intergenerational differences that extend far beyond what is normally understood as a "generation gap".

The factors described above have also contributed significantly to the generational differences observed in values in Czechia; they are related not only to the intergenerational discontinuity in worldviews in general society, but also to their transmission within families. For example, in a cross-cultural study of intergenerational transmission of work values between parents and their offspring in young adulthood, Sümer et al. (2019) found Czech families to demonstrate a lower parent-child similarity in work values compared to their Turkish and Spanish counterparts. Changes in sets of beliefs in general Czech society have also been indicated in older sociological studies. Spousta (2002) notes that Czech society significantly changed in the area of religious beliefs, by moving from the traditional Christian dogmatic or atheistic ideology towards more religious syncretism, spirituality, and Far East inspirations. Rabušic (2001) draws attention to the different life principles of people born in the 1970s and 1980s, who tend to demonstrate more 'rational' attitudes to family, work, childbearing and gender roles in general compared to older generations in Czech society.

A more recent study by Slezackova et al. (2018a) explored the hierarchy of life values in relation to the level of subjective well-being among Czech adults: The most important values were found to be family relationships, intimate relationships and friends, and social life. It also showed that life satisfaction was significantly associated with the perceived importance of family relationships. These results are in line with previous findings showing that happy family relationships were ranked among the most important hopes and personal wishes among Czech adults: those who were satisfied with the quality of their relationships also reported greater life satisfaction (Slezackova & Krafft, 2016). The significant impact of interpersonal values, such as family and friends, on subjective well-being is also in agreement with findings suggesting that quality of close relationships plays an important role in well-being (Delle Fave et al., 2016; Diener & Seligman, 2002).

7.1.1.2 Macrosocial Changes in Poland

The number of major socio-political changes occurring since the Second World War have also affected Poland: the country lived under a totalitarian regime ruled by the Soviet Union, which led to suppression of human rights in domains ranging from mobility, education, and justice to the free market, lifestyle, and religion. An important role at that time was played by the Roman Catholic Church. Its representatives played a vital role in fighting against communism, boosting public national-catholic identity and maintaining traditions (Marody & Mandes, 2017).

Like Czechia, Poland underwent a key political transformation associated with the Round Table Agreement in 1989, i.e., at the same time as the Czechoslovak Velvet Revolution, and joined NATO (in 1999) and the EU (in 2004) at around the same time; these changes opened a new chapter of European integration and resolved similar socioeconomic challenges such as unemployment, economic migration, late motherhood, or low fertility rate (Genowska et al., 2018). Having access to the European labor market resulted in one of the largest waves of economic migration to Western European countries. These new challenges were connected with economic growth, boosting globalization, and increasing the number of younger Poles completing higher education, suggesting that the risk to democracy and further prosperity was rather low.

Still, like in Czechia, certain groups (i.e., working class, retired) found themselves somewhat disadvantaged in the post-communist system. Not surprisingly, the government escalated top down polarization, using populist, national-conservative propaganda, stoking frustrations, mutual hostility, and redistributing certain goods to lower class groups (Żuk, 2017). Right-wing political movements contributed, first and foremost, to divisions within society (within-generation gap), as well as the erosion of the democratic state, with various threats to freedom, and the sense of a civil and inclusive society (Tworzecki, 2019). Overall, the current macrosocial situation in Poland could be expressed in terms of transition, and can be discussed through the lens of global changes in society, post-communist transformation in Central Europe, contemporary transitions in religiosity or domestic sociopolitical strains.

Following the number of macrosocial changes in Poland, there have been intergenerational differences in worldviews that are partially related to the processes that affected the Czech community. On the ethnic and religious maps of the world, Poland could be characterized as one of the most homogeneous societies. However, there are many examples of individualization of morality, with national surveys conducted between 2014–2015 indicating high approval of sex before marriage (74%), acceptance of in vitro fertilization (76%), and positive attitudes towards the liberalization of abortion regulations (84%) (Borowik, 2017). The value change process could also be represented by the transition from a traditional family lifestyle to the emancipation of women or the increase in the number of informal relationships. Still, pro-family values seem to be shared traditionally or selectively across generations (Mariański, 2015). Positive views on further European integration and pro-Western orientation, indicated by more than 80% of Polish respondents in favor of remaining in the European Union (Balcer et al., 2016), could be attributed to, among others, acquired benefits such as financial gains, free movement of people, and employment availability (Kołodziejczyk, 2016). The current macrosocial situation may have moved society towards a more materialistic orientation, represented, for example by consumer behavior in various age groups, including older adults (Zalega, 2016). Concerning political participation, an indicator of the level of democratization and one that reflects the structure of civic attitudes, Polish society shows lower political activism than western democracies such as Germany (Vecchione et al., 2015).

A person-centered approach by Bojanowska and Piotrowski (2019) identified different sets of values among the young generation of Poles and analyzed their relationships with psychological well-being. They found that individuals with different value hierarchies, i.e., those valuing conservation and self-transcendence- vs. those with a higher valuation of openness and self-enhancement, differed in terms of psychological well-being. However, those with 'healthier' sets of beliefs report lower indices of well-being in some aspects, such as positive relationships, compared to people who share traditional spiritual worldviews (conservation, self-transcendence).

7.1.1.3 Religiosity

Religion can be defined as a system of beliefs and rituals by means of which people acknowledge God, a greater-than-human power or non-empirical dimension of reality (Golan, 2006). It plays a potentially important role in psychological adaptation, affecting coping with stress mechanisms, emotion regulation (Abu-Raiya & Pargament, 2015), and the process of discovering purpose and meaning in life (Krok, 2009). Keyes (2002) states that spiritual well-being can positively affect both the emotional, psychological, and social components of mental health.

Religion and religious beliefs are also known to be associated with negative phenomena, such as in-group and out-group effects, intolerance, military conflicts, or certain acts of violence within its institutions (Cairns et al., 2006; Toft, 2007; Tombs, 2014). Emmons (1999) emphasizes that spiritual yearnings are aimed at fulfilling various important personal needs, such as those related to ethics, end-of-life purpose, identifying more complex parts of reality, seeking manifestations of transcendence in everyday situations, and discovering the mystery of life. All countries may express and manifest hope in different ways depending on their culture, which comprises shared beliefs. Discovering the nature of hope, especially its transcendent aspect, provides possible pathways toward understanding human religiousness and spirituality (Krafft et al., 2018). For instance, the spiritual-religious dimension of hope might play a more central role or manifest itself differently in countries known as religious, with long-term traditions of prayer or worship. In contrast, Emmons humanistic-existential view emphasizes the universal character of spiritual strivings; this is similar to considering the concept of hope as something related to other people, the universe, or a transcendent power (Krafft & Walker, 2018a). The integrative approach to hope by Scioli et al. (2011, p. 82) identifies its spiritual subsystem; however, they clarify that 'faith does not have to be religious in nature'. Exploring religiosity and spirituality collectively may allow a deeper insight into understanding the holistic and transcendent nature of hope and the possible cultural differences of its structure. This view is supported by previous studies showing significant differences in religiosity between Czechia and Poland (Biolcati et al., 2020).

As mentioned above, Poland and Czechia share a lot in common, such as their culture, modern history, and language, but they significantly differ in religiosity (Biolcati et al., 2020; Halman et al., 2011). According to IndexMundi (2011, 2017), 10.4% of Czechs declared themselves Roman Catholics, 1.1% Protestants, 54% other and unspecified, and 34.5% had no religion (2011 est.); in contrast, in Poland, 85.9% were Roman Catholics, 12.1% unspecified, 1.3% Orthodox, 0.4% Protestant, and the other 0.4% included Jehovah's Witness, Buddhist, Hare Krishna, Muslim, Jewish, and Mormon (2017 est.).

During the 1990s, significant changes occurred in the attitudes of the Czech population in their religious beliefs. Many people distanced themselves from religious institutions and developed a rather noninstitutional approach to religious beliefs, a so-called 'alternative religiosity' (Hamplová, 2013; Spousta, 2002; Václavík, 2010). According to the International Social Survey Program (ISSP, 2008), 40% of respondents claimed they did not believe in God, which made Czechia one of the most secular European countries, in terms of the share of the population professing a religion, attending services, and trusting churches. However, distrust of churches does not automatically mean distrust of Christianity as such: 71% of those who expressed sympathy for Christianity claimed that they did not trust churches (Hamplová, 2013). The data from the ISSP 2008 also showed that only 6% of Czechs do not believe in the existence of God and at the same time strongly reject the existence of other supernatural phenomena, while more than 80% admitted the existence of at least one supernatural phenomenon.

The post-communist period was also associated with the change in religious attitudes in Poland. Recent years events suggest that the instrumental and fundamentalistic use of religious, conservative, and superpatriotic ideology by the Polish government and the political involvement of the domestic catholic church have exacerbated the existing intergenerational gap, which is typical for changing societies (Silbereisen & Tomasik, 2008). An example of this phenomenon is the progress in laicization of Polish society in the last two decades, especially among adolescents and young adults (Stachowska, 2019). Older generations raised in more hostile environments are generally still more religious, while people born after 1990 seem not to believe that the Church gives relevant answers to their moral or social problems or the needs of the individual (Halman et al., 2011; Marody & Mandes, 2017). However, despite the increasing number of young Poles becoming alienated from the Church, as reflected in the European Values Study, this country is still considered as one of the most religious in Europe (Marody & Mandes, 2017).

Previous studies have found that religiosity and spirituality are connected with personal well-being. For example, Slezackova and Janstova (2016) indicate a significant relationship between positive mental health and spiritual intelligence conceptualized by King and DeCicco (2009). Of the four dimensions of spiritual intelligence (i.e., critical existential thinking, personal meaning production, transcendental awareness, and conscious state expansion), the strongest predictor of mental health was personal meaning production. This is in alignment with the conclusions of King (2010), who emphasizes the importance of the ability to find meaning in difficult situations to effectively cope with life difficulties. The crucial role played by meaningfulness in psychological well-being and mental health has also been highlighted elsewhere (Byron & Miller-Perrin, 2009; Delle Fave et al., 2011; Emmons, 2005).

7.1.2 Positive and Negative Indicators of Mental Health

7.1.2.1 Mental Health

Before incorporating positive indicators of well-being, traditional mental health models offered a one-sided approach, focusing on negative symptoms. Since then, several positive models (Diener, 1984; Masten et al., 1990; Seligman, 2012) have been empirically confirmed to present an accurate picture of the state of psychological well-being and to predict impaired functioning (Joseph & Wood, 2010). Combined models, such as the dual-factor model of positive mental health (DFM) (Greenspoon & Saklofske, 2001), also known as the complete state model of mental health (Keyes, 2005), conceptualize mental health on two interrelated continua (negative indicators—psychopathology and positive indicators—subjective well-being). Although DFM is not restricted to a particular list of indicators, it stresses the possible negative outcomes of incomplete mental health (low well-being and low psychopathology) (Antaramian et al., 2010) and languishing (low end in two continua) (Wang et al., 2011).

7.1.2.2 Dispositional and Perceived Hope

Snyder's (Snyder, 2000) cognitive theory of hope construes *dispositional hope* as a positive motivational state that focuses and maintains goal-directed behavior. From this perspective, dispositional hope is directly related to personal goals and the sense of control necessary to achieve these goals through one's own efforts. In contrast, *perceived hope* is a broader concept that particularly accounts for phenomena that are beyond human control. Perceived hope is the sense of deep trust that things will turn out well, regardless of the outcome of one's personal strivings (Krafft et al., 2017).

Both dispositional and perceived hope showed significant relationships with various factors of positive psychosocial functioning. Multiple studies have established a positive relationship between dispositional hope and various aspects of mental health (e.g., Alarcon et al., 2013; Grigg, 2017). Perceived hope is more related to experiencing meaning in life, enjoying close and trusted relationships, and spiritual or religious experience (Krafft et al., 2018). Slezackova and Krafft (2016) report significant positive interrelationships among perceived hope, dispositional hope, life satisfaction, and meaning in life in a large sample of Czech adults. Both types of hope served as independent predictors of life satisfaction, with perceived hope being the strongest predictor. Similarly, in a study among Swiss and German populations, perceived hope showed stronger predictive power with respect to life satisfaction and happiness than dispositional hope (Krafft et al., 2017). Perceived hope has recently been confirmed to be related to subjective well-being in an Indian sample (Krafft & Choubisa, 2018).

In a recent study among samples of Czech and South African adults, perceived hope was found to serve as an independent predictor of harmony in life, which is a more holistic and flexible perspective on well-being, emphasizing peaceful acceptance over satisfaction. Furthermore, perceived hope mediated the relationship between positive feelings and harmony in life (Slezackova et al., 2021). While research on perceived hope has been expanding, there is still a need for studies on the dynamics of perceived hope in diverse contexts and cultures.

Hope is closely interconnected with mental health—it is not only a significant predictor, but it is also predicted by various characteristics of mental health. For example, a comparative study explored the psychosocial correlates and predictors of perceived hope among Czech and Maltese adults (Slezackova et al., 2018b). In both samples, a key predictor of perceived hope was dispositional optimism, a characteristic responsible for one's positive outlook on life. However, the predictive capacity of the varying predictors in relation to perceived hope was shown to be culturally dependent: while higher perceived hope was predicted by higher generativity and lower loneliness in the Czech sample, the second independent predictor of perceived hope was found to be spirituality in the Maltese sample.

7.1.2.3 Depression and Anxiety

Positive and negative emotions reflect the affective component of subjective well-being (Lucas & Diener, 2015). Positive emotions are consistently associated with higher levels of well-being, psychological resilience, and better mental and physical health (Le Nguyen & Fredrickson, 2018; Pressman et al., 2019). Experiencing negative emotions in response to daily stressors could have a long-term negative effect on well-being and health (Leger et al., 2018). Evidence suggests that cultural differences may exist in the psychological meanings and value ascribed to positive and negative emotions and feelings (Diener et al., 2017; Tsai et al., 2006; Wirtz et al., 2009). Therefore, we consider it important to explore possible differences in the experience of negative emotions in this study.

7.1.2.4 Social Relationships and Loneliness

Evidence suggests that poor social relationships have a negative effect on mental health outcomes, such as psychological well-being and psychological distress, including depressive symptoms and anxiety (Kawachi & Berkman, 2001). Perceived emotional and instrumental support and diverse social networks were confirmed to show significant protective effects on depression in the general population (Santini et al., 2015). A better quality of relationships with others was repeatedly associated with higher levels of psychological well-being (Diener et al., 2017; Diener & Seligman, 2002). The importance of social relationships has been confirmed also in relation to dispositional hope (Lopez, 2013) and perceived hope (Krafft et al., 2017; Slezackova, 2017; Slezackova & Krafft, 2016).

Lack of social and intimate relationships can lead to loneliness (Betts & Bicknell, 2011; Cacioppo et al., 2006a). Loneliness has been identified as a key predictor of mental and physical health (Cacioppo et al., 2002) and one of the significant factors increasing the risk of depression among elderly (Golden et al., 2009). Studies show that loneliness also has negative effects on mental health among adolescents and young adults (Goosby et al., 2013; Mahon et al., 2006). Longitudinal studies revealed that loneliness increases the risk of developing depression (Stessman et al., 2013) and exacerbates mental health problems among people who are already depressed (Wang et al., 2018). Moreover, loneliness and depression influence each other, i.e., those who are lonely are more likely to become depressed, and reciprocally, their depression increases their loneliness (Cacioppo et al., 2006b). A population-based survey on a representative sample of individuals aged 16 to 102 years described a shallow U-shaped distribution of loneliness, with higher rates of loneliness among young people and the elderly (Lasgaard et al., 2016).

Similar results were found in a recent study that included Czech adults: loneliness was negatively associated with life satisfaction, perceived hope, optimism, and positive relationships. Furthermore, lower loneliness along with higher optimism and generativity predicted higher levels of perceived hope (Slezackova et al., 2018b).

7.2 Objectives of the Study

A relatively small body of literature focusing on Czech and Polish cultures identified similarities between Czech and Polish cultures in the framework of Hofstede's model. Although a larger power distance and a more individualistic and short-term orientation were reported in Czechia, those patterns did not vary substantially between Czech and Polish societies (Kolman et al., 2003). Another study based on the Inglehart value change model (Inglehart, 1990) indicated that Czech society estimated work-life and religion as less desirable domains, while leisure time and relationships were considered more important and worthwhile (Swadźba, 2015). Considering all of this evidence for differences between Czech and Polish societies, one may be concerned that these countries may vary in terms of well-being and mental health. However, there is a lack of research investigating possible differences in the domains of psychological well-being and mental health between these two countries. To address this research gap, the present article stemmed from the theory and empirical findings presented and reviewed in the text above and focuses on the influence of hope on negative and positive indicators of mental health. It also examines whether the generation effect interacts with these relationships.

Our research aims were as follows: First, considering the intercultural variability of the structure of hope, the aim of the study was to determine whether the Czech and Polish participants differ in their levels of dispositional and perceived hope. Second, it compares positive and negative indicators of positive mental health, satisfaction with the past year and views on the upcoming year between the studied generations, controlled for cultural background, religious, and spiritual beliefs. The study also investigates whether dispositional and perceived hope are related both to negative and positive mental health indicators (controlled for cultural background). Finally, it examines whether the Czech and Polish participants vary in their predictors of positive mental health.

7.3 Method

7.3.1 Sample

Participants for online collection of data were recruited through national newspapers, social networks, and announcements on university websites. Participation was completely voluntary and anonymous. The entire sample consisted of 1007 adult persons; of these, 526 (52.2%) participants were from Czechia and 481 (47.8%) were from Poland (Table 7.1). Data was collected during November 2019 in both countries simultaneously. The two samples were comparable with respect to sample size, gender distribution, and parenthood. The Czech participants were slightly older ($t = 2.81$, $df = 945.67$, $p < 0.01$, Glass' $\Delta = -0.22$), with a lower level of education ($\chi^2 = 39.19$, $df = 2$, $p < 0.001$, Cramer's $V = 0.20$), more often single ($\chi^2 = 28.76$,

Table 7.1 Sample characteristics

		Czechia				Poland			
Variable	Characteristics	*n*	%	*M*	*SD*	*n*	%	*M*	*SD*
Age	–	526	100	33.91	15.34	481	100	31.58	10.82
Sex	Males	174	33.1			140	29.1		
	Females	352	66.9			341	70.9		
Education	High school without leaving exam or less	31	5.9			17	3.5		
	High school with leaving exam	304	57.8			195	40.5		
	University	191	36.3			269	55.9		
Current family status	Single	206	36.2			156	32.5		
	In partnership	131	24.9			144	29.8		
	Married	144	27.4			166	34.5		
	Divorced	37	7			14	2.9		
	Widowed	8	1.5			1	0.2		
Current employment status	Studying	236	44.9			144	29.9		
	Employed	240	45.6			302	62.8		
	On parental leave	15	2.9			18	3.7		
	Unemployed	2	0.4			7	1.5		
	Retired	33	6.3			10	2.1		

$df = 5$, p < 0.001, Cramer's V = 0.17), and more often studying ($\chi^2 = 44.77$, $df = 5$, $p < 0.001$, Cramer's $V = 0.21$) compared to the Polish participants.

7.3.2 Measures

Age groups: In alignment with the socio-historical background of Czechia and Poland, we divided both samples into three age groups. *New generation* = 18 to 29 years (people born after macrosocial changes in the 1990s in Czechia and Poland); *transition generation* = 30 to 50 years (people born during the totalitarian regime in both countries but growing up after macrosocial changes); and *the oldest generation* = 51+ years (people living most of their lives during the totalitarian regime).

Religiosity-Spirituality: We identified three groups according to religious affiliation: *Christians* = persons affiliated with Catholic, Protestant, or other Christian churches; *spiritual but not religious* = spiritually grounded persons who do not profess any traditional world religion; and *atheists* = people without religion or belief.

Perceived hope: The Perceived Hope Scale (PHS; Krafft et al., 2017; Czech version Slezackova et al., 2020; Polish version was translated for this study) consists of six items rated on a 6-point Likert-type scale (0 = *strongly disagree*; 5 = *strongly agree*). The scale measures the self-reported level of perceived hope.

Dispositional hope: The Adult Dispositional Hope Scale (ADHS; Snyder et al., 1991; Czech version Ocisková et al., 2016; Polish version Łaguna et al., 2005) consists of 12 items. In this study we used 6-point Likert-type scale (0 = *strongly disagree*; 5 = *strongly agree*). The scale measures a cognitive model of hope comprised of two dimensions: agency (goal-directed energy; measured by four items) and pathways (planning to meet goals; measured by four items). Four items (distractors) are not included in the total score.

Depression and anxiety: The Patient Health Questionnaire (PHQ-4; Kroenke et al., 2009; Czech and Polish translations were created for this study) is a brief, 4-item scale to measure depression and anxiety. Items are rated on a 4-point Likert-type scale in which participants indicate how often they experience a certain situation or state (0 = *not at all*; 3 = *nearly every day*).

Positive mental health: The Mental Health Continuum-Short Form (MHC-SF; Keyes, 2005; Czech version Singh et al., 2016; Polish version Karaś et al., 2014) measures the emotional, psychological and social aspects of subjective well-being. It allows the identification of the presence and absence of mental health. In the tool, 14 items are rated on a 6-point Likert-type scale in which participants indicate how often they experience a certain situation or state (1 = *never*; 6 = *every day*).

Loneliness: The Loneliness Scale from The National Institute of Health Adult Toolbox Social Relationship Scales (Cyranowski et al., 2013; Czech and Polish translations were created for this study) assesses the level of loneliness in five items rated on a 5-point Likert-type scale (1 = *never*; 5 = *always*).

Life satisfaction in the past year: Life satisfaction in the year 2019 was assessed in five life domains: personal life, national politics, national economy, current social issues, and climate and environment. They were measured by a single item for each life domain rated on a 5-point Likert scale (1 = *very unsatisfied*; 5 = *very satisfied*).

Expectations for the upcoming year: The expectations for the upcoming year 2020 were assessed in the same five domains of life: private life, national politics, national economy, current social issues, and climate and environment. They were measured by a single item for each life domain rated on a 5-point Likert-type scale (1 = *very pessimistic*; 5 = *very optimistic*).

7.3.3 Data Analysis

Descriptive analyses, correlation and regression analyses, and group comparisons were performed using IBM SPSS Statistics. The internal consistencies of all scales were assessed using Cronbach's alpha, and the scale distribution was assessed by skewness and kurtosis. Since the scales measuring life satisfaction in various life domains in the current year and expectations for the upcoming year consisted of a single item each, their levels of internal consistency were not computed. Differences in the studied variables according to age group or religiosity and country were tested by factorial ANOVA with Bonferroni *post hoc* tests. The significance of the differences of correlation coefficients was compared between Czech and Polish samples according to Eid et al. (2011). Predictors of mental health were assessed using regression analysis for each sample separately. Since some of the were slightly skewed, analyses including these variables were checked against nonparametric versions (where applicable). The results of the nonparametric analyses are only reported in cases when their results differed from those of the parametric analyses.

7.4 Results

7.4.1 Descriptive Analysis

The descriptive statistics are shown in Table 7.2. Since the values of skewness indicated positive skewness in Depression/anxiety and Loneliness in the Czech sample and negative skewness in Life satisfaction in personal life and Expectations for personal life in both samples, the analyses including these variables were cross-checked with nonparametric versions of the used tests. Reliability analysis revealed acceptable values of internal consistency coefficients for all studied scales.

7.4.2 Comparison of Czech and Polish Samples in General

In addition to the differences in demographic characteristics between the Czech and Polish samples described in the Sample section, other studied characteristics were also included in the analysis. In *life satisfaction in the past year*, significant differences were found in the national economy and social issues: the Czech participants were more satisfied in both areas compared to the Polish sample (national economics: $t = 5.62$, $df = 933.28$, $p < 0.001$, Glass' $\Delta = -0.36$; social issues: $t = 5.50$, $df = 989.22$, $p < 0.001$, Glass' $\Delta = -0.34$). Participants in both countries were similarly satisfied in the other three domains (personal life, national politics, and climate and environment).

In *life expectations for the upcoming year*, the Czech participants were more optimistic about national politics ($t = 3.36$, $df = 1005$, $p < 0.001$, Cohen's $d = -0.21$), national economy ($t = 4.47$, $df = 971.32$, $p < 0.001$, Glass' $\Delta = -0.28$), social issues ($t = 5.58$, $df = 970.62$, $p < 0.001$, Glass' $\Delta = -0.34$), and climate and environment problems ($t = 3.31$, $df = 1005$, $p < 0.001$, *Cohen's* $d = -0.21$) than the Polish participants. They did not differ only in expectations in personal life.

The Czech and Polish participants differed in *perceived and dispositional hope, positive mental health, depression and anxiety, and loneliness*: the Czech respondents reported higher perceived hope ($t = 2.99$, $df = 1005$, $p < 0.01$, Cohen's $d = -0.19$) and positive mental health ($t = 2.81$, df $= 962.19$, $p < 0.01$, Glass' $\Delta = -0.15$). In contrast, the Polish participants scored higher in dispositional hope measure

Table 7.2 Descriptive statistics and internal consistency of measured characteristics for both countries

	Czechia					Poland				
Variable	*M*	*SD*	α	Skewness	Kurtosis	*M*	*SD*	α	Skewness	Kurtosis
Perceived hope	20.66	5.83	0.88	−0.82	0.78	19.54	5.96	0.90	−0.68	0.24
Dispositional hope	27.68	6.50	0.88	−0.75	0.75	28.57	6.76	0.89	−0.64	0.11
Depression and anxiety	3.25	3.14	0.88	1.17	0.72	4.05	3.21	0.86	0.94	0.10
Positive mental health	53.84	13.27	0.92	−0.35	−0.39	51.34	14.99	0.93	−0.18	−0.71
Loneliness	10.00	4.13	0.88	1.15	1.24	11.97	4.68	0.92	0.42	−0.41
Life satisfaction in										
Private life	3.83	1.04	–	−1.05	0.35	3.86	1.09	–	−1.04	0.49
National politics	2.16	0.89	–	0.67	0.24	2.16	1.07	–	0.64	−0.45
National economy	2.94	0.97	–	−0.09	−0.73	2.59	1.00	–	0.18	−0.56
Social issues	2.47	0.90	–	0.35	−0.22	2.15	0.96	–	0.63	−0.18
Environment	2.31	1.04	–	0.62	−0.57	2.20	1.05	–	0.55	−0.57
Expectations for										
Private life	3.92	0.94	–	−1.22	1.27	3.92	0.95	–	−1.09	0.98
National politics	2.54	0.92	–	0.37	−0.84	2.33	1.04	–	0.55	−0.54
National economy	2.82	0.91	–	0.07	−0.82	2.55	1.01	–	0.28	−0.70
Social issues	2.73	0.93	–	0.26	−0.72	2.39	1.03	–	0.44	−0.72
Environment	2.78	1.09	–	0.06	−1.35	2.55	1.14	–	0.23	−1.02

($t = 2.13$, $df = 1005$, $p < 0.01$, Cohen's $d = -0.13$), depression and anxiety ($t = 4.03$, $df = 1005$, $p < 0.001$, Cohen's $d = -0.25$), and loneliness ($t = 7.13$; df $= 961.92$; $p < 0.001$, Glass' $\Delta = -0.48$).

7.4.3 Comparison of Czech (CZ) and Polish (PL) Samples According to Age Groups

As reported above, the participants were divided into three age groups: the *new generation* (18–29 years old; $N_{CZ} = 282$, $N_{PL} = 246$), the *transition generation* (30–50 years old; $N_{CZ} = 154$, $N_{PL} = 246$) and *the oldest generation* (51 years old and older; $N_{CZ} = 90$, $N_{PL} = 42$). Although the size of the new generation was similar in both samples, the transition generation group was slightly larger in the Polish sample and the oldest generation group was slightly larger in the Czech sample ($\chi^2 = 22.33$, $df = 2$, $p < 0.001$, Cramer's $V = 0.15$).

The results of 2 × 3 (country × age group) factorial ANOVA showed that neither country nor age group had a significant effect on *satisfaction with personal life*. However, there was a significant interaction effect ($F(2, 1005) = 3.19$, $p < 0.05$, $\eta_p^2 = 0.005$), with the Polish transition generation scoring higher and the oldest generation scoring lower in *satisfaction with personal life* compared to the Czech groups. No effects (main or interaction) were found among the Czech and Polish age groups in *satisfaction with national politics*. Czech participants had higher *satisfaction with the national economy* and *satisfaction with social issues* (national politics: $F(1, 1006) = 11.62$, $p < 0.001$, $\eta_p^2 = 0.010$; social issues: $F(1, 1006) = 10.69$, $p < 0.001$, $\eta_p^2 = 0.009$). Finally, in *satisfaction with climate and environment,* Czech participants in general scored higher ($F(1, 1006) = 4.03$, $p < 0.05$, $\eta_p^2 = 0.005$) and young people from the new generation scored lower ($F(2, 1005) = 8.91$, $p < 0.001$, $\eta_p^2 = 0.008$). A significant interaction effect was also observed, indicating that Czech participants from the transition and oldest generations scored higher compared to the Polish sample ($F(2, 1005) = 5.31$, $p < 0.01$, $\eta_p^2 = 0.005$).

Factorial ANOVA revealed several significant results in *expectations for the upcoming year*; however, in the case of *expectations for personal life*, only a significant main effect of the age group ($F(2, 1005) = 4.80$, $p < 0.01$, $\eta_p^2 = 0.008$) with the oldest generation scoring significantly lower compared to the transition generation. No significant main effect was observed for the country or interaction effect (country x age group). In *expectations for national politics, social issues*, and *climate and environment,* Czech participants were more optimistic than Polish participants (politics: $F(1, 1006) = 5.36$, $p < 0.05$, $\eta_p^2 = 0.005$; social issues: $F(1, 1006) = 16.40$, $p < 0.001$, $\eta_p^2 = 0.016$; climate and environment: $F(1, 1006) = 6.41$, $p < 0.05$, $\eta_p^2 = 0.006$). No significant results were observed for different age groups or for the interaction effect of the country x age group. On the contrary, for *expectations for national economy*, the results of factorial ANOVA indicate that the country had a significant main effect (Czech participants scored higher than Polish participants: $F(1, 1006) = 8.79, p < 0.01, \eta_p^2 = 0.009$) as did the age group (the youngest group scored lower than the two older groups: $F(2, 1005) = 3.26, p < 0.05, \eta_p^2 = 0.007$). However, similarly to previous expectations, we did not find any significant interaction effect of the country and age group.

In *perceived hope, the* country was found to have significant main effects (Czechs scored higher than Poles: $F(1, 1006) = 7.42, p < 0.01, \eta_p^2 = 0.007$) as did the age group (new generation had the lowest and the oldest generation had the highest level of perceived hope: $F(2, 1005) = 20.01, p < 0.001, \eta_p^2 = 0.038$); however, no significant interaction effect was observed. Regarding *dispositional hope,* the results showed that members of the transition generation scored higher than members of the new or oldest generation ($F(2, 1005) = 11.27, p < 0.001, \eta_p^2 = 0.022$). The country did not demonstrate any significant main effect or any interaction effect. *Loneliness* was higher in the Polish sample ($F(1, 1006) = 42.38, p < 0.001, \eta_p^2 = 0.041$) and in young people from new generation ($F(2, 1005) = 21.14, p < 0.001, \eta_p^2 = 0.041$). However, neither country nor age group demonstrated any significant interaction effect. Similarly, the level of *depression and anxiety* was higher in Polish participants ($F(1, 1006) = 21.51, p < 0.001, \eta_p^2 = 0.021$) and the youngest in the new generation group. The results of the factorial ANOVA also showed a significant interaction effect: members of Polish oldest generation had a higher level of depression and anxiety than their Czech counterparts ($F(2, 1005) = 2.93$, $p = 0.05$, $\eta_p^2 = 0.006$). On the other hand, *positive mental health* was higher in the Czech sample ($F(1, 1006) = 8.08, p < 0.01, \eta_p^2 = 0.008$) and in participants from transition and the oldest generation ($F(2, 1005) = 8.33, p < 0.001, \eta_p^2 = 0.016$). No significant interaction effect was observed for the country x age group.

7.4.4 Comparison of Czech and Polish Samples According to Religiosity and Spirituality

Participants were divided into three groups with regard to religiosity and spirituality: Christians ($N_{CZ} = 151$, $N_{PL} = 323$), spiritual but not religious ($N_{CZ} = 155$, $N_{PL} = 50$), and atheists ($N_{CZ} = 134$, $N_{PL} = 96$). The Chi-square test revealed significant differences in religiosity: There were more Christians and less 'spiritual but not religious' participants in the Polish sample compared to the Czech sample ($\chi^2 = 121.67$, $df = 2$, $p < 0.001$, Cramer's $V = 0.37$).

The results of 2 × 3 (country × religiosity-spirituality) factorial ANOVA in *satisfaction with personal life* did not indicate that the country had any significant main effect or interaction effect; however, a significant main effect was observed for religiosity: Christians were more *satisfied with their personal life* than atheists ($F(2, 1005) = 3.04, p < 0.05, \eta_p^2 = 0.007$). On the other hand, country and religiosity demonstrated significant main effects in *satisfaction with national politics* (higher in the Czech sample: $F(1, 1006) = 5.78, p < 0.05, \eta_p^2 = 0.006$; higher in

Christians compared to atheists: $F(2, 1005) = 5.67$, $p < 0.01$, $\eta_p^2 = 0.012$); in addition, a significant interaction effect was found (country x religiosity) indicating that Czech atheists scored higher than Polish atheists ($F(2, 1005) = 15.86$, $p < 0.001$, $\eta_p^2 = 0.034$).

Czech participants were more *satisfied with the national economy, social issues* and *climate and environment* compared to Polish participants (economy: $F(1, 1006) = 32.76$, $p < 0.001$, $\eta_p^2 = 0.035$; social issues: $F(1, 1006) = 34.41$, $p < 0.001$, $\eta_p^2 = 0.037$; environment: $F(1, 1006) = 5.54$, $p < 0.05$, $\eta_p^2 = 0.006$) and Czech atheists also obtained higher scores than Polish atheists (economy: $F(2, 1005) = 3.52$, $p < 0.05$, $\eta_p^2 = 0.008$; social issues: $F(2, 1005) = 12.13$, $p < 0.001$, $\eta_p^2 = 0.026$; environment: $F(2, 1005) = 9.24$, $p < 0.001$, $\eta_p^2 = 0.020$). Furthermore, in general, Christians were more satisfied with social issues than atheists ($F(2, 1005) = 8.10$, $p < 0.001$, $\eta_p^2 = 0.018$). No significant main effect was observed between religiosity-spirituality groups in general and *satisfaction with national economy, environment, and climate*.

Factorial ANOVA also revealed several significant results in *the expectations for the upcoming year*: the Czech participants were more optimistic about *national politics* and *national economy* than Polish participants (politics: $F(1, 1006) = 15.06$, $p < 0.001$, $\eta_p^2 = 0.016$; economy: $F(1, 1006) = 18.03$, $p < 0.001$, $\eta_p^2 = 0.020$), as well as Christians compared to atheists (in politics: $F(2, 1005) = 11.59$, $p < 0.001$, $\eta_p^2 = 0.025$) or spiritual but not religious compared to atheists (in economy: $F(2, 1005) = 4.05$, $p < 0.05$, $\eta_p^2 = 0.009$). The results of the interaction effect showed that Czech atheists had more optimistic expectations for national politics and national economy than Polish atheists (politics: $F(2, 1005) = 4.92$, $p < 0.01$, $\eta_p^2 = 0.011$; economy: $F(2, 1005) = 3.64$, $p < 0.05$, $\eta_p^2 = 0.008$). Similarly, in the area of *expectations for social issues* and *climate and environment*, the Czech sample scored higher than the Polish sample (social issues: $F(1, 1006) = 28.85$, $p < 0.001$, $\eta_p^2 = 0.031$; environment: $F(1, 1006) = 15.36$, $p < 0.001$, $\eta_p^2 = 0.017$), and atheists scored lower than both the Christian and the spiritual but not religious group (social issues: $F(2, 1005) = 17.14$, $p < 0.001$, $\eta_p^2 = 0.037$; environment: $F(2, 1005) = 6.48$, $p < 0.01$, $\eta_p^2 = 0.014$). In line with previous areas of expectations, Czech atheists showed more optimistic expectations in these areas compared to Polish atheists (social issues: $F(2, 1005) = 6.71$, $p < 0.001$, $\eta_p^2 = 0.015$; environment: $F(2, 1005) = 8.83$, $p < 0.001$, $\eta_p^2 = 0.019$). On the contrary, in *expectations for personal life,* the analysis revealed neither any significant main effects (country, religiosity-spirituality) nor any interaction effect (country x religiosity-spirituality).

Regarding differences in *perceived hope* in the context of country and religiosity-spirituality, the results of factorial ANOVA showed a significant main effect for the country (higher in Czechia: $F(1, 1006) = 15.90$, $p < 0.001$, $\eta_p^2 = 0.017$) and religiosity (lower in atheists: $F(2, 1005) = 19.03$, $p < 0.001$, $\eta_p^2 = 0.040$) but without significant interaction effect. In *dispositional hope*, *loneliness* and *depression and anxiety,* only the main effect of the country was significant (all characteristics were higher in Poland; dispositional hope: $F(1, 1006) = 7.20$, $p < 0.01$, $\eta_p^2 = 0.008$; loneliness: $F(1, 1006) = 40.51$, $p < 0.001$, $\eta_p^2 = 0.043$; negative emotivity: $F(1, 1006) = 14.91, p < 0.001, \eta_p^2 = 0.016$). On the other hand, *positive mental health* was higher among Czech participants ($F(1, 1006) = 11.91, p < 0.001, \eta_p^2 = 0.013$), the Christian and the spiritual but not religious groups (compared to atheists; $F(2, 1005) = 7.64, p < 0.001, \eta_p^2 = 0.017$). No significant interaction effect was found for any of the variables.

7.4.5 Relationships Between Hope, Loneliness, Negative Emotivity, and Mental Health in Czech and Polish Samples

The next stage of our analysis examines the variables relationships between the studied variables in the Czech and Polish samples using correlation analysis (Table 7.3). Since we wanted to compare both samples, correlation analyses were run for the Czech and Polish samples separately. The results for the Czech sample are reported below the diagonal line, and the results for the Polish sample above the diagonal line.

The results of the correlation analysis revealed very similar patterns of relationships between variables in both samples. A comparison of the correlation coefficients between the Czech and Polish samples showed only a single significant difference; a stronger correlation was observed between depression/anxiety and positive mental health in the Polish sample ($r_{CZ} = -0.52$, $r_{PL} = -0.59$, $p < 0.001$; Fischer $z = 1.60$; $p = .05$; Cohen $q = 0.10$).

To test whether perceived hope, dispositional hope, loneliness, and depression/anxiety would predict mental health differently in the Czech and Polish samples, we conducted a regression analysis for each sample separately. The results are shown in Table 7.4.

The two national samples demonstrate very similar structures regarding the predictors of positive mental health: While perceived hope and dispositional hope positively predicted mental health, depression/anxiety and loneliness negatively

Table 7.3 Correlations between measures of hope, loneliness, depression and anxiety and positive mental health in the Czech and Polish samples ($n_{CZ} = 526$; $n_{PL} = 481$)

Variable	1	2	3	4	5
1. Perceived hope	–	0.57***	−0.51***	0.63***	−0.42***
2. Dispositional hope	0.53***	–	−0.44***	0.60***	−0.36***
3. Depression and anxiety	−0.55***	−0.37***	–	−0.59***	0.54***
4. Positive mental health	0.62***	0.58***	−0.52***	–	−0.54***
5. Loneliness	−0.46***	−0.33***	0.60***	−0.55***	–

Note: $^{***}p < 0.001$, $^{**}p < 0.01$, $^{*}p < 0.05$ after applying Bonferroni correction for familywise Type I error

Results for the Czech sample are displayed below the diagonal; those for the Polish sample are displayed above the diagonal

Table 7.4 Results of regression of positive mental health in the Czech and Polish samples

	Predictors of mental health									
	Czechia					Poland				
		95% CI of *B*					95% CI of *B*			
Predictors	*B*	*LL*	*UL*	*SE*	β	*B*	*LL*	*UL*	*SE*	β
Perceived hope	0.65	0.48	0.83	0.09	0.29^{***}	0.69	0.50	0.88	0.10	0.27^{***}
Dispositional hope	0.62	0.48	0.76	0.07	0.30^{***}	0.61	0.45	0.76	0.08	0.28^{***}
Depression and anxiety	−0.38	−0.72	−0.05	0.17	-0.09^{*}	−1.00	−1.35	−0.64	0.18	-0.21^{***}
Loneliness	−0.83	−1.07	−0.59	0.12	-0.26^{***}	−0.69	−0.92	−0.46	0.12	-0.22^{***}
Total R^2	0.54^{***}					0.58^{***}				
n	526					481				

Note: $^{*}p < 0.05$, $^{**}p < 0.01$, $^{***}p < 0.001$
CI = confidence interval; *LL* = lower limit; *UL* = upper limit

predicted mental health. The only difference between the samples was in the level of depression and anxiety: although it was a significant negative predictor in both samples, the effect was much stronger in the Polish sample than in the Czech sample.

7.5 Discussion

The present study compares various aspects of psychosocial functioning (i.e. satisfaction with different life domains in the past year and expectations in these domains for the upcoming year) demonstrated by groups from the Czech and Polish populations. It also looks at the differences between them in the levels of various concepts of hope (dispositional and perceived) and indicators of positive mental health. To account for the macrosocial framework, it explores these differences between different age groups: each group represents people with different life experiences in societies that underwent major macrosocial transition in the last couple of decades. These differences were controlled not only for cultural background or age, but also for religious and spiritual beliefs. Finally, it reveals the structure of the relationships between dispositional and perceived hope and positive mental health indicators in the Czech and Polish groups separately.

7.5.1 Satisfaction with the Past Year and Expectations for the Upcoming Year

Firstly, the study focused on the general cultural differences in *satisfaction with the past year*. The results showed that both Czech and Polish respondents were highly satisfied with their personal life, in addition, both samples were equally satisfied with the national politics, climate and environmental issues. However, the Czech respondents were significantly more satisfied with their national economy and social issues in the past year than the Polish participants. This might be explained by the economic and macrosocial differences between the two countries. Recent estimations conducted by Bertelsmann Stiftung (Sustainable Governance Indicators, 2020) suggest that political trust in Poland has declined rapidly between 2014 and 2020 due to the downfall in quality of democratic governance, which has been placed in the bottom rank in the EU. Another possible explanation may be that Czechia has better economic indicators, such as unemployment rate, inflation, or GDP per inhabitant, and better overall quality of life than Poland (Eurostat, 2021a, 2021b). Our findings indicating stronger dissatisfaction with politics and more pessimistic expectations towards the future in the Polish sample suggest that the current socio-political transformations could be vital agents of prospective hope.

Satisfaction with the past year might also affect expectations for the future. Both the Czech and Polish participants were equally highly optimistic about their personal lives for the upcoming year. Similar results regarding the transmission of optimistic or pessimistic expectations towards the future were obtained in a recent study by Slezackova et al. (2018b), who note that Czech adult respondents were most satisfied with their personal life in the past year and, at the same time, they were most optimistic about the same domain for the forthcoming year. These findings are also in line with the results obtained in previous studies on larger samples of Swiss and German respondents (Krafft & Walker, 2018b). This could be explained either by the effect of the optimistic bias, which postulates that people tend to believe that their future will be better than the future of others (Weinstein, 1980), or it can be also related to the fact that people tend to show higher perceived control over their personal life than over the broader circumstances such as politics, economy, and social issues.

Secondly, the study examined the general cultural differences and similarities regarding expectations for the next year. Our findings indicate that both the Czech and Polish groups shared a generally low level of optimism about their national politics. This appears to be related to a shared perceived lack of trust in political leaders and public institutions, which seems to be common in many post-communist countries (Eurostat, 2020). The higher social economic and political expectations towards the future observed in the Czech sample could be better understood when comparing our results to the recent data (Sustainable Governance Indicators, 2020): they show that Czechia scores generally better in democracy quality (civil rights, access to information, rule of law, electoral process) compared to Poland. Low community-related expectations towards the future in Poland could also be attributed to the intensification of social polarization by populist right-wing movements and the Catholic church through anti-abortion discourse or stigmatization policies, i.e., introducing 'LGBT-free' zones or anti-gender campaigns (Koralewska & Zielińska, 2021; Korolczuk, 2020).

7.5.2 Cultural Differences in the Positive and Negative Indicators of Mental Health

Further analyses revealed significant differences between the Czech and Polish participants in the positive and negative indicators of mental health: The Czech group showed higher levels of perceived hope and positive mental health, and lower levels of dispositional hope, negative emotivity and loneliness than Poles. This is to some extent congruent with the findings of Slezackova et al. (2018b), which revealed that Czech adult respondents scored significantly higher in perceived hope, optimism, life satisfaction, and perceived importance of spirituality compared to participants from other countries (i.e. Malta). These results can also be supported by the World Happiness Report 2019, which showed that Czechia (the 20th happiest country out of 156 countries) was higher in the happiness ranking of happiness than Poland (the 40th happiest country). Both countries showed similar values for positive affect, however, Poland reported higher values for negative affect (Helliwell et al., 2019).

In general, the Czech group showed higher levels of positive characteristics, apart from dispositional hope, which was higher among the Polish group, together with greater loneliness and negative emotivity. Although this result may seem paradoxical at first glance, growing evidence from research studying dispositional and perceived hope has suggested that the two may form different relationships with other positive and negative characteristics, such as life satisfaction, self-efficacy, resilience, happiness, optimism, gratitude or depression and anxiety (Krafft et al., 2017, 2021; Krafft & Walker, 2018a; Slezackova et al., 2020; Slezackova & Krafft, 2016). The overall comparison shows that while Snyder's concept of dispositional hope is rather self-concerned and it is very close to the construct of self-efficacy, with an emphasis on personal control and active involvement in problem-solving, perceived hope emphasizes the emotional, social, and spiritual aspects of hope in the sense of self-transcendence (Krafft & Walker, 2018b; Slezackova, 2017).

7.5.3 Generational Differences in Psychosocial Functioning

The study also compared studied characteristics according to three *age groups*, which were formed according to the specific macrosocial context in Czechia and Poland: a *new generation* born after macrosocial transitions, a *transition generation* born in a totalitarian regime but growing up in democratic society, and the *oldest generation* born in a totalitarian regime and living most of their lives in this regime. These age groups also reflect different parts of adulthood—young adulthood, middle to older adulthood, and old age. The findings show relatively consistently that the youngest group reported more negative characteristics: low satisfaction with climate and environment, pessimistic expectations for the national economy, low levels of perceived hope and positive mental health, and high levels of loneliness, anxiety, and depression. These results are in line with several previous studies indicating that older adults report higher well-being, life satisfaction, and more positive views toward the future than their younger counterparts (e.g., Carstensen et al., 2011; Chopik et al., 2020; Chowdhury et al., 2014). One of the possible explanations is brought by socioemotional selectivity theory suggesting that people tend to select emotionally more relevant and satisfying goals as they grow older (Carstensen et al., 1999). Similarly, growing research on dispositional and perceived hope suggests that both types tend to increase even in old age (Krafft & Walker, 2018b; Perrig-Chiello et al., 2018; Slezackova et al., 2020; Slezackova et al., 2018b).

These findings suggest that age differences could be assigned to general developmental trends throughout life. In terms of the *macrosocial context*, our results show that the Czech and Polish samples differed in many studied domains mentioned in the text above. Although they share many common areas in terms of modern social development, especially in the second half of the twentieth century, i.e., several decades of a totalitarian regime followed by its disintegration in the late 1980s and transformation into a democratic society, in both cases, their functioning is also influenced by current macrosocial characteristics which are also reflected in their individual functioning, as suggested by Bronfenbrenner's bioecological theory (Bronfenbrenner, 2005).

It is possible that macrosocial factors, such as the current political and economic situation mentioned in the text above, could have a significant influence on these results. Therefore, an analysis was performed on the three age groups in Czechia and Poland separately. However, only a few differences were found in a couple of areas (satisfaction with personal life, satisfaction with climate and environment, and negative emotivity), and these differences did not follow any specific trend. The patterns of the results suggest that either country or age has a general significance, without any interaction effect: The studied characteristics may be influenced by the country where a person lives, but they tend to increase or decrease in a similar way during the lifespan.

7.5.4 *Cultural Differences in the Context of Religiosity and Spirituality*

The differences in religiosity and spirituality observed between the Czech and Polish samples are similar to those observed elsewhere and reflect the religious specificity of those two countries (IndexMundi, 2011, 2017). Therefore, the study examined the predictive value of religiosity and spirituality for three characteristics: positive expectations for the upcoming year, satisfaction with the past year in different life domains, and positive mental health. Our findings suggest that religious participants were more satisfied with politics and social issues, and that atheists tended to report lower satisfaction with economy and social issues. Similarly, religiousness was found to have a positive association with expectations for the next year in politics. It is possible, therefore, that religious individuals are generally more satisfied with different life domains and can share more positive expectations towards certain domains of the proximal future. This should be explained with caution: Religious engagement is associated with conservative attitudes and is known to determine the political involvement of citizens. However, a recent Polish study did not indicate any straightforward connection between being religious and developing populist attitudes favored by the government or Catholic Church (Turska-Kawa & Wojtasik, 2020). Rather, it suggests that our present findings linking religiousness with positive expectations towards the future in the political domain could not be explained only by identification with nationalist-conservative state policy. Religiousness could also be interpreted as a factor including various norms, values, and beliefs producing more optimistic expectations towards different aspects of the future.

Our results also show that both the Christian group and those considering themselves spiritual scored higher in different aspects of well-being, suggesting that these groups report better mental health. Religion and spirituality could be defined both as an idiosyncratic system allowing the search for meaning and one related to the self, other people, the universe and the sacred. Previous research has suggested many possible pathways to explain this effect, including the positive influence of religion and spirituality on the ability to cope with stressful life events, the promotion of positive emotions, and the facilitation of hope and a sense of meaning (Abu-Raiya & Pargament, 2015; Krok, 2009). Regarding the relationship between religiousness and negative indicators of mental health, Krok (2014) found little evidence that religious orientation is negatively associated with somatic symptoms but not with other mental health problems (anxiety, insomnia, social dysfunction, depression). This suggests that both religion and spirituality appear to have a moderate positive impact on positive mental health and a rather weak effect on negative indicators of mental health.

Regardless of cultural background, the religious participants displayed higher levels of perceived hope, suggesting that religion may act as an important source of perceived hope; however, the Czech participants reported a higher level of perceived hope, despite being a nonreligious country. These results may indicate that there might be cultural differences between Czechia and Poland regarding the variability of sources of perceived hope. This research problem remains unsolved and could be studied in further Hope Barometer studies. It should also be noted that any generalizations on how cultural differences correspond to the structure of hope based on our present findings should be made with caution, particularly considering the convenience sampling method employed and cultural diversity of each studied country.

7.5.5 Relationships Between Hope, Loneliness, Negative Emotivity, and Mental Health in a Cultural Context

In addition to the expected strong positive correlations between perceived hope, dispositional hope and positive mental health, significant negative relationships were observed between the two concepts of hope, depression and anxiety, and loneliness. These results revealed very similar patterns of relationships in both national samples. A similar structure was found for the predictors of positive mental health: While perceived hope and dispositional hope positively predicted mental health, negative emotivity and loneliness negatively predicted mental health. The only difference between the groups was in depression and anxiety: Although it served as an independent negative predictor in both samples, the effect was much stronger in the Polish sample than in the Czech sample. From the macrosocial point of view, it is not surprising that the structure of relationships in Czech and Polish samples is similar: even though the level of psychosocial characteristics *per se* can be influenced by macrosocial characteristics (for further discussion see Silbereisen & Chen, 2010), the structure of the relationship is generally quite constant, regardless of the country and macrosocial situation.

Our empirically confirmed observations establishing similarities between Czech and Polish samples can also enrich the understanding of national autostereotypes, heterostereotypes and their relevance with real personality traits of people in Central Europe. Hřebíčková and Graf (2014) determined that the Polish national autostereotype is similar both to that of Czech and to self-reporting ratings; however, Polish respondents have considered themselves slightly more anxious and depressive than Czechs (in line with our results). In contrast, national heterostereotypes were not consistent with real personality traits, suggesting that cross-cultural comparisons can sometimes overrate differences between countries due to the individual's tendency to achieve a sense of distinct social identity.

Our findings are to some extent in line with previous studies, which found perceived hope to be significantly positively related with life satisfaction and negatively with loneliness (Slezackova et al., 2018b). It was also found that perceived hope predicted most of the variance in psychological well-being operationalized as harmony in life, and, furthermore, perceived hope mediated the relationship between positive feelings and harmony in life (Slezackova et al., 2021).

7.6 Limitations and Perspectives on Future Research

The main limitation of our study consists in the cross-sectional design and the use of convenience sampling, resulting in nonrepresentative samples and slightly uneven demographic data distribution in each of the research samples. Further bias might have been caused by factors such as self-presentation and lack of introspection.

A longitudinal study would shed more light on a deeper understanding of the investigated variables and the dynamics of the relations between them. Interesting results about the dynamics between current life satisfaction, short-term future expectations, and experiencing different aspects of hope (cognitions on capability to pursue goals, belief in self and others, sensing hope or positive general expectations towards future) could be delivered using a repeated-measures design or cross-sectional comparisons from the past Hope Barometer waves with the forthcoming data collection. We acknowledge that our findings are preliminary: further cross-national comparisons with more countries involved and waves of data collection might contribute to better understanding of the role played by current sociopolitical changes (including COVID pandemic) in experiencing hope and positive mental health.

7.7 Conclusion

The present study contributes to the discussion about the complexity of the relationships between life satisfaction, future expectations, positive mental health, negative emotivity and different manifestations of hope in the Czech and Polish populations. The findings are discussed in the context of intergenerational differences, the cultural, religious, and spiritual diversity of Poland and Czechia, and the framework of macrosocial changes in Central Europe.

The experience of hope is implicitly reflected in life satisfaction over the past year and the expectations for the upcoming year. Satisfaction with the past year and optimism related to different aspects of life in the upcoming year varied between the Czech and Polish samples; however, the two groups demonstrated similar contentment and positive expectations towards their personal life. Lower satisfaction with national politics and environment could be attributed to psychological factors, such as low sense of control in areas of life they are not personally involved, or to social factors, i.e., the context of macrosocial changes in this region. Our results support previous findings that indicate the transmission of negative or positive satisfaction with the proximal past to reflections on the near future.

Our findings highlight the differences in positive and negative indicators of mental health between the Czech and Polish populations. It is possible that the lower perceived hope observed among Polish participants could be explained by higher indices of loneliness, anxiety and depression in this group. Among atheists, the Czech group demonstrated higher perceived hope than its Polish counterparts, suggesting that the religiosity-spirituality domain does not solely explain the variability of hope in its transcendental aspects. We conclude that this issue should be discussed with respect to the different trajectories of transformations that Polish and Czech society underwent, particularly concerning religious beliefs. Furthermore, our findings seem to reveal that the Polish sample may experience hope differently, associating it with optimistic beliefs about self and the capability to set future-oriented goals.

Despite the non-experimental design of the study, our findings may also suggest that growing older is associated with becoming happier, more hopeful, less depressed and lonely; however, in both samples, the young generation also appeared to display difficulties in developing a complete state of mental health, as manifested by lower indices of hope and well-being, or more negative emotivity symptoms. Therefore, policies aimed at boosting positive mental health should acknowledge that particularly young adults suffer from insufficiencies regarding their trust in themselves and other people, goal-oriented motivation, self-efficacy, emotional experience of hope or psychological well-being, making this subpopulation more vulnerable to macrosocial changes. The young generation is a potential target population for implementing preventive mental health interventions, focusing on negative indicators of mental health, such as depression and anxiety.

References

Abu-Raiya, H., & Pargament, K. I. (2015). Religious coping among diverse religions: Commonalities and divergences. *Psychology of Religion and Spirituality, 7*(1), 24–33. https://doi.org/10.1037/a0037652

Alarcon, G. M., Bowling, N. A., & Khazon, S. (2013). Great expectations: A meta-analytic examination of optimism and hope. *Personality and Individual Differences, 54*(7), 821–827. https://doi.org/10.1016/j.paid.2012.12.004

Antaramian, S. P., Huebner, E., Hills, K. J., & Valois, R. F. (2010). A dual-factor model of mental health: Toward a more comprehensive understanding of youth functioning. *American Journal of Orthopsychiatry, 80*(4), 462–472. https://doi.org/10.1111/j.1939-0025.2010.01049.x

Balcer, A., Buras, P., Gromadzki, G., & Smolar, E. (2016). *Polacy wobec UE: Koniec konsensusu [Poles vs. EU: The end of consensus]*. Fundacja im. Stefana Batorego.

Betts, L. R., & Bicknell, A. S. A. (2011). Experiencing loneliness in childhood: Consequences for psychosocial adjustment, school adjustment, and academic performance. In S. J. Be-vinn (Ed.), *Psychology of loneliness* (pp. 1–28). Nova Science Publishers.

Biolcati, F., Lomazzi, V., Molteni, F., Quandt, M., & Vezzoni, C. (2020). Church attendance and religious change pooled European dataset (CARPE). *Archivio Istituzionale della Ricerca, 56*, 1729. https://doi.org/10.7802/2040

Bojanowska, A., & Piotrowski, K. (2019). Values and psychological well-being among adolescents–are some values 'healthier' than others? *European Journal of Developmental Psychology, 16*(4), 402–416. https://doi.org/10.1080/17405629.2018.1438257

Borowik, I. (2017). Religion, politics and social attitudes in transforming Poland: A conclusion. In S. P. Ramet & I. Borowik (Eds.), *Religion, politics, and values in Poland* (pp. 313–324). Palgrave Macmillan. https://doi.org/10.1057/978-1-137-43751-8_11

Bronfenbrenner, U. (2005). The bioecological theory of human development (2001). In U. Bronfenbrenner (Ed.), *Making human beings human: Bioecological perspectives on human development* (pp. 3–15). Sage Publications.

Bronfenbrenner, U., & Morris, P. A. (1998). The ecology of developmental process. In W. Damon & R. M. Lerner (Eds.), *Handbook of child psychology* (Vol. 1. Theoretical models of human development, 5th ed., pp. 993–1028). Wiley.

Byron, K., & Miller-Perrin, C. (2009). The value of life purpose: Purpose as a mediator of faith and well-being. *The Journal of Positive Psychology, 4*(1), 64–70. https://doi.org/10.1080/17439760802357867

Cacioppo, J. T., Hawkley, L. C., Crawford, L. E., Ernst, J. M., Burleson, M. H., Kowalewski, R. B., Malarkey, W. B., Van Cauter, E., & Berntson, G. G. (2002). Loneliness and health: Potential mechanisms. *Psychosomatic Medicine, 64*(3), 407–417. https://doi.org/10.1097/00006842-200205000-00005

Cacioppo, J. T., Hawkley, L. C., Ernst, J. M., Burleson, M., Berntson, G. G., Nouriani, B., & Spiegel, D. (2006a). Loneliness within a nomological net: An evolutionary perspective. *Journal of Research in Personality, 40*, 1054–1085. https://doi.org/10.1016/j.jrp.2005.11.007

Cacioppo, J. T., Hughes, M. E., Waite, L. J., Hawkley, L. C., & Thisted, R. A. (2006b). Loneliness as a specific risk factor for depressive symptoms: Cross-sectional and longitudinal analyses. *Psychology and Aging, 21*(1), 140–151. https://doi.org/10.1037/0882-7974.21.1.140

Cairns, E., Kenworthy, J., Campbell, A., & Hewstone, M. (2006). The role of in-group identification, religious group membership and intergroup conflict in moderating in-group and out-group affect. *British Journal of Social Psychology, 45*(4), 701–716. https://doi.org/10.1348/014466605X69850

Carstensen, L. L., Isaacowitz, D. M., & Charles, S. T. (1999). Taking time seriously: A theory of socioemotional selectivity. *American Psychologist, 54*(3), 165–181. https://doi.org/10.1037/0003-066X.54.3.165

Carstensen, L. L., Turan, B., Scheibe, S., Ram, N., Ersner-Hershfield, H., Samanez-Larkin, G. R., Brooks, K. P., & Nesselroade, J. R. (2011). Emotional experience improves with age: Evidence based on over 10 years of experience sampling. *Psychology and Aging, 26*(1), 21–33.

Chaloupková, J. (2006). Dohromady, nebo každý zvlášť? Hospodaření s příjmy manželských a nesezdaných párů. [Joint or separate? Income management among married and cohabiting couples]. *Sociologický časopis/Czech Sociological Review, 42*, 971–986.

Chopik, W. J., Kim, E. S., Schwaba, T., Krämer, M. D., & Smith, J. (2020). Changes in optimism and pessimism in response to life events: Evidence from three large panel studies. *Journal of Research in Personality, 88*, 103985. https://doi.org/10.1016/j.jrp.2020.103985

Chowdhury, R., Sharot, T., Wolfe, T., Düzel, E., & Dolan, R. J. (2014). Optimistic update bias increases in older age. *Psychological Medicine, 44*(9), 2003–2012. https://doi.org/10.1017/S0033291713002602

Cyranowski, J. M., Zill, N., Bode, R., Butt, Z., Kelly, M. A., Pilkonis, P. A., Salsman, J. M., & Cella, D. (2013). *Health Psychology, 32*(3), 293–301. https://doi.org/10.1037/a0028586

Delle Fave, A., Brdar, I., Freire, T., Vella-Brodrick, D., & Wissing, M. P. (2011). The eudaimonic and hedonic components of happiness: Qualitative and quantitative findings. *Social Indicators Research, 100*(2), 185–207. https://doi.org/10.1007/s11205-010-9632-5

Delle Fave, A., Brdar, I., Wissing, M. P., Araujo, U., Castro, S. A., Freire, T., Hernández-Pozo, M., Jose, P., Martos, T., Nafstad, H. E., Nakamura, J., Singh, K., & Soosai-Nathan, L. (2016). Lay definitions of happiness across nations: The primacy of inner harmony and relational connectedness. *Frontiers in Psychology, 7*. https://doi.org/10.3389/fpsyg.2016.00030

Diener, E. (1984). Subjective well-being. *Psychological Bulletin, 95*(3), 542–575. https://doi.org/10.1037/0033-2909.95.3.542

Diener, E., & Seligman, M. E. P. (2002). Very happy people. *Psychological Science, 13*(1), 81–84. https://doi.org/10.1111/1467-9280.00415

Diener, E., Heintzelman, S. J., Kushlev, K., Tay, L., Wirtz, D., Lutes, L. D., & Oishi, S. (2017). Findings all psychologists should know from the new science on subjective well-being.

Canadian Psychology/Psychologie Canadienne, 58(2), 87–104. https://doi.org/10.1037/cap0000063

Eid, M., Gollwitzer, M., & Schmitt, M. (2011). *Statistik und Forschungsmethoden* (2nd ed.). Beltz.

Elder, G. H., Jr. (1998). The life course as developmental theory. *Child Development, 69*(1), 1–12. https://doi.org/10.1111/j.1467-8624.1998.tb06128.x

Emmons, R. A. (1999). *The psychology of ultimate concerns: Motivation and spirituality in personality*. Guilford Press.

Emmons, R. A. (2005). Striving for the sacred: Personal goals, life meaning, and religion. *Journal of Social Issues, 61*(4), 731–745. https://doi.org/10.1111/j.1540-4560.2005.00429.x

Eurostat. (2015). *Mean age of women at birth of first child, 1995, 2000, 2005 and 2012*. Accessed March 2, 2021, from http://ec.europa.eu/eurostat/statistics-explained/index.php?title=File:Mean_age_of_women_at_birth_of_first_child,_1995,_2000,_2005_and_2012_(years)_BYIE15.png&oldid=228653

Eurostat. (2018). *Population by educational attainment level, sex and age*. Accessed March 2, 2021, from http://appsso.eurostat.ec.europa.eu/nui/submitViewTableAction.do

Eurostat. (2020). *Quality of life indicators - governance and basic rights*. Accessed June 15, 2021, from https://ec.europa.eu/eurostat/statistics-explained/index.php?title=Quality_of_life_indicators_-_governance_and_basic_rights&oldid=420994#Trust_in_the_political_and_legal_systems

Eurostat. (2021a). *Economic indicators*. Accessed March 2, 2021, from https://ec.europa.eu/eurostat/cache/infographs/economy/desktop/index.html

Eurostat. (2021b). *Quality of life*. Accessed June 15, 2021, from https://ec.europa.eu/eurostat/cache/infographs/qol/index_en.html

Genowska, A., Szafraniec, K., Polak, M., Szpak, A., Walecka, I., & Owoc, J. (2018). Study on changing patterns of reproductive behaviours due to maternal features and place of residence in Poland during 1995-2014. *Annals of Agricultural and Environmental Medicine, 25*(1), 137–144. https://doi.org/10.26444/aaem/75544

Golan, Z. (2006). Pojęcie religijności [Religiousness]. In S. Głaz (Ed.), *Podstawowe zagadnienia psychologii religii [Basic concepts of psychology of religion]* (pp. 71–79). Wydawnictwo WAM.

Golden, J., Conroy, R. M., Bruce, I., Denihan, A., Greene, E., Kirby, M., & Lawlor, B. A. (2009). Loneliness, social support networks, mood and wellbeing in community-dwelling elderly. *International Journal of Geriatric Psychiatry, 24*(7), 694–700. https://doi.org/10.1002/gps.2181

Goosby, B. J., Bellatorre, A., Walsemann, K. M., & Cheadle, J. E. (2013). Adolescent loneliness and health in early adulthood. *Sociological Inquiry, 83*(4), 505–536. https://doi.org/10.1111/soin.12018

Greenspoon, P. J., & Saklofske, D. H. (2001). Toward an integration of subjective well-being and psychopathology. *Social Indicators Research, 54*(1), 81–108. https://doi.org/10.1023/A:1007219227883

Grigg, S. (2017). Hope and mental health in young adult college students: An integrative review. *Journal of Psychosocial Nursing and Mental Health Services, 55*(2), 28–35. https://doi.org/10.3928/02793695-20170210-04

Halman, L., Sieben, I., & van Zundert, M. (Eds.). (2011). *Atlas of European values. Trends and traditions at the turn of the century*. Brill.

Hamplová, D. (2013). *Náboženství v české společnosti na prahu 3. tisíciletí [Czech religion at the beginning of the 3rd Millennium]*. Charles University.

Helliwell, J., Layard, R., & Sachs, J. (2019). *World happiness report 2019*. Sustainable Development Solutions Network. Accessed May 17, 2021, from https://worldhappiness.report/ed/2019/

Hnilica, K. (2007). Vývoj a změny hodnot v dospělosti [Development and change in values in adulthood]. *Československá psychologie, 51*(5), 437–463.

Hofäcker, D., Buchholz, S., & Blossfeld, H.-P. (2010). Globalization, institutional filters and changing life course. Patterns in modern societies: A summary of the results from the

GLOBALIFE-project. In R. K. Silbereisen & X. Chen (Eds.), *Social change and human development: Concept and results* (pp. 101–124). Sage.

Hřebíčková, M., & Graf, S. (2014). Accuracy of National Stereotypes in Central Europe: Outgroups are not better than ingroup in considering personality traits of real people. *European Journal of Personality., 28*(1), 60–72. https://doi.org/10.1002/per.1904

IndexMundi. (2011). Retrieved from http://www.indexmundi.com/

IndexMundi. (2017). Retrieved from http://www.indexmundi.com/

Inglehart, R. (1990). *Culture shift in advanced industrial society*. Princeton University Press.

Joseph, S., & Wood, A. (2010). Assessment of positive functioning in clinical psychology: Theoretical and practical issues. *Clinical Psychology Review, 30*(7), 830–838. https://doi.org/10.1016/j.cpr.2010.01.002

Karaś, D., Cieciuch, J., & Keyes, C. L. M. (2014). The Polish adaptation of the mental health continuum-short form (MHC-SF). *Personality and Individual Differences, 69*, 104–109. https://doi.org/10.1016/j.paid.2014.05.011

Kawachi, I., & Berkman, L. F. (2001). Social ties and mental health. *Journal of Urban Health, 78*(3), 458–467. https://doi.org/10.1093/jurban/78.3.458

Keyes, C. L. M. (2002). The mental health continuum: From languishing to flourishing in life. *Journal of Health and Social Behavior, 43*(2), 207–222. https://doi.org/10.2307/3090197

Keyes, C. L. M. (2005). Mental illness and/or mental health? Investigating the axioms of the complete state model of health. *Journal of Consulting and Clinical Psychology, 73*(3), 539–548. https://doi.org/10.1037/0022-006X.73.3.539

King, D. B. (2010). Personal meaning production as a component of spiritual intelligence. *International Journal of Existencial Psychology and Psychotherapy, 3*(1), 1–5.

King, D. B., & DeCicco, T. L. (2009). A viable model and self-report measure of spiritual intelligence. *International Journal of Transpersonal Studies, 28*(1), 68–85. https://doi.org/10.24972/ijts.2009.28.1.68

Klicperová, M., Feierabend, I. K., & Hofstetter, C. R. (1997). In the search for a post-communist syndrome. A theoretical framework and empirical assessment. *Journal of Community and Applied Social Psychology, 7*(1), 39–52. https://doi.org/10.1002/(SICI)1099-1298(199702)7:1<39::AID-CASP398>3.0.CO;2-1

Knafo, A., & Schwartz, S. H. (2012). Relational identification with parents, parenting, and parent–child value similarity among adolescents. *Family Science, 3*(1), 13–21. https://doi.org/10.1080/19424620.2011.707794

Kolman, L. K., Noorderhaven, N. G., Hofstede, G., & Dienes, E. (2003). Cross-cultural differences in Central Europe. *Journal of Managerial Psychology, 18*(1), 76–88. https://doi.org/10.1108/02683940310459600

Kołodziejczyk, K. (2016). Poland in the European Union. Ten years of membership. *Revista UNISCI, 39*(January), 9–26. https://doi.org/10.5209/rev_RUNI.2016.n40.51803

Koralewska, I., & Zielińska, K. (2021). 'Defending the unborn','protecting women'and 'preserving culture and nation': Anti-abortion discourse in the Polish right-wing press. *Culture, Health & Sexuality, 24*(5), 673–687. https://doi.org/10.1080/13691058.2021.1878559

Korolczuk, E. (2020). The fight against 'gender and 'LGBT ideology': New developments in Poland. *European Journal of Politics and Gender, 3*(1), 165–167. https://doi.org/10.1332/251510819X15744244471843

Krafft, A., & Choubisa, R. (2018). Hope in the Indian psychology context: Philosophical foundations and empirical findings. In A. Krafft, P. Perrig-Chiello, & A. Walker (Eds.), *Hope for a good life. Results of the Hope-barometer international research program* (pp. 131–163). Springer.

Krafft, A. M., & Walker, A. (2018a). Exploring the concept and experience of hope - theoretical and methodological foundations. In A. M. Krafft, P. Perrig-Chiello, & A. Walker (Eds.), *Hope for a good life. Results of the Hope-barometer international research program* (pp. 3–19). Springer.

Krafft, A. M., & Walker, A. (2018b). Exploring the concept and experience of hope – Empirical findings and the virtuous circle of hope. In A. M. Krafft, P. Perrig-Chiello, & A. Walker (Eds.),

Hope for a good life. Results of the Hope-barometer international research program (pp. 21–61). Springer.

Krafft, A. M., Martin-Krumm, C., & Fenouillet, F. (2017). Adaptation, further elaboration, and validation of a scale to measure hope as perceived by people: Discriminant value and predictive utility vis-à-vis dispositional hope. *Assessment, 24*, 1–16. https://doi.org/10.1177/1073191117700724

Krafft, A. M., Perrig-Chiello, P., & Walker, A. (Eds.). (2018). *Hope for a good life. Results of the Hope-barometer international research program*. Springer.

Krafft, A. M., Guse, T., & Maree, D. (2021). Distinguishing perceived hope and dispositional optimism: Theoretical foundations and empirical findings beyond future expectancies and cognition. *Journal of Well-Being Assessment*. Advance online publication, *4*, 217–243. https://doi.org/10.1007/s41543-020-00030-4

Kroenke, K., Spitzer, R. L., Williams, J. B. W., & Löwe, B. (2009). An ultra-brief screening scale for anxiety and depression: The PHQ-4. *Psychosomatics, 50*(6), 613–621. https://doi.org/10.1176/appi.psy.50.6.613

Krok, D. (2009). Religijność a duchowość–różnice i podobieństwa z perspektywy psychologii religii [Religiousness and spirituality - differences and similarities from the perspective of psychology of religion]. *Polskie Forum Psychologiczne, 14*(1), 126–141.

Krok, D. (2014). Religiousness and social support as predictive factors for mental health outcomes. *Archives of Psychiatry and Psychotherapy, 4*, 65–76. https://doi.org/10.12740/APP/31319

Łaguna, M., Trzebiński, J., & Zięba, M. (2005). *Kwestionariusz nadziei na sukces: podręcznik. [Adult Dispositional Hope Scale: manual]*. Pracownia Testów Psychologicznych Polskiego Towarzystwa Psychologicznego [Psycholocial Test Laboratory of the Polish Psychological Association].

Lasgaard, M., Friis, K., & Shevlin, M. (2016). "Where are all the lonely people?" a population-based study of high-risk groups across the life span. *Social Psychiatry and Psychiatric Epidemiology, 51*(10), 1373–1384. https://doi.org/10.1007/s00127-016-1279-3

Le Nguyen, K. D., & Fredrickson, B. L. (2018). Positive emotions and well-being. In D. S. Dunn (Ed.), *Frontiers of social psychology. Positive psychology: Established and emerging issues* (pp. 29–45). Routledge/Taylor & Francis Group.

Leger, K. A., Charles, S. T., & Almeida, D. M. (2018). Let it go: Lingering negative affect in response to daily stressors is associated with physical health years later. *Psychological Science, 29*(8), 1–8. https://doi.org/10.1177/0956797618763097

Lopez, S. J. (2013). *Making hope happen: Create the future you want for yourself and others*. Atria Books.

Lucas, R. E., & Diener, E. (2015). Personality and subjective well-being: Current issues and controversies. In M. Mikulincer, P. R. Shaver, M. L. Cooper, & R. J. Larsen (Eds.), *APA handbook of personality and social psychology* (Vol. 4, pp. 577–599). American Psychological Association.

Mahon, N. E., Yarcheski, A., Yarcheski, T. J., Cannella, B. L., & Hanks, M. M. (2006). A meta-analytic study of predictors for loneliness during adolescence. *Nursing Research, 55*(5), 308–315. https://doi.org/10.1097/00006199-200609000-00003

Mariański, J. (2015). Małżeństwo i rodzina w świadomości Polaków - analiza socjologiczna [Marriage and family in the perception of the Polish people: A sociological analysis]. *Zeszyty Naukowe KUL, 58*(4), 77–103.

Marody, M., & Mandes, S. (2017). Polish religious values as reflected in the European values study. In S. P. Ramet & I. Borowik (Eds.), *Religion, politics, and values in Poland: Continuity and change since 1989* (pp. 231–255). Palgrave Macmillan. https://doi.org/10.1057/978-1-137-43751-8_11

Masten, A. S., Best, K. M., & Garmezy, N. (1990). Resilience and development: Contributions from the study of children who overcome adversity. *Development and Psychopathology, 2*(4), 425–444. https://doi.org/10.1017/S0954579400005812

Millová, K., Blatný, M., & Jelínek, M. (2015). Factors of positive social functioning in the context of transforming societies: Results of the Brno longitudinal study on life-span human development. *Československá psychologie, 59*(Supplement 1), 47–55.

Ocisková, M., Sobotková, I., Praško, J., & Mihál, V. (2016). Standardizace české verze Škály dispoziční naděje pro dospělé [Standardization of the Czech version of the Snyder's adult dispositional hope scale]. *Psychologie a její kontexty, 7*(1), 109–123.

OECD. (2018). *How's life in Czech Republic?* Accessed March 2, 2021, from https://www.oecd.org/statistics/Better-Life-Initiative-country-note-Czech-Republic.pdf

Perrig-Chiello, P., Spahni, S., & Margelisch, K. (2018). The older, the better? The role of hope for the regulation of subjective well-being over life-span. In A. M. Krafft, P. Perrig-Chiello, & A. M. Walker (Eds.), *Hope for a good life. Results of the Hope-Barometer international research program* (pp. 79–94). Springer.

Pressman, S. D., Brooke, N. J., & Moskowitz, J. T. (2019). Positive affect and health: What do we know and where next should we go? *Annual Review of Psychology, 70*, 627–560. https://doi.org/10.1146/annurev-psych-010418-102955

Rabušic, L. (2001). Value change and demographic behaviour in the Czech Republic. *Sociologický časopis/Czech Sociological Review, 9*(1), 99–122. https://doi.org/10.2307/41133175

Ranieri, S., & Barni, D. (2012). Family and other social contexts in the intergenerational transmission of values. *Family Science, 3*(1), 1–3. https://doi.org/10.1080/19424620.2012.714591

Sagiv, L., & Schwartz, S. H. (2000). Value priorities and subjective well-being: Direct relations and congruity effects. *European Journal of Social Psychology, 30*(2), 177–198. https://doi.org/10.1002/(SICI)1099-0992(200003/04)30:2<177::AID-EJSP982>3.0.CO;2-Z

Santini, Z. I., Koyanagi, A., Tyrovolas, S., Mason, C., & Haro, J. M. (2015). The association between social relationships and depression: A systematic review. *Journal of Affective Disorders, 175*, 53–65. https://doi.org/10.1016/j.jad.2014.12.049

Schwartz, S. H. (2012). An overview of the Schwartz theory of basic values. *Online Readings in Psychology and Culture, 2*(1). https://doi.org/10.9707/2307-0919.1116

Scioli, A., Ricci, M., Nyugen, T., & Scioli, E. R. (2011). Hope: Its nature and measurement. *Psychology of Religion and Spirituality, 3*(2), 78–97. https://doi.org/10.1037/a0020903

Seligman, M. E. (2012). *Flourish: A visionary new understanding of happiness and well-being*. Simon and Schuster.

Silbereisen, R. K., & Chen, X. (Eds.). (2010). *Social change and human development: Concepts and results*. Sage.

Silbereisen, R. K., & Tomasik, M. J. (2008). Berlin—Warsaw—Jena: A journey with Glen H. Elder through sites of social change. *Research in Human Development, 5*(4), 244–258. https://doi.org/10.1080/15427600802494005

Singh, K., Jain, A., Kaur, J., Junnarkar, M., & Slezáčková, A. (2016). Cross-cultural differences on Gunas and other well-being dimensions. *Asian Journal of Psychiatry, 24*, 139–146. https://doi.org/10.1016/j.ajp.2016.09.001

Slezackova, A. (2017). *Hope and well-being: Psychosocial correlates and benefits*. University of Malta, Centre for Resilience & Socio-Emotional Health.

Slezackova, A., & Janstova, E. (2016). Vztah spirituální inteligence a duševního zdraví: význam nalézání osobního smyslu a duchovní praxe [Spiritual intelligence and positive mental health: The value of personal meaning production and spiritual practice]. *E-psychologie, 10*(2), 18–33.

Slezackova, A., & Krafft, A. (2016). Hope: A driving force of optimal human development. In J. Mohan & M. Sehgal (Eds.), *Idea of excellence: Multiple perspectives* (pp. 1–12). Panjab University.

Slezackova, A., Cefai, C., Čejková, E., & Gassman, S. (2018a). The role of life values in subjective well-being among Czech and Maltese university students. *Horizons of Psychology/Psihološka obzorja, 27*, 35–47. https://doi.org/10.20419/2018.27.483

Slezackova, A., Cefai, C., & Prosek, T. (2018b). Psychosocial correlates and predictors of perceived hope across cultures: A study of Czech and Maltese contexts. In A. M. Krafft, P. Perrig-Chiello,

& A. M. Walker (Eds.), *Hope for a good life. Results of the Hope-Barometer international research program* (pp. 165–197). Springer.

Slezackova, A., Prošek, T., Malatincová, T., & Krafft, A. M. (2020). Psychometrické vlastnosti české verze škály prožívané naděje: faktorová struktura a vnitřní konzistence [Psychometric characteristics of the Czech version of The Perceived Hope Scale: Factor structure and internal consistency]. *Československá psychologie, 64*(3), 288–305.

Slezackova, A., Guse, T., & Prosek, T. (2021). The role of perceived hope in harmony in life among Czech and South African adults. In R. K. Pradhan & U. Kumar (Eds.), *Emotion, well-being and resilience: Theoretical perspectives and practical applications* (pp. 77–94). Apple Academic Press.

Snyder, C. R. (2000). The past and possible futures of hope. *Journal of Social and Clinical Psychology, 19*(1), 11–28. https://doi.org/10.1521/jscp.2000.19.1.11

Snyder, C. R., Harris, C., Anderson, J. R., Holleran, S. A., Irving, L. M., Sigmon, S. T., Yoshinobu, L., Gibb, J., Langelle, C., & Harney, P. (1991). The will and the ways: Development and validation of an individual-differences measure of hope. *Journal of Personality and Social Psychology, 60*(4), 570–585. https://doi.org/10.1037/0022-3514.60.4.570

Spousta, J. (2002). Changes in religious values in the Czech Republic. *Sociologický časopis /Czech Sociological Review, 38*(3), 345–363. https://doi.org/10.13060/00380288.2002.38.3.06

Stachowska, E. (2019). Religijność młodzieży w Europie - perspektywa socjologiczna. Kontynuacje [Religiousness among young people in Europe - the sociological perspective. Continuations]. *Przegląd Religioznawczy/The Religious Studies Review, 273*(3), 77–94.

Stessman, J., Rottenberg, Y., Shimshilashvili, I., Ein-Mor, E., & Jacobs, J. (2013). Loneliness, health, and longevity. *The Journals of Gerontology: Series A., 69*(6), 744–750. https://doi.org/10.1093/gerona/glt147

Sümer, N., Pauknerová, D., Vancea, M., & Manuoğlu, E. (2019). Intergenerational transmission of work values in Czech Republic, Spain, and Turkey: Parent-child similarity and the moderating role of parenting behaviors. *The Annals of the American Academy of Political and Social Science, 682*(1), 86–105. https://doi.org/10.1177/0002716219830953

Sustainable Governance Indicators. (2020). *Quality of democracy. Bertelsmann Stiftung. SGI 2020 survey*. Accessed April 20, 2021, from https://www.sgi-network.org/2020/Democracy/Quality_of_Democracy

Švejnar, J. (1999). Labor markets in the transitional central and east European economies. In O. Ashenfelter & D. Card (Eds.), *Handbook of labor economics* (Vol. 3B, pp. 2810–2857). Elsevier Science B.V.

Swadźba, U. (2015). Różnice i podobieństwa. Miejsce religii i rodziny w systemie wartości społeczeństwa polskiego, czeskiego i słowackiego [Differences and similarities. Religion and the family in the value systems of the Polish, Czech and Slovak societies]. *Górnośląskie Studia Socjologiczne, 6*, 101–122.

Titma, M., & Tuma, N. B. (2005). Human agency in the transition from communism: Perspectives on the life course and aging. In K. W. Schaie & G. Elder (Eds.), *Historical influences on lives and aging* (pp. 108–143). Springer Publishing.

Toft, M. D. (2007). Getting religion? The puzzling case of Islam and civil war. *International Security, 31*(4), 97–131. https://doi.org/10.1162/isec.2007.31.4.97

Tombs, D. (2014). Silent no more: Sexual violence in conflict as a challenge to the worldwide church. *Acta Theologica, 34*(2), 147–165. https://doi.org/10.4314/actat.v34i2.9

Tsai, J. L., Knutson, B., & Fung, H. H. (2006). Cultural variation in affect valuation. *Journal of Personality and Social Psychology, 90*(2), 288–307. https://doi.org/10.1037/0022-3514.90.2.288

Turska-Kawa, A., & Wojtasik, W. (2020). The importance of religiosity in the formation of populist attitudes: The case of Poland. *Journal for the Study of Religions and Ideologies, 19*(55), 34–52.

Tworzecki, H. (2019). Poland: A case of top-down polarization. *The Annals of the American Academy of Political and Social Science, 681*(1), 97–119. https://doi.org/10.1177/0002716218809322

Václavík, D. (2010). *Náboženství a moderní česká společnost [Religion and modern Czech society]*. Grada.
Vecchione, M., Schwartz, S. H., Caprara, G. V., Schoen, H., Cieciuch, J., Silvester, J., Bain, P., Bianchi, G., Kirmanoglu, H., Baslevent, C., Mamali, C., Manzi, J., Pavlopoulos, V., Posnova, T., Torres, C., Verkasalo, M., Lönnqvist, J. E., Vondráková, E., Welzel, C., & Alessandri, G. (2015). Personal values and political activism: A cross-national study. *British Journal of Psychology, 106*(1), 84–106. https://doi.org/10.1111/bjop.12067
Wang, X., Zhang, D., & Wang, J. (2011). Dual-factor model of mental health: Surpass the traditional mental health model. *Psychology, 2*(8), 767–772. https://doi.org/10.4236/psych.2011.28117
Wang, J., Mann, F., Lloyd-Evans, B., Ma, R., & Johnson, S. (2018). Associations between loneliness and perceived social support and outcomes of mental health problems: A systematic review. *BMC Psychiatry, 18*(1), 156. https://doi.org/10.1186/s12888-018-1736-5
Weinstein, N. D. (1980). Unrealistic optimism about future life events. *Journal of Personality and Social Psychology, 39*(5), 806–820. https://doi.org/10.1037/0022-3514.39.5.806
Wirtz, D., Chiu, C. Y., Diener, E., & Oishi, S. (2009). What constitutes a good life? Cultural differences in the role of positive and negative affect in subjective well-being. *Journal of Personality, 77*(4), 1167–1196. https://doi.org/10.1111/j.1467-6494.2009.00578.x
Zalega, T. (2016). *Segment osób w wieku 65+ w Polsce. Jakość życia - Konsumpcja - Zachowania konsumenckie [Segment of persons aged 65+ in Poland. Quality of life - consumption - consumer behavior]*. Wydawnictwo Naukowe Wydziału Zarządzania Uniwersytetu Warszawskiego.
Żuk, P. (2017). Non-alternative reality? On the misery of the left in Eastern Europe: The case of Poland. *Journal of Contemporary Central and Eastern Europe, 25*(1), 63–84. https://doi.org/10.1080/0965156X.2017.1339976

Alena Slezackova, Ph.D., is an Associate Professor of Psychology and a Vice Head of the Dept. of Medical Psychology and Psychosomatics, Faculty of Medicine, Masaryk University, in Brno, Czech Republic. Her scientific interests include mainly hope, mental health, and well-being. She also has a special interest in the research and practice of mindfulness. Alena is a founder and director of the Czech Positive Psychology Centre (CPPC), a member of the Advisory Council of the International Positive Psychology Association (IPPA), and a member of the Executive Board of the European Network for Positive Psychology (ENPP). She has been a member of several international research projects, and she serves on the editorial boards of five academic psychological journals. Alena is the author of the first comprehensive monograph on positive psychology in the Czech language and dozens of scientific publications in positive psychology and health psychology.

Patryk Stecz, a psychologist, is an assistant professor at the Institute of Psychology, University of Lodz, Poland. From 2014–2017 and 2021–2025, he was elected to the Executive Board of the Polish Suicidology Association. Dr Stecz completed his Ph.D. at the Medical University of Lodz. He published approx. 40 scientific works related to applied clinical psychology (attitudes towards suicide, positive suicidology, religious coping, well-being predictors in clinical and non-clinical populations, risk behavior in students with visual impairment, studies on hope). Dr Stecz has been serving psychological support at the Academic Counseling Centre (Technical University of Lodz) for students and employees with disabilities and special needs since 2008. Dr Stecz was aged 31 when he received the Medical University Rector's Scientific Award. Currently he is finishing a four-year post-graduate Clinical Psychology Specialization Program (Center of Postgraduate Medical Education).

Katarina Millova, Ph.D. (born in 1983) attended Masaryk University (Brno, Czech Republic), where she earned her M.A. (2006) and Ph.D. (2012) degree in psychology. She worked as a research associate at the Institute of Psychology of the Czech Academy of Sciences, where she focused on longitudinal research. At Masaryk University, where she worked as an assistant professor, she taught courses on developmental psychology and psychology of personality. Currently she works as assistant professor at the University of Ostrava. In her research, she focuses on successful development in general, lifespan psychology, and adult development, especially on established adulthood and quarter-life crisis.

Chapter 8
Hope and Flourishing: A Cross-Cultural Examination Between Spanish and South African Samples

Valle Flores-Lucas, Raquel Martínez-Sinovas, Raúl López-Benítez, and Tharina Guse

Abstract This chapter explores the commonalities and differences in hope between Spanish ($N = 206$) and South African ($N = 100$) samples based on data collected with the Hope Barometer in November 2018. Furthermore, we investigate similarities and differences in the sources of hope between the two samples, as reflected in the activities that people engage in to fulfil their hopes and to attain the hoped-for targets (hope activities). Finally, we examine these activities as predictors of hope. Since hope is an important predictor of flourishing, we also analyze the predictive power of hope and its dimensions on flourishing in both samples, using two different measures and conceptualizations of hope (perceived hope and dispositional hope). Finally, we explore the role of sociodemographic indicators as predictors of hope and flourishing. Our results indicated that South African participants had higher levels of hope than the Spanish sample. We also found differences and commonalities in terms of endorsement of specific hope activities. The results indicated that perceived hope was a strong predictor of flourishing in both samples, supporting the idea that perceived hope may be a universal motivational need applicable across cultures. These findings highlight the need to carry out more cross-cultural studies on hope and paves the way for further cross-cultural understanding of this important human resource.

V. Flores-Lucas (✉) · R. López-Benítez
Department of Psychology, University of Valladolid, Valladolid, Spain
e-mail: mariavalle.flores@uva.es

R. Martínez-Sinovas
Department of Health Sciences (Psychological Area), European University Miguel de Cervantes, Valladolid, Spain

T. Guse
Department of Psychology, University of Pretoria, Pretoria, South Africa

A. M. Krafft et al. (eds.), *Hope across cultures*, Cross-Cultural Advancements in Positive Psychology 14, https://doi.org/10.1007/978-3-031-24412-4_8

8.1 Introduction

With the expansion of the field of positive psychology, there is increasing interest in the role of cultural variables in positive psychological functioning. Evidence suggests that western conceptualizations of positive psychology constructs may differ from those in non-Western contexts (Oishi & Gilbert, 2016). However, most studies have focused on differences between western and eastern cultures, and less is known about similarities and differences among western and other contexts, such as African contexts. This chapter reports on hope and flourishing among South African and Spanish adults, and examines correlates and mechanisms of these constructs, taking socio-demographic variables into account.

Research examining the applicability of positive psychological constructs from western cultures to other cultures, such as eastern cultures, are expanding. Specifically, the role of cultural differences in the relationships between constructs such as flourishing, well-being, hope, emotions, forgiveness, etc., are gaining attention. Diverse studies reported cultural differences in the assessments or perceived relevance of some of the main constructs of positive psychology like flourishing (Węziak-Białowolska et al., 2019), hope, life satisfaction, positive affect, and emotions (An et al., 2017; Hutz et al., 2014). Furthermore, cross-cultural research is also focussing on the possible effect of cultural differences in the relationship between some of those variables and flourishing, personal well-being or quality of life (Bernardo et al., 2018a, 2018b; Hutz et al., 2014).

The above brief review shows the increasing relevance of cross-cultural research in positive psychology; therefore, it seems relevant to engage in more cross-cultural comparative studies to broaden knowledge of the universal vs cultural value of theories, models and relationships of central elements of Positive Psychology. One of the constructs which has shown to be central to well-being is hope. Many authors have identified hope as a key resource in our lives because of its role in our mental and physical health, and in our well-being (Bailey et al., 2007; Scioli et al., 2016). However, most of the research has focused on the positive effect of hope on one of the elements of well-being, i.e. life satisfaction (Alarcon et al., 2013; Bailey et al., 2007; Du et al., 2015; Krafft et al., 2021; Peterson et al., 2007, among others) and less research has examined the relationship between hope and flourishing, which is another main element of well-being.

Considering the role of culture, some studies have shown that some aspects of hope are universal across cultures (Bernardo et al., 2018a, 2018b; Ling et al., 2016). However, although hope is relevant in all cultures, the conceptualization of hope, its central elements, and the sources or targets of hope would be different in different cultures (Bernardo, 2010). Due to the important role of hope and flourishing in our well-being, we considered it valuable to examine and understand possible cultural differences in the conceptualization and elements of hope and in its role in flourishing.

In this chapter we report a cross cultural comparison of hope between samples from a Mediterranean European country (Spain) and an African country with multicultural roots, including North European roots (South Africa). As previously indicated, there is a lack of comparative positive psychological research between European and African countries. The current study could therefore extend knowledge on similarities and differences in hope and flourishing in these two contexts. We also explore the possible cross-cultural differences in sources of hope. Finally, we analyze the possible differences and common aspects in the role of hope in flourishing in both countries.

8.2 Hope and Flourishing

Hope has been defined and conceptualized in several ways. Most of the theories agree in conceptualizing hope as a positive expectation about future outcomes (Krafft & Walker, 2018a; Krafft et al., 2019), but there are also several differences in the conceptualization and theoretical models of hope. In fact, there is not a single, unified conceptualization of hope, as some authors conceptualize hope as a multidimensional psychological construct (Dufault & Martocchio, 1985; Herth, 1992) others highlight hope as an emotion (Averill et al., 1990) while others conceptualize it as a cognitive mind-set (Snyder, 1994, 2000, 2002).

Despite those discrepancies, Snyder's hope model and the dispositional hope scale (DHS) (Snyder et al., 1991) is one of the most widely used in research. It is consistently discussed in the literature on hope and its relationship with other variables, and it is used in measuring hope among different populations and in various languages (Bernardo, 2010; Lopez et al., 2003). In Snyder's model, hope is seen as a motivational resource to plan and perform actions in order to achieve goals; it is like a cognitive evaluation by individuals of their ability to achieve their goals (Snyder, 1994). This involves various elements: goal setting, agency thoughts and pathways to achieve those goals (Snyder, 2000).

However, Snyder's model has received some criticism regarding its lack of accounting for possible cultural differences, especially between western and eastern cultures, mainly about the role of other significant people such as family or even other significant spiritual beliefs as sources of hope (Bernardo, 2010). Another important criticism of this model concerns its excessive emphasis on the cognitive nature of hope, minimizing the role of the other elements of hope such as the emotional or spiritual components (Bruininks & Howington, 2018; Scioli et al., 2011).

Accordingly, another conceptualization and measurement of hope have been put forward. Krafft et al. (2019) developed the Perceived Hope Scale (PHS) in order to assess hope as it is perceived by ordinary people. These authors proposed a concise hope measure to "assess hope directly in order to gain access to individuals' unfiltered judgment of their own level of hopefulness..." (Krafft et al., 2019, pp. 1597). Furthermore, the PHS aims to assess hope free of cognitive and spiritual bias, and could be used in different populations and cultures, as well as among people with different belief systems. In that sense, the Perceived Hope Scale (PHS) was designed in order to have a hope assessment scale that fulfil those requirements.

Despite the controversies and difficulties of its conceptualization and measure, there is no doubt that hope plays an important role in achieving positive outcomes in different fields such as academic, work, and social spheres, and it is also central to our well-being. Previous research has shown that hope is positively related to subjective well-being, specifically the hedonic elements such as life satisfaction (Bailey & Snyder, 2007; Diener & Chan, 2011; Rand et al., 2011, among others). However, other theories focus more on eudaimonic aspects of well-being, broadly referred to as psychological well-being (Ryff, 1995). Recent research suggests that there is considerable overlap among these facets of well-being and points to the need to integrate these two components in understanding well-being (Díaz et al., 2015; Disabato et al., 2016; Ryan & Deci, 2001, among others). More recent conceptualizations of psychological well-being propose a more integrated view of these two perspectives on well-being and define psychological well-being as a multidimensional construct composed by emotional elements—hedonic components like life satisfaction—and the eudaimonic component -as the optimal functioning and flourishing- (Kern et al., 2014).

The concept of human flourishing has its origins in antiquity, specifically in Aristotle who described flourishing as the ultimate end or goal of a good life, which he also referred to as "good spirit" (Levin, 2020). Flourishing has been related to the sense of purpose in life, hope, and many positive emotions like happiness (Gunderman, 2008), also with clear goals in life and positive emotions such as optimism (Keyes, 2007). In that sense, flourishing is about optimal psychological functioning, which includes positive relationships, feelings of competence, and meaning and purpose in life (Diener et al., 2010).

Concerning the relationship between hope and flourishing, some authors such as Cohn and Fredrickson (2009) pointed out that hope could be considered a part of the eudaimonic component of flourishing. However, as previously stated, while there is evidence of the association between hope and life satisfaction (Alarcon et al., 2013; Bailey & Snyder, 2007; Rand et al., 2011), less is known about the relationship between hope and flourishing.

The limited research has shown some evidence that hope is a major predictor of flourishing, above resilience (Munoz et al., 2020). In another study, Khodarahimi (2013) reported that high levels of hope were related to a sense of flourishing. This study also found evidence for the association between hope and flourishing with emotions. Specifically, higher levels of hope and flourishing were related to more positive emotions, and conversely, low levels of hope and flourishing were related with more negative emotions. These results are consistent with research suggesting that both variables, hope and flourishing, are related to life satisfaction (Diener & Chan, 2011; Gunderman, 2008; Keyes, 2007; Snyder et al., 1991, 1994, 2000). There is also some evidence about the mediating role of hope in the relationship between flourishing and fear of happiness (Belen et al., 2020).

These results show that it is important to explore the relationship between hope and flourishing in more depth, in order to better understand their dynamics in our well-being and fulfilment. Additionally, more research is needed to explore possible cultural differences in these relationships. Finally, we have to highlight that most existing studies have implemented Snyder's hope measures, and more research is needed using other measures and conceptualizations of hope. In that sense, using a more comprehensive conceptualization of hope, namely perceived hope (Krafft et al., 2019) could be useful to understanding the dynamics of flourishing. Additionally, more research is required to confirm the cross-cultural applicability of the PHS.

8.3 Hope and Flourishing in Cross-Cultural Context

8.3.1 Cross-Cultural Research on Hope

Snyder's Hope model (Snyder, 1994, 2002) has been widely applied to behavioural and psychological studies. The function of hope and its relationship to other personal variables and behaviour seems to be the same in different cultures (Chang & Banks, 2007). Most studies agree in the applicability and reliability of Snyder's dispositional hope scale (DHS) and conclude that it has cross-cultural applicability (Chang & Banks, 2007; Flores-Lucas et al., 2018; Li et al., 2018). However, as we pointed out earlier, recent studies reported subtle cross-cultural differences in some of the components of hope, like in pathways (Li et al., 2018). Other studies, such as the one carried out by Tang (2019) among Chinese people in the United Kingdom, show that there are other factors, like certain cultural traits, that mediate the relationship between hope and agency development. Furthermore, cultural and social context elements mediate the role of hope in its effects on recovery (Matsuoka, 2015; Mattingly, 2010).

Probably one of the main critical reviews of Snyder's Hope Model in relation to cultural differences is Bernardo's (2010) extension to Snyder's hope theory. This author stated that, in conjoint cultures in which there is a contextual sense of self, such as Asian cultures, the influence and the interdependence of others such as the family would be stronger than in disjoint cultures. Thus, his conjoint model of agency assumes that definition and motivational thoughts related to goals are defined interpersonally, not only individually (Bernardo, 2010; Bernardo et al., 2018b). In that sense, he proposed his four-factor locus-of-hope model (one internal and three externals—family, friends and spirituality) loci of hope and it has been verified in various Asian cultural groups (Bernardo & Estrellado, 2014; Bernardo & Nalipay, 2016; Bernardo et al., 2016). Several studies have shown that there is a significant relation between those external loci of hope and well-being indicators in adults, high school and university students (Bernardo, 2015; Bernardo & Estrellado, 2017a, 2017b; Bernardo et al., 2017). However, as Bernardo and Mendoza (2020) said, the locus-of-hope model does not mean that Snyder's hope theory is not cross-culturally valid; he only argues that it is incomplete because people in different cultures might have different agency (personal or shared) in goal related thoughts. In that sense, using other measures of hope with a broader hope conceptualization would be useful in order to explore hope in a more comprehensive way across different cultures.

Regarding perceived hope, there are only a few cross-cultural comparisons reported to date, with inconclusive results. Krafft and Choubisa (2018) found no significant differences in levels of perceived hope between a sample of Indian and German participants. However, there were significant differences in the levels of perceived hope between Czech and Maltese participants, with the Czech sample showing significant higher levels of perceived hope (Slezackova et al., 2018). Further, a sample of young Indian participants showed significantly higher levels of perceived hope compared to their Spanish counterparts (Flores-Lucas et al., 2018). It is evident that more research on perceived hope is required in cross-cultural contexts.

In relation to other elements of hope, partially related with Bernardo's (2010) proposal of different loci of hope, Krafft and Walker (2018b) proposed that there are different hope providers and different activities which people do in order to achieve hope, and that those could be different in different cultures. Krafft and Choubisa (2018) and Flores-Lucas et al. (2018) found significant differences between German and Indian samples regarding hope providers and hope activities, and between German, Indian and Spanish young people regarding hope providers respectively.

Therefore, we consider it relevant to analyze in depth the possible cross-cultural commonalities and differences in a more global way and assess hope using the PHS, as well as the DHS. We also deem it important to explore possible cross-cultural differences in hope providers or hope activities. This will enable us to obtain a more comprehensive understanding of hope across cultures and the multidimensional nature of the concept of hope.

8.3.2 Cross-Cultural Research on Flourishing

Numerous studies have pointed out the positive impact of flourishing on individuals. In this sense, flourishing people report healthier relationships, higher levels of life satisfaction or greater job satisfaction, among other benefits (i.e., Keyes, 2004; Seligman, 2011). However, to date, the study of flourishing across nations has received less attention. Some research has attempted to clarify the effect of flourishing variability by comparing different countries.

A recent line of cross-cultural research on flourishing has focused on determining its impact in populations as well as exploring differences among them through diverse perspectives. For example, some studies have focused on cross-culturally testing theoretical models on flourishing and making comparisons between the levels of flourishing between different countries. In this vein, Huppert and So (2013) proposed a conceptual delimitation of flourishing through the combination of a series of indicators linked to well-being such as competence, optimism, or emotional stability, among others. Subsequently, they analyzed flourishing in 22 European countries, which were divided into 3 regions: Northern Europe, Southern/Western Europe and Eastern Europe. The results showed a high consistency between regions, as well as differences between countries, regarding both the prevalence of flourishing and characteristics that defined it. In general, the Nordic countries showed the highest levels of flourishing while the Eastern countries showed the lowest. In a similar line, and employing a sample composed of US, Sri Lankan, Cambodian, Chinese and Mexican participants, Węziak-Białowolska et al. (2019) observed differences between cultures on the different dimensions of flourishing analysed. Specifically, Chinese participants showed high levels in flourishing social relations and health dimensions, Cambodian individuals in satisfaction with life and characters and virtues and the Mexican population on purpose in life. Regarding their levels on the flourishing index, Cambodian and Chinese participants scored highest, followed by Mexicans, whereas the US and Sri Lankan samples obtained the lowest scores. Santini et al. (2020) also reported differences in flourishing between Canadian, Danish and Dutch samples. In particular, they found higher prevalence rates of flourishing for Canadians, followed by Danish and Dutch individuals. It is evident that more research is needed in order to expand knowledge of cross-cultural differences associated with flourishing.

Surprisingly, to the best of our knowledge, there is a lack of research on the relationship between hope and flourishing across cultures. To address this gap, we intended to examine the role of hope, conceptualized as perceived hope as well as dispositional hope, and flourishing across two different countries: Spain and South Africa, a European country, and an African country.

8.4 Hope and Flourishing in Spain and South Africa

South Africa and Spain are two countries that share some characteristics, but they are also quite different on various levels. Despite the fact that both have a European heritage, there are also several cultural and ethnic differences, which may contribute to differences in hope and flourishing.

8.4.1 The South African Context

South Africa is a multicultural country with four main ethnic groups. A total of 80. 9% of the population is of African ethnicity. The remaining three population groups are Coloured (8.8%), White (7.8%) and Indian (2.5%). The term "coloured" is officially used in the South African census and refers to individuals from mixed-race ancestry (IndexMundi, 2020). It is also a reasonably young democracy, with the first democratic elections involving all South Africans taking place in 1994. However, after 27 years the majority of the population remains less affluent than the minority white group (Adams et al., 2016). There are consistent concerns about the political and economic situation (Guse, 2018), further fuelled by an unemployment rate of 26.6%, which temporarily reached 30% during 2020 (Statistics South Africa,

2018, 2020). In sum, South Africa is an unequal society, which has implications for people's hopes, expectations and well-being.

Research on hope and flourishing in the South African context is only starting to emerge. Existing studies revealed relatively high levels of dispositional and perceived hope among adults (Guse, 2018; Guse & Shaw, 2018; Guse & van Zyl, 2019; Slezackova et al., 2021). However, these findings should be interpreted with caution, as some studies question the validity of existing hope measures in African contexts (Abler et al., 2017; Hansen et al., 2020). In addition, social class and perceived social standing seem to be associated with lower levels of hope among South Africans (Boyce & Harris, 2013).

In terms of flourishing, several studies examined levels of optimal functioning or flourishing among South African adults and adolescents. Most research conceptualized flourishing using Keyes' (2002, 2005) model of the mental health continuum. Existing cross-cultural studies reported that a South African sample showed higher levels of social and psychological well-being in comparison to samples from the Netherlands and Iran (Joshanloo et al., 2013).

Studies using the Flourishing Scale (Diener et al., 2010) reported mean scores reflecting relatively high levels of flourishing (Coetzee & Oosthuizen, 2017; Mason, 2019; Nel, 2019). However, these studies were mainly conducted in work contexts or among university students and more research is needed in community samples. Research on the dynamics between hope and flourishing in the South African context indicated that higher levels of hope are associated with higher levels of flourishing or well-being (Guse & Shaw, 2018; Guse & Vermaak, 2011). Still, more research among adults is needed to confirm these findings.

8.4.2 The Spanish Context

Spain is a country with different autonomous regions; some of them have their own language in addition to Castilian (Spanish), and their own cultural heritage. However, there are also wide communal roots, history, and culture. Spain has been receiving an increasing number of people from other countries in recent years. In fact, since the turn of the century, Spain has experienced great social change due to massive immigration (Del Pueblo, 2019). According the 2020 report on immigration by the governmental Permanent Immigration Observatory (2020), the number of legal immigrants was 5,800,468 people in December of 2020, most of them (61%) from European Union Countries. Most of the migrants from countries not in the EU come from Morocco, China, Venezuela and Ecuador. This is a significant change, not only in terms of the number of migrants, but also qualitatively in terms of cultural and social diversity that it has generated (Del Pueblo, 2019).

The economic situation is relatively good, but unemployment in Spain is higher in comparison with other countries of the EU. In 2020, unemployment stood at 15.5%, although it is more severe among young people: in the population under 25 years old unemployment rose to 38.3% by the end of that year according to the data from the National Statistics Institute (INE, 2020a). In sum, Spain is a relatively culturally diverse country, economically developed but with a high rate of unemployment and increasing levels of poverty and inequality and with growing disaffection towards and lack of trust in politicians.

Regarding the research into hope in Spain, as far as we know there are very few studies on the subject. It is of growing interest among researchers in positive psychology, but research into hope is still scarce. Some studies among adolescents indicated that hope is associated with a better self-perception of general health (Esteban-Gonzalo et al., 2020). Furthermore, few recent studies have related hope with resilience during the COVID-19 pandemic, but results were inconclusive (Robles-Bello et al., 2020). There is also some evidence of hope as a predictor of quality of life among the Spanish population (Flores-Lucas & Martínez-Sinovas, 2019). There are even fewer cross-cultural hope studies of Spain and other countries. In our previous study, Flores-Lucas et al. (2018), we found some subtle differences in sources of hope (providers) between Spanish, Indian and German university students, and, more interestingly, we did not find differences in dispositional hope. However, we found significant differences in perceived hope between Indian and Spanish students: in our samples, Spanish students had significantly lower levels of perceived hope than Indian students. However, the limited number of studies and the limitations of these studies, like our cross-cultural study, obliged us to be cautions with our conclusions and engage in more research among Spanish participants as well as cross-cultural comparisons.

Regarding flourishing, Huppert and So (2013) compared 22 European countries, including Spain, on a flourishing scale, which combined multiple positive features. Spain was in 13th position of 22 on global flourishing criteria, above Portugal and France, for example, and below countries like Cyprus, Belgium, and Germany. However, the most striking feature was that Spain showed extreme variations from highest to lowest scores throughout the different features, being one of the countries with more extreme variability along with France and Bulgaria. Regarding the different features assessed in this flourishing survey, Spain is the country with the highest scores in self-esteem and the country with the lowest scores in competence and vitality.

As there are limited studies on hope among Spanish adults, we cannot yet draw conclusions about the dynamics of hope and flourishing in the Spanish context. Thus, more research is warranted.

8.4.3 Rationale for Comparing South Africa and Spain on Hope and Flourishing

Although Spain and South Africa are two countries that share not only some characteristics but also a European heritage, they are also very different. Despite the fact that both have a European heritage as common ground, they are culturally different. Spain, although a European country, differs from North European countries, as it has a Mediterranean culture with some particular characteristics that set it apart from Northern European countries. However, the European heritage of South Africa comes from Northern European countries. Thus, both countries also differ in areas of their common European heritage. They further differ in terms of age of the population, language, geography, and social and political indicators. For example, where Spain is a more homogenous country in terms of language (even though there are four official languages which are spoken in specific regions), South Africa has 11 official languages spoken by four main population groups. South Africa also has a very young population, with a median age of 28 years, while in Spain it is 43.9 years (IndexMundi, 2020). Spain is about half of the size of South Africa, but has almost the same size of population, which means it has a higher population density (My life elsewhere, n.d.). In terms of economy and quality of life, Spain yielded higher scores in most of the economic indicators (GDP, GDP per capita, unemployment, etc.) (countryeconomy.com, n.d.). Furthermore, the countries differ in terms of the United Nations' Human Development Index (which measures life expectancy, education and income) with South Africa scoring lower than Spain. South Africa has also worse indicators for inequality and human security (such as murder and suicide rates, UNDP, 2020).

Comparing South Africa and Spain could also be understood using Hofstede's (2001) cultural dimensions. The countries share some common features, for example, both countries have high scores on the dimension of power distance, so they accept a hierarchical society. Both are also seen as individualistic societies (although in the South African context this may only be true for the White population group). However, there were contradictory findings: Minkov et al. (2017) reported Spain to be a more individualistic country than South Africa, while Hofstede (2001) reported the opposite. Moreover, in comparison to other Europeans countries (except Portugal), Spain is a more collectivist country (Hofstede, 2001; Hofstede, n.d.). However, while there are inconsistent findings regarding dimensions of collectivism-individualism in the two countries, it is evident that they may differ to some extent.

Spain and South Africa also seem to differ on the dimension of uncertainty avoidance and pessimism, with Spain scoring much higher in this aspect. On the other hand, Spain scored lower on masculinity and indulgence. This means that Spanish people have a great aversion to uncertainty, which generates a great deal of anxiety. They need rules for everything, even when they are obliged break them if they make life more difficult. Regarding masculinity, Spanish society is not driven by achievement or competition. Spain is less competitive and looks for more cooperation and balance. Spanish people do not like excessive competitiveness and they do not have a conception of success defined by being a winner or the best in the field. Finally, Spain is a restrained society, which is related to a pessimistic view of the life and the future. Spanish people feel that their actions are restrained by social norms and that self-indulgence is a bad thing (Hofstede, 2001; Hofstede, n.d.). We believe that comparing hope and flourishing among samples from South Africa and Spain could contribute to cross-cultural understanding of these positive psychological characteristics.

8.5 The Current Study

The broad research goal of our research is to examine possible differences in hope between South African and Spanish samples and to explore the role of perceived hope in flourishing in these countries.

The specific research aims are:

1. To examine the significance of differences in hope and flourishing between a sample of South African and Spanish adults.
2. To identify the most important sources of hope, as reflected in activities that generate hope, for the two samples.
3. To examine the predictive power of these hope activities in explaining perceived hope for the two samples.
4. To examine the predictive power of hope in explaining flourishing in the two samples.
5. To analyze the predictive power of demographic variables in explaining hope and flourishing in the two samples.

8.6 Methods and Measurements

8.6.1 Participants

Our sample consisted of 206 adults from the general population, of which 100 were South African and 106 were Spanish. The mean age of the participants was 39.58 ($SD = 13.29$) years for the Spanish sample and 42.65 ($SD = 13.57$) years for the South African sample. The majority of the participants in both samples were female, namely 79 (74,5%) of the Spanish sample and 81 (81%) of the South African sample. The samples were equivalent in terms of age ($t = 1.637$; $p = 0.103$) and gender (contingency analysis Chi square = 1.243; $p = 0.265$). Additional sociodemographic variables that were considered for the study are described in Table 8.1 below. The majority of both samples obtained a higher education qualification, held full-time employment, and endorsed a religion.

8.6.2 Measures

We used the following scales to assess the variables of comparison in this study. The South African sample completed the English versions, while the Spanish sample completed the adapted Spanish versions.

Table 8.1 Demographic information of all samples

Variable	Sample 1: South Africa *n* (%)	Sample 2: Spain *n* (%)	Total sample *n* (%)
Total	100 (100)	106 (100)	206 (100)
Gender			
Male	19 (19.0)	27 (25.5)	46 (22.3)
Female	81 (81.0)	79 (74.5)	160 (77.7)
Age (years)			
18 to 29	18 (18.0)	30 (28.3)	48 (23.3)
30 to 39	28 (28.0)	21 (19.8)	49 (23.8)
40 to 49	20 (20.0)	24 (22.6)	44 (21.4)
50 to 59	22 (22.0)	23 (21.7)	45 (21,8)
60 to 69	10 (10.0)	8 (7.5)	18 (8.7)
70 and older	2 (2.0)	–	2 (1.0)
Education			
Primary school	–	2 (1.9)	2 (1.0)
High School up to grade 10	1 (1.0)	2 (1.9)	3 (1.5)
High School up to grade 12	11 (11.0)	9 (8.5)	20 (9.7)
Diploma	11 (11.0)	5 (4.7)	16 (7.8)
Higher education (University degree, professional education)	77 (77.0)	88 (83)	165 (80.1)
Main Activity			
In education or training (student)	16 (16.0)	26 (24.5)	42 (20.4)
Household/raising children	4 (4.0)	5 (4.7)	9 (4.4)
Part-time job	11 (11.0)	7 (6.6)	18 (8.7)
Fulltime job	64 (64.0)	62 (58.5)	126 (61.2)
Unemployed	–	3 (2.8)	3 (1.5)
Retired	5 (5.0)	3 (2.8)	8 (3.9)
Professional Status			
No position in an organization	10 (10.0)	16 (15.1)	26 (12.6)
In education/training	21 (21.0)	20 (18.9)	41 (19.9)
Employee	25 (25.0)	36 (34.0)	61 (29.6)
Junior/Middle management	10 (10.0)	12 (11.3)	22 (10.7)
Senior management/Board of directors	11 (11.0)	11 (10.4)	22 (10.7)
Entrepreneur/Business owner	23 (23.0)	11 (10.4)	34 (16.5)
Family Status			
Still living with parents	6 (6.0)	20 (18.9)	26 (12.6)
Single, unmarried	12 (12.0)	16 (15.1)	28 (13.6)
Living in a partnership but in separate households	10 (10.0)	2 (1.9)	12 (5.8)
Living together in a partnership	6 (6.0)	13 (12.3)	19 (9.2)
Married	57 (57.0)	43 (40.6)	100 (48.5)
Divorced/separated	6 (6.0)	10 (9.4)	16 (7.8)
Widowed	3 (3.0)	2 (1.9)	5 (2.4)

(continued)

Table 8.1 (continued)

Variable	Sample 1: South Africa *n* (%)	Sample 2: Spain *n* (%)	Total sample *n* (%)
Religion			
Religion	92 (92.0)	79 (74.5)	171 (83.0)
No religion	8 (8.0)	27 (25.5)	35 (17.0)

Perceived Hope Scale (PHS)
This is a scale to assess hope, as it is perceived by ordinary people, it is formed by 6 items rated on a Likert scale ranging from 0–5 (where 0 is "strongly disagree" and 5 is "strongly agree") (Krafft et al., 2019). Validation studies reported Cronbach alpha values of 0.87–0.94 (Krafft et al., 2019, 2021; Marujo et al., 2021). In the current study the Cronbach alpha values were 0.89 and 0.86 for the South African and Spanish samples, respectively.

Adult Dispositional Hope Scale (DHS)
This scale assesses hope according Snyder's hope model. It has eight items and two subscales: Agency thinking and Pathways thinking (Snyder et al., 1991). Items are scored on a 6-point Likert scale with an answer 0–5 rank (where 0 "is strongly disagree" and 5 is "strongly agree"). The DHS has been implemented in many international studies and demonstrated acceptable reliability indices (Krafft et al., 2021). The Cronbach alpha value for the overall DHS ranged from 0.74 to 0.84; from 0.71 to 0.76 for the Agency subscale, and from 0.63 to 0.80 for the Pathways subscale (Snyder et al., 1991). In the current study, the Cronbach alpha values were 0.82 for the overall DHS score for both samples, for the Agency scale 0.71 and 0.68 for the South African and Spanish samples respectively and for Pathways subscale, 0.82 for both samples.

Flourishing Scale
This scale assesses positive human functioning or flourishing. It is an eight-item scale, and 7-point answer Likert scale with a rank of answers from 0 to 7 (where 0 is "strongly disagree" and 7 is "strongly agree") (Diener et al., 2010). The reported Cronbach alpha value was 0.87. In our samples, the Cronbach alpha values were 0.87 for the South African sample and 0.86 for the Spanish sample.

Additionally, we also used 13 questions to obtain information about the activities that people engage in to fulfil their hopes and to attain the hoped-for targets (Hope activities) with a Likert scale of 4 points with an answer rank from 0 (not at all) to 3 (very often). These questions are classified in four dimensions: Cognitive-rational dimension; Social-relational dimension; Spiritual-religious dimension, and motivational/agency dimension (Krafft & Walker, 2018a). Additionally, we obtained sociodemographic information such as educational level, marital status, and employment status, among others.

8.6.3 Procedure

Our study is a cross-sectional international survey and is part of the International Hope Barometer Survey, as described by Krafft in an earlier chapter in this book. Data collection took place in November 2018. Data were obtained by distributing the survey through different communication media (social networks, webpages, radio stations, email, etc.) in order to get the widest variety of participants in the samples. Participants completed the survey anonymously online.

8.6.4 Ethical Considerations

Participants voluntarily participated in the study and were informed of the aims of the study and the confidential treatment of the data; thus, the study was in accordance with the principles of the 1964 Declaration of Helsinki and its later addenda.

8.6.5 Data Analysis

We used the Mplus 8.6 software to conduct the invariance analysis of the Perceived Hope Scale between the two samples in order to check the viability of making meaningful comparisons between the two samples using this scale. Additionally, we used the SPSS statistical package version 23 to calculate descriptive statistics and perform additional analyses. First, we calculated the descriptive statistics of the sociodemographic characteristics of the sample to describe the two samples. In order to analyse the possible differences between the two samples on the main variables, we conducted a T-test mean differences analysis. Additionally, to identify the most important sources of hope, we ranked the relevance that participants gave to the different hope activities using the mean scores. To analyse the possible differences in the relevance given to those activities between the two samples, we used a T-test comparison analysis. Finally, in order to examine the predictive power of the main variables in perceived hope and flourishing in each sample we used a bivariate correlational analysis and later a stepwise multiple regression analysis.

8.7 Results

8.7.1 Invariance Analysis

As a first step before carrying out the rest of the analyses, we checked the measurement invariance of the Perceived Hope Scale (PHS) to test that data from both samples were comparable. To do that, we applied confirmatory factor analysis in a stepwise incremental manner, moving from configurational invariance to scalar invariance, which is considered the most restricted model to obtain invariance between samples. In this case, we used the Maximum Likelihood Method (MLR estimator) as well as the following indices: Root Mean Square Error of Approximation (RMSEA), Comparative Fit Index (CFI), Tucker Lewis Index (TLI) and Standardized Root Mean Residual (SRMR).

First, we applied a Confirmatory Factor Analysis (CFA) to the total sample. As can be seen in Table 8.2, fix indices for the one-factor model showed a good model fit (RMSEA and SRMR values lower than 0.08 and CFI and TLI values higher than 0.90). Second, after confirming the structure of the scale, we checked the configural, metric, and scalar invariance between the Spanish and South African samples (see Table 8.2). Results did no show statistically significant differences in the model fit between the configural and the metric models ($p = 0.20$), the metric and the scalar models ($p = 0.07$), and the configural and the scalar model ($p = 0.07$).

In addition, and similar to the total sample, the equal form (configurational invariance) provided an adequate fit (see Table 8.2). Furthermore, employing the configural model as baseline, and following the recommended threshold values (Chen, 2007) to test the measurement invariance, we observed, except for the SRMR parameter, an acceptable goodness of fit indices for metric invariance (Δ RMSEA = 0.005; Δ CFI = 0.004; ΔTLI = – 0.004; ΔSRMR=–0.047) and for scalar invariance (Δ RMSEA = 0.002; Δ CFI = 0.012; ΔTLI = – 0.002; ΔSRMR = – 0.055). Therefore, in general, our data showed strong measurement invariance between Spanish and South African populations for the Perceived Hope Scale.

Table 8.2 Measurement invariance of the perceived Hope scale among Spanish and South African samples

Variable	X^2	*Df*	RMSEA	CFI	TLI	SRMR
Total sample	383.905	15	0.016	0.999	0.998	0.020
Configurational Invariance	33.254	18	0.091	0.976	0.959	0.034
Metric (weak) Invariance	40.530	23	0.086	0.972	0.963	0.081
Scalar (strong) Invariance	50.593	28	0.089	0.964	0.961	0.089

8.7.2 Mean Differences in Levels of Hope and Flourishing Between the Two Samples

As reflected in Table 8.3, there were statistically significant differences between the South African and Spanish samples in hope. Specifically, the South African sample showed significantly higher levels of perceived hope ($p = 0.04$) and dispositional hope ($p < 0.001$). However, the effect size for perceived hope was small ($d = 0.28$) and medium for dispositional hope ($d = 0.53$). The difference in flourishing between the two samples was not significant.

8.7.3 Mean Values and Rank Orders for Hope Activities Among the Two Samples

In Table 8.4 we report on the most important sources of hope, i.e., the activities that people engage in to generate hope.

For both samples, the three most important hope-generating activities were similar, although slightly different in rank order. There were statistically significant differences in the mean scores for endorsing specific hope-generating activities between the two samples. Specifically, the South African sample showed statistically significant higher scores for the following activities: "I pray, meditate" ($t_{(204)} = 8.057; p < 0.001$; IC95% [0.856; 1.410]), "I take responsibility and commit myself" ($t_{(186,192)} = 3.809; p < 0.001$; IC95% [0.123; 0.388]), "I go to church/other place of worship" ($t_{(178,095)} = 5.951; p < 0.001$; IC95% [0.605; 1.206]), "I donate money to the object of my hopes" ($t_{(204)} = 4.236; p < 0.001$; IC95% [0.293; .802]), "I trust in God" ($t_{(204)} = 8.275; p < 0.001$; IC95% [0.944; 1.534]) and "I talk about my hopes with my spouse/partner" ($t_{(200,761)} = 3.668$; $p < 0.001$; IC95% [0.239; 0.794]). Large effect sizes were evident for "I pray, meditate" ($d = 0.978$) and "I trust in God" ($d = 1.002$); medium effect sizes were discovered for "I take responsibility and commit myself" ($d = 0.518$), "I go to church/other place of worship"

Table 8.3 Means, standard deviations and *t*-tests of Hope and flourishing variables for South African and Spanish samples

	South Africa		Spain					
Variable	*M*	*SD*	*M*	*SD*	*t*	*df*	*p*	*d*
Perceived Hope	3.692	0.922	3.443	0.843	2.018	0.248	0.045*	0.279
Dispositional Hope	4.015	0.580	3.692	0.599	3.927	0.323	0.000**	0.529
Agency	4.088	0.630	3.672	0.667	4.589	0.415	0.000**	0.611
Pathways	3.943	0.709	3.712	0.690	2.362	0.230	0.019**	0.326
Flourishing	5.889	0.778	5.815	0.708	0.713	0.104	0.074	0.098

* $p < 0.05$
** $p < 0.01$
d—Cohen's effect size

Table 8.4 Mean values, rank orders and t-test for hope activities for the South African and Spanish samples

Variable	South Africa			Spain			t-test for equality of means			
	R	*M*	*SD*	*R*	*M*	*SD*	*t*	*df*	*p*	*d*
I take responsibility and commit myself	1	2.85	0.386	1	2.59	0.565	3.809	0.256	0.000**	0.518
I inform myself (read widely, use internet, etc.)	2	2.65	0.626	3	2.47	0.679	1.961	0.178	0.051	0.274
I think a lot and analyze circumstances	3	2.61	0.549	2	2.53	0.650	0.972	0.082	0.332	0.133
I motivate my family	4	2.48	0.689	5	2.37	0.695	1.162	0.112	0.246	0.159
I talk about my hopes with my spouse/partner	5	2.46	0.915	8	1.94	1.103	3.668	0.517	0.000**	0.497
I trust in God	6	2.39	1.053	11	1.15	1.094	8.275	1.239	0.000**	1.001
I motivate my friends	7	2.38	0.693	4	2.37	0.622	0.132	0.012	0.895	0.015
I pray, meditate	8	2.18	1.048	12	1.05	0.970	8.057	1.133	0.000**	0.978
I have a job that allows me to fulfil my hopes	9	2.17	0.911	9	1.82	1.058	2.532	0.349	0.012*	0.349
I save money	10	2.08	0.907	7	1.95	0.898	1.011	0.127	0.313	0.144
I engage myself entrepreneurially	11	1.95	0.845	6	2.14	0.723	−1.751	−.192	0.082	0.241
I donate money to the object of my hopes	12	1.84	0.896	10	1.29	0.956	4.236	0.548	0.000**	0.570
I go to church/other place of worship	13	1.50	1.251	13	0.59	0.892	5.951	0.906	0.000**	0.778

* $p < 0.05$
** $p < 0.01$
d—*Cohen's effect size*

($d = 0.778$) and "I donate money to the object of my hopes" ($d = 0.570$); and small effect size was observed for "I talk about my hopes with my spouse/partner" ($d = 0.497$).

8.8 Predictors of Perceived Hope

Correlational analysis and multiple linear regression analyses were carried out to study the predictive power of hope activities and sociodemographic variables on perceived hope.

8.8.1 Hope Activities as Predictors of Perceived Hope

The correlational analysis showed some statistically significant relationships for: "I pray, meditate" ($r = 0.342$; $p < 0.001$), "I go to church/other place of worship" ($r = 0.298$; $p = 0.001$) and "I have a job that allows me to fulfil my hopes" ($r = 0.310$; $p = 0.001$) for the South African sample. In the Spanish sample, the hope activities that significantly correlated with perceived hope were: "I motivate my friends" ($r = 0.249$; $p = 0.005$), "I go to church/other place of worship" ($r = 0.279$; $p = 0.002$), "I have a job that allows me to fulfil my hopes" ($r = 0.426$; $p < 0.001$), "I save money" ($r = 0.315$; $p = 0.001$), "I trust in God" ($r = 0.300$; $p = 0.001$) and "I talk about my hopes with my spouse/partner" ($r = 0.271$; $p = 0.002$).

The stepwise multiple regression analysis showed that, in the South African sample, perceived hope was predicted through the following hope activities (see Table 8.5): "I pray, meditate" (*beta* = 0.274; $p = 0.004$), "I talk about my hopes with spouses/partner" (*beta* = 0.217; $p = 0.018$) and "I have a job that allows me to fulfil my hopes" (*beta* = 0.224; $p = 0.019$). The regression model for the South African sample was significant [$F_{(3)} = 8.865$; $p < 0.001$] and explained 21.7% of the variance of perceived hope ($R = 0.466$; $R^2 = 0.217$; R^2 *adjusted* = 0.192). In the Spanish sample (see Table 8.6), the hope activities that were significant predictors of the perception of hope were: "I have a job that allows me to fulfil my hopes" (*beta* = 0.364; $p < 0.001$), "I trust in God" (*beta* = 0.221; $p = 0.012$) and "I

Table 8.5 Hope activities as predictors of perceived Hope for the South African sample

Variable	Order	*B*	*SE*	*β*	*P*	Tolerance	VIF
I pray, meditate	1	0.241	0.082	0.274	0.004**	0.935	1.070
I talk about my hopes with spouses/partner	2	0.219	0.091	0.217	0.018*	0.993	1.007
I have a job that allows me to fulfil my hopes	3	0.227	0.095	0.224	0.019*	0.932	1.073

* $p < 0.05$
** $p < 0.01$

Table 8.6 Hope activities as predictors of perceived Hope for the Spanish sample

Variable	Order	*B*	*SE*	*β*	*P*	Tolerance	VIF
I have a job that allows me to fulfil my hopes	1	0.290	0.069	0.364	0.001**	0.957	1.045
I trust in God	2	0.170	0.066	0.221	0.012*	0.965	1.036
I motivate my friends	3	0.259	0.116	0.191	0.027*	0.984	1.016

* $p < 0.05$
** $p < 0.01$

Table 8.7 Sociodemographic predictors of perceived hope for the Spanish sample

Variable	*B*	*SE*	*β*	*P*	Tolerance	VIF
Age	0.015	0.006	0.236	0.015*	1.000	1.000

* $p < 0.05$

motivate my friends" (*beta* = 0.191; p = 0.027). The model was significant [$F_{(3)} = 12.516$; $p < 0.001$] and explained 26.9% of the variance of perceived hope ($R = 0.519$; $R^2 = 0.269$; R^2 *adjusted* = 0.248).

8.8.2 Sociodemographic Predictors of Perceived Hope

Demographic characteristics of the participants were previously presented in Table 8.1. Here, we present the findings from the regression analyses.

The correlational analysis showed the following significant differences in correlations with perceived hope: For the South African sample it was gender ($r = 0.171$; $p = 0.045$) and for the Spanish sample they were age ($r = 0.236$; $p = 0.007$), religion ($r = -0.169$; $p = 0.042$) and main activity ($r = 0.205$; $p = 0.017$).

Regarding the predictive power of sociodemographic variables (age, gender, family status, education level and professional status, main activity, and religion) in hope, we did not find any predictive significant regression model for the South African sample. Regarding the Spanish sample, age (*beta* = 0.236; $p = 0.015$) was the only significant predictor in the multiple linear regression analysis (see Table 8.7). This regression model was significant [$F_{(1)} = 6.119$; $p < 0.05$] and explained 5.6% of the variance of perceived hope ($R = 0.236$; $R^2 = 0.056$; R^2 *adjusted* = 0.046).

8.8.3 Perceived Hope and Dispositional Hope as Predictors of Flourishing

In order to analyse the predictive power of Perceived Hope and Dispositional Hope on Flourishing, we firstly carried out bivariate correlations which showed strong positive relationships between all variables (see Tables 8.8 and 8.9).

In a second step, we did linear regression analyses for both samples. For the South African sample (see Table 8.10), flourishing was strongly predicted by perceived hope (*beta* $= 0.505$; $p < 0.001$) and moderately predicted by agency (*beta* $= 0.312$; $p < 0.001$). Dispositional hope and pathways were no predictors for flourishing. The linear regression model for the South African sample was significant [$F_{(2)} = 42.982$; $p < 0.001$] and explained 47% of the variance of flourishing ($R = 0.685$; $R^2 = 0.470$; R^2 *adjusted* $= 0.459$).

The multiple linear regression analysis for the Spanish sample (see Table 8.11) identified agency (*beta* $= 0.443$; $p < 0.001$) and perceived hope (*beta* $= 0.305$;

Table 8.8 Bivariate correlations among flourishing and hope variables for the South African sample

Variable	Flourishing	Perceived Hope	Dispositional Hope	Agency	Pathways
Flourishing	1	–	–	–	–
Perceived Hope	0.621**	1	–	–	–
Dispositional Hope	0.535**	0.501**	1	–	–
Agency	0.501**	0.373**	0.848**	1	–
Pathways	0.431**	0.488**	0.882**	0.499**	1

$^{**}p < 0.001$

Table 8.9 Bivariate correlations among flourishing and hope variables for the Spanish sample

Variables	Flourishing	Perceived Hope	Dispositional Hope	Agency	Pathways
Flourishing	1	–	–	–	–
Perceived Hope	0.556**	1	–	–	–
Dispositional Hope	0.536**	0.613**	1	–	–
Agency	0.616**	0.567**	0.878**	1	–
Pathways	0.335**	0.515**	0.887**	0.558**	1

$^{**}p < 0.001$

Table 8.10 Predictors of flourishing for the South African sample

Variable	Order	*B*	*SE*	*β*	*P*	Tolerance	VIF
Perceived hope	1	0.426	0.067	0.505	0.000**	0.861	1.162
Agency	2	0.386	0.098	0.312	0.000**	0.861	1.162

** $p < 0.01$

Table 8.11 Predictors of flourishing for the Spanish sample

Variable	Order	*B*	*SE*	*B*	*P*	Tolerance	VIF
Agency	1	0.470	0.095	0.305	0.000**	0.679	1.473
Perceived hope	2	0.257	0.305	0.445	0.001**	0.679	1.473

** $p < 0.01$

Table 8.12 Sociodemographic variables as predictors of flourishing for the South African sample

Variable	*B*	*SE*	*β*	*P*	Tolerance	VIF
Education level	0.242	0.107	0.224	0.025*	1.000	1.000

* $p < 0.05$

Table 8.13 Sociodemographic variables as predictors of flourishing for the Spanish sample

Variable	*B*	*SE*	*β*	*P*	Tolerance	VIF
Professional Status	0.015	0.006	0.236	0.015*	1.000	1.000

* $p < 0.05$

$p < 0.001$) as predictors of flourishing. For this sample, dispositional hope and pathways variables were not found as significant predictors for flourishing. The model was significant [$F_{(2)} = 40.868; p < 0.001$] and explained 44% of the variance of flourishing ($R = 0.655$; $R^2 = 0.442$; R^2 *adjusted* = 0.432).

8.8.4 *Sociodemographic Variables as Predictors of Flourishing*

For the South African sample (see Table 8.12), the multiple stepwise regression analysis showed that education level was the only predictor of flourishing (*beta* = 0.224; $p = 0.025$). This regression model was significant [$F_{(1)} = 5.163$; $p = 0.025$] and explained 5% of the variance ($R = 0.224$; $R^2 = 0.050$; R^2 *adjusted* = 0.040). For the Spanish sample (see Table 8.13) the only predictor of flourishing was professional status (*beta* = 0.236; $p = 0.015$). The model was significant [$F_{(1)} = 5.847$; $p = 0.015$] and explained 5.3% of the variance of flourishing ($R = 0.231$; $R^2 = 0.053$; R^2 *adjusted* = 0.044).

8.9 Discussion

The main aim of our study was to examine and compare hope and flourishing between South African and Spanish adults. We first examined the measurement invariance of the Perceived Hope Scale (PHS) in order to engage in meaningful comparisons between the two groups. Our results showed that the PHS met the invariance criteria and that we could continue to compare the two samples with this scale.

The first research aim was to investigate the significance of differences in perceived hope, dispositional hope and flourishing between the two samples. Our results showed that the South African sample showed a significantly higher level of perceived hope than the Spanish sample but with a small effect size. Similarly, the South African sample showed higher levels of dispositional hope than the Spanish sample. These results are concordant with previous studies indicating that Spanish young people showed significantly lower levels of perceived hope than Indian young people, but not different from German young people (Flores-Lucas et al., 2018). Similarly, Slezackova et al. (2021) found that a South African sample scored significantly higher on perceived hope than a Czech sample. Thus, despite the fact that South Africa is a developing country and economically less advantaged than Spain, the sample in this study was more hopeful than the Spanish sample. Some reasons for these differences in hope may be offered.

Overall, we can consider cultural differences between the two countries in terms of Hofstede's (2001) dimensions of culture. According to Hofstede (2001), South Africa scored low on the dimension of uncertainty avoidance, whereas Spain scored high. This means that South African culture is more relaxed, flexible, and tolerant of ambiguity, while Spanish culture seems to prefer rules and are concerned about undefined situations (Hofstede, n.d.). Research suggests that higher levels of hope are associated with a higher tolerance for uncertainty (Balen & Merluzzi, 2021; Sancam et al., 2020) which could partly explain the higher mean hope score for the South African sample. Another dimension of culture which could be considered is that of indulgence. This dimension is broadly defined as the extent to which individuals control their impulses, based on their upbringing. According to Hofstede's (2001) survey, South African culture reflects higher endorsement of indulgence, and therefore holds more positive and optimistic attitudes. Conversely, Spanish culture seems to be less indulgent and to have a tendency towards cynicism and pessimism (Hofstede n.d.). Several studies suggest that higher levels of optimism are associated with higher levels of hope (see Krafft et al., 2021 for a recent review). Therefore, the difference in levels of hope between the two samples may also partly be due to the fact that South African culture is generally an optimistic culture. Hofstede's scores on the dimensions of culture for South Africa was based on research among mostly White adults, as was the sample in the current study. However, findings should be interpreted cautiously as it may not reflect the diversity of cultures in South Africa.

There was no statistically significant difference in mean scores for flourishing between the South African and Spanish samples, which indicates that the two groups experienced similar levels of socio-psychological prosperity, or overall psychological well-being, from a subjective point of view (Diener et al., 2010). This was a surprising finding, given that Spain ranked much higher (36) than South Africa (105) in the 2018 World Happiness Report (WHR) (Sachs et al., 2018). However, the WHR evaluates subjective well-being through a single question, and may not adequately assess other dimensions of well-being such as relationships, self-esteem, purpose, and optimism.

The second research aim was to identify the most important sources of hope, as reflected in activities that generate hope, for the two samples. Although both samples pointed out the same activities as the three most important hope activities, our results indicate that South African and Spanish adults differed significantly in endorsing some activities that generate hope (here referred to as hope activities). There were statistically significantly differences in mean scores for endorsing activities with religious/spiritual dimensions. Specifically, the South African sample was more likely to "trust in God", "pray; meditate" or "to go to church/other place to worship" as means to generate hope. In addition, the South African sample seem more likely to donate to others as a way to increase hope. Further, the two samples differed in endorsing activities with motivational/agency dimensions, as South African participants were more likely to take responsibility for generating their own hope and to find hope in having a job. On the social-relational dimension of hope activities, South African participants more often indicated that they would talk about their hopes with a spouse. We did not find any significant difference in any items from the cognitive-rational dimension. In terms of overall ranking of activities, both samples indicated that taking responsibility for generating hope themselves was the most important source of hope.

South Africa is a very religious country, with most people considering God important to their lives (Kollamparambil, 2020; Loubser & Kotzé, 2017). It can be expected that South African adults would endorse spiritual/religious activities as very important in generating hope in South African people. Spain is a country in which a majority of people identify themselves as Catholic, but when asked if they practise religious activities like going to church, praying, etc., most Spanish people answer that they do not practise any religious activity (Centre of Sociological Research (CIS), 2018, 2021). Thus, it seems that Spanish people may hold religious beliefs but they do not practise any specific religious activity. This difference between the two countries in their religious activities may explain the differences in the role of these activities in their different levels of perceived hope. In fact, according to a previous study among German and Swiss samples, the activities which have more predictive value on perceived hope were those from religious/spiritual; motivational/agency and relational dimensions (Krafft & Walker, 2018b). This lends some support to our idea that differences in the hope activities found in our study could partially explain the differences in perceived hope found between the two countries.

Further, given the high rate of unemployment in South Africa, having a job may sustain hope and this activity may be more important to South African than Spanish participants. The findings that the South African sample was more likely to talk to a spouse as a hope activity is difficult to explain in a cross-cultural context. Existing research supports the notion that effective communication is key to relationship satisfaction and ultimately well-being in general (see du Plooy & de Beer, 2018, for a review), but it is unclear whether cultural differences between the two samples may have contributed to our findings.

The third aim of our study was to investigate the predictive power of these hope activities in explaining perceived hope for the two samples. The linear multiple regression analysis showed that the strongest hope activities predictors of perceived hope in South African sample were "I pray/meditate"; "I talk about my hopes to my spouse/partner"; and "I have a job that allows me fulfil my hopes". In the Spanish sample the strongest predictors were "I have a job that allows me fulfil my hopes"; "I trust in God" and "I motivate my friends". Overall, although there were differences in the specific activities predicting hope for the two samples, for both the South African and Spanish participants these activities entailed motivational/agency, the religious/spiritual and relational dimensions, similar to Krafft and Walker's (2018b) findings among Swiss and Germans participants. As indicated previously, the fact the spiritual/religious dimension ("I pray/meditate") was the strongest predictor of perceived hope for the South African sample is in line with the religious nature of South African society (see Loubser & Kotzé, 2017). Because Spanish people consider themselves as believers but do not practise any religious activity, it seems reasonable that for this sample "trust in God" was one of the most powered predictors of hope; but, unlike the South African sample, religious activities like "pray" have no effect on Spanish people's hope levels.

Further, having a job is extremely important to South Africans owing to difficult economic circumstances and high levels of unemployment. Thus, being employed may support positive future expectancies and consequently perceived hope. This seems similar to the Spanish context, as Spain has one of the highest rates of unemployment among European countries. In fact, the CIS (2018) data showed that the majority of Spanish people viewed unemployment as the main problem of the country. Thus, as in the South African sample, having a job is a powerful predictor of hope and of positive future expectations.

As far as relational sources of hope are concerned, Krafft and Walker (2018b) similarly reported that these activities are very important predictors of perceived hope among Swiss and German samples. For the South African sample in our study, talking to a spouse was one of the strongest predictors and for Spanish people another relational source of hope "I motivate my friends" was a relevant predictor of hope. This is congruent with the consideration of Spain as a very sociable country in which relationships with friends are an important part of the Spanish lifestyle, and thus in line with Krafft and Walker's (2018b) findings.

The fourth aim of our study was to examine the role of perceived hope and dispositional hope in predicting flourishing in the two samples. Regarding the relationship between perceived hope and flourishing, our regression analysis indicated that perceived hope was a significant predictor of flourishing for both groups. In terms of dispositional hope, only agency was a significant predictor of perceived hope for both samples. The other components of Snyder's model (global dispositional hope and pathways thinking) were not significant predictors. The only difference between the South African and Spanish regression models were the different prediction values of these variables. Specifically, agency was the strongest predictor of flourishing for the Spanish sample, while we found an inverse pattern for the South African sample. Therefore, our results suggest that flourishing is predicted by the same hope-related variables for participants from these different cultures. However, results should be interpreted with caution because we only confirmed measurement invariance of the PHS between the two samples, and not the DHS. Overall, the results seem to point to the universality of hope as an existential human need that is central to the experience of well-being (see Krafft et al., 2021 for a recent review).

While a large body of existing research reported that dispositional hope is a good predictor of flourishing (Munoz et al., 2020) and specifically of life satisfaction (Diener & Chan, 2011; Gunderman, 2008; Keyes, 2007; Snyder, 1994, 2000; Snyder et al., 1991), our findings seem to indicate the possibility that other conceptualizations of hope could add to understanding flourishing. Specifically, perceived hope contributed to predicting flourishing in both samples in the current study, in addition to only one component of dispositional hope. Our results thus support Krafft et al.'s (2021) finding that perceived hope might be an important underlying factor in understanding well-being, regardless of cultural context.

Finally, regarding our last goal, sociodemographic variables in our data showed that in the South African sample the only predictor in the multiple regression model was the educational level, but in Spain the only predictor was professional status. This difference may be due partially to the fact that in Spain most people below 50 years old have at least high school education level, and a large part of this population has a university degree (National Statistical Institute (INE), 2020b) which could mean that educational level is not a good predictor of flourishing because it is not a good discriminant variable in the Spanish population. In the South African context, university education is still not accessible to the majority of the population partly due socio-economic factors and problematic basic education (Walton et al., 2015). It can thus be expected that educational level would be a strong predictor of flourishing in this context.

Despite potentially valuable findings, we acknowledge some limitations of our study. First, we had a limited number of participants, which may have made it impossible to investigate the measurement invariance of the DHS. Consequently, any comparison between the two samples using this scale has to be taken with caution and further research is needed to confirm our results. Second, in both samples the majority of participants were female, which limits generalization. Finally, the participants in the South African sample were not demographically representative of the South African population, which is predominately Black. The results should therefore not be generalized to the South African population as a whole. However, our study has also some strengths. It is one of the few studies to examine hope and its role in well-being in two different countries, and it is the first between Spain and South Africa. This study also implemented more than one conceptualization of hope and considered the complementarity of both. This is has allowed us to understand and explore in more depth possible cultural differences and communalities in the dynamics of hope and flourishing. Finally, by identifying the important sources of hope for both samples, it provides some guidance for developing interventions to strengthen hope in each cultural context.

8.10 Conclusion

In this study, we found higher levels of hope in a South African sample in comparison to a Spanish sample. We also found that the two samples differed in terms of endorsement of specific hope activities, but that for both samples, spiritual, motivational and relational activities were important predictors of hope. Perceived hope and agency were both significant predictors of flourishing for the two samples. Since perceived hope was a strong predictor of flourishing for both samples, our study supports the notion that perceived hope may be a universal motivational need applicable across cultures. Our results also suggest that, while there may be differences in levels of hope between the South African and Spanish samples, hope remains an important construct in the experience of human flourishing. This adds to extant knowledge on universal and specific characteristics of hope and paves the way for further cross-cultural understanding of this important human need.

References

Abler, L., Hill, L., Maman, S., DeVellis, R., Twine, R., Kahn, K., et al. (2017). Hope matters: Developing and validating a measure of future expectations among young women in a high HIV prevalence setting in rural South Africa (HPTN 068). *AIDS and Behavior, 21*(7), 2156–2166. https://doi.org/10.1007/s10461-016-1523-6

Adams, B. G., Abubakar, A., Van de Vijver, F. J., De Bruin, G. P., Arasa, J., Fomba, E., Omri, G., Hapunda, G., Looh, J., Mazrui, L., & Murugami, M. (2016). Ethnic identity in emerging adults in sub-Saharan Africa and the USA, and its associations with psychological well-being. *Journal of Community and Applied Social Psychology, 26*(3), 236–252. https://doi.org/10.1002/casp.2247

Alarcon, G. M., Bowling, N. A., & Khazon, S. (2013). Great expectations: A meta-analytic examination of optimism and hope. *Personality and Individual Differences, 54*(7), 821–827. https://doi.org/10.1016/j.paid.2012.12.004

An, S., Ji, L. J., Marks, M., & Zhang, Z. (2017). Two sides of emotion: Exploring positivity and negativity in six basic emotions across cultures. *Frontiers in Psychology, 8*, 1–14. https://doi.org/10.3389/fpsyg.2017.00610

Averill, J. R., Catlin, G., & Chon, K. K. (1990). *Rules of hope*. Springer.

Bailey, T. C., & Snyder, C. R. (2007). Satisfaction with life and hope: A look at age and marital status. *The Psychological Record, 57*, 233–240. https://doi.org/10.1007/BF03395574

Bailey, T. C., Eng, W., Frisch, M. B., & Snyder, C. R. (2007). Hope and optimism as related to life satisfaction. *The Journal of Positive Psychology, 2*(3), 168–175. https://doi.org/10.1080/17439760701409546

Balen, N. S., & Merluzzi, T. V. (2021). Hope, uncertainty, and control: A theoretical integration in the context of serious illness. *Patient Education and Counselling, 104*(11), 2622–2627. https://doi.org/10.1016/j.pec.2021.07.029

Belen, H., Yildirim, M., & Belen, F. S. (2020). Influence of fear of happiness on flourishing: Mediator roles of hope agency and hope pathways. *Australian Journal of Psychology, 72*(2), 165–173. https://doi.org/10.1111/ajpy.12279

Bernardo, A. B. I. (2010). Extending hope theory: Internal and external locus of trait hope. *Personality and Individual Differences, 49*, 944–949. https://doi.org/10.1016/j.paid.2010.07.036

Bernardo, A. B. I. (2015). Hope in early adolescence: Measuring internal and external locus-of-hope. *Child Indicators Research, 8*(3), 699–715. https://doi.org/10.1007/s12187-014-9254-6

Bernardo, A. B. I., & Estrellado, A. F. (2014). Measuring hope in the Philippines: Validating the short version of the Locus-of-Hope Scale in Filipino. *Social Indicators Research, 119*(3), 1649–1661. https://doi.org/10.1007/s11205-013-0573-7

Bernardo, A. B. I., & Estrellado, A. F. (2017a). Locus-of-hope and help-seeking intentions of Filipino battered women victims of intimate partner violence. *Current Psychology, 36*, 66–75. https://doi.org/10.1007/s12144-015-9385-z

Bernardo, A. B. I., & Estrellado, A. F. (2017b). Well-being of Filipino women who experienced intimate partner violence: A person-centered analysis. *International Journal for the Advancement of Counselling, 39*, 360–376. https://doi.org/10.1007/s10447-017-9303-1

Bernardo, A. B. I., & Mendoza, N. B. (2020). Measuring hope during the COVID-19 outbreak in the Philippines: Development and validation of the state locus-of-Hope scale short form in Filipino. *Current Psychology, 40*, 1–10. https://doi.org/10.1007/s12144-020-00887-x

Bernardo, A. B. I., & Nalipay, M. (2016). Social axioms as social foundations of locus-of-hope: A study in three Asian cultural groups. *Personality and Individual Differences, 95*, 110–113. https://doi.org/10.1016/j.paid.2016.02.046

Bernardo, A. B. I., Salanga, M. G. C., Khan, A., & Yeung, S. S. (2016). Internal and external loci-of-hope predict use of individual and collaborative learning strategies: Evidence from university learners in four Asian cities. *The Asia-Pacific Education Researcher, 25*, 367–376. https://doi.org/10.1007/s40299-015-0249-y

Bernardo, A. B. I., Wang, T. Y., Pesigan, I. J. A., & Yeung, S. S. (2017). Pathways from collectivist coping to life satisfaction among Chinese: The roles of locus-of-hope. *Personality and Individual Differences, 106*, 253–256. https://doi.org/10.1016/j.paid.2016.10.059

Bernardo, A. B. I., Khan, A., & Salanga, M. G. C. (2018a). Hope and satisfaction with life: Testing the mediating roles of self-esteem in three Asian cultures [Esperanza y satisfacción con la vida: Probando los roles mediadores de la autoestima en tres culturas asiaticas]. *Acción Psicológica, 15*(2), 69–82. https://doi.org/10.5944/ap.15.2.23456

Bernardo, A. B., Yeung, S. S., Resurreccion, K. F., Resurreccion, R. R., & Khan, A. (2018b). External locus-of-hope, well-being, and coping of students: A cross-cultural examination within Asia. *Psychology in the Schools, 55*(8), 908–923. https://doi.org/10.1002/pits.22155

Boyce, G., & Harris, G. (2013). Hope the beloved country: Hope levels in the new South Africa. *Social Indicators Research, 113*(1), 583–597. https://doi.org/10.1007/s11205-012-0112-y

Bruininks, P., & Howington, D. E. (2018). Hopeful + hoping = Hope: Unique experiential features in the measurement of emotion. *The Journal of Positive Psychology, February*, 1–13. https://doi.org/10.1080/17439760.2018.1437465

Centre of Sociological Research (CIS). (2018). *Barómetro de Marzo de 2018*. Retrieved from http://www.cis.es/cis/export/sites/default/-Archivos/Marginales/3200_3219/3207/es3207mar.pdf

Centre of Sociological Research (CIS). (2021). *Barómetro de Octubre de 2021*. Retrieved from https://www.cis.es/cis/opencms/ES/NoticiasNovedades/InfoCIS/2021/Documentacion_3337.html.

Chang, E. C., & Banks, K. H. (2007). The colour and texture of hope: Some preliminary findings and implications for hope theory and counselling among diverse racial/ethnic groups. *Scholarship, 13*(2), 94–103. https://doi.org/10.1037/1099-9809.13.2.94

Coetzee, M., & Oosthuizen, R. M. (2017). Work-role psychosocial flourishing: Its mediation role on workplace bullying and employee turnover intention. *Journal of Psychology in Africa, 27*(3), 211–215.

Cohn, M. A., & Fredrickson, B. L. (2009). Positive emotions. In S. J. Lopez & C. R. Snyder (Eds.), *Oxford handbook of positive psychology* (pp. 13–24). Oxford University Press.

Countryeconomy.com. (n.d.) *Countries data. Demographics and economy. Country comparison Spain vs South Africa*. Retrieved June 22, 2021, from https://countryeconomy.com.

Del Pueblo, D. (2019). *La situación demográfica en España. Efectos y.* consecuencias.

Díaz, D., Stavraki, M., Blanco, A., & Gandarillas, B. (2015). The eudaimonic component of satisfaction with life and psychological well-being in Spanish cultures. *Psicothema, 27*(3), 247–253. https://doi.org/10.7334/psicothema2015.5

Diener, E., & Chan, M. Y. (2011). Happy people live longer: Subjective well-being contributes to health and longevity. *Applied Psychology: Health and Well-Being, 3*, 1–43. https://doi.org/10.1111/j.1758-0854.2010.01045.x

Diener, E., Wirtz, D., Tov, W., Kim-Prieto, C., Choi, D. W., Oishi, S., & Biswas-Diener, R. (2010). New well-being measures: Short scales to assess flourishing and positive and negative feelings. *Social Indicators Research, 97*(2), 143–156. https://doi.org/10.1007/s11205-009-9493-y

Disabato, D. J., Goodman, F. R., Kashdan, T. B., Short, J. L., & Jarden, A. (2016). Different types of well-being? A cross-cultural examination of hedonic and eudaimonic well-being. *Psychological Assessment, 28*(5), 471–482. https://doi.org/10.1037/pas0000209

Du Plooy, K., & De Beer, R. (2018). Effective interactions: Communication and high levels of marital satisfaction. *Journal of Psychology in Africa, 28*(2), 161–167. https://psycnet.apa.org/doi/10.1080/14330237.2018.1435041

Du, H., Bernardo, A. B. I., & Yeung, S. S. (2015). Locus of-hope and life satisfaction: The mediating roles of personal self-esteem and relational self-esteem. *Personality and Individual Differences, 83*, 228–233. https://doi.org/10.1016/j.paid.2015.04.026

Dufault, K., & Martocchio, B. C. (1985). Hope: Its spheres and dimensions. *Nursing Clinics of North America, 20*, 379–391.

Esteban-Gonzalo, S., Esteban-Gonzalo, L., Cabanas-Sánchez, V., Miret, M., & Veiga, O. L. (2020). The investigation of gender differences in subjective wellbeing in children and adolescents: The UP & DOWN study. *International Journal of Environmental Research and Public Health, 17* (8), 2732. https://doi.org/10.3390/ijerph17082732

Flores-Lucas, V. & Martínez-Sinovas, R. (2019). *Predictors of psychological quality of life in the Spanish population: The role of hope, vitality and other characteristics*. Paper presented at the 17th ISQLS Conference, Granada, Spain, September 2019.

Flores-Lucas, V., Martínez-Sinovas, R., & Choubisa, R. (2018). Hope and education: Role of psychological capital and cultural differences. In A. Krafft, P. Perrig-Chiello, & A. Walker (Eds.), *Hope for a good life. Results of the Hope-Barometer international research program* (pp. 63–77). Springer.

Gunderman, R. B. (2008). Authentic flourishing. In E. L. Ealy (Ed.), *Conversation philanthropy: An interdisciplinary series of reflections and research* (Philanthropy and the pursuit of happiness) (Vol. V, pp. 49–560). Donors Trust.

Guse, T. (2018). *Hope among South African adults: Preliminary findings from the Hope-Barometer Survey 2017*. Paper presented at the 9th European Conference on Positive Psychology, Budapest, Hungary, June.

Guse, T., & Shaw, M. (2018). Hope, meaning in life and well-being among a group of young adults. In A. Krafft, P. Perrig-Chiello, & A. Walker (Eds.), *Hope for a good life. Results of the Hope-Barometer international research program* (pp. 63–77). Springer.

Guse, T., & van Zyl, C J.J. (2019). *The role of hope in the relationship between benevolence, universalism and flourishing in a South African sample*. Paper presented at the 17th ISQLS Conference, Granada, Spain, September 2019.

Guse, T., & Vermaak, Y. (2011). Hope, psychosocial well-being and socioeconomic status among a group of South African adolescents. *Journal of Psychology in Africa, 21*(4), 527–533. https://doi.org/10.1080/14330237.2011.10820493

Hansen, C. H., Lees, S., Kapiga, S., Seeley, J., & Barnett, T. (2020). Measuring hope amongst Tanzanian women who participate in microfinance: An evaluation of the Snyder hope scale. *Global Public Health, 15*(3), 402–413. https://doi.org/10.1080/17441692.2019.1682027

Herth, K. (1992). Abbreviated instrument to measure hope: Development and psychometric evaluation. *Journal of Advanced Nursing, 17*(10), 1251–1259. https://doi.org/10.1111/j.1365-2648.1992.tb01843.x

Hofstede, G. (2001). *Culture's consequences: Comparing values, behaviors, institutions and organizations across nations*. Sage.

Hofstede. (n.d.) *Country comparisons*. Retrieved June 21, 2021, from https://www.hofstede-insights.com/country-comparison/south-africa,spain/.

Huppert, F. A., & So, T. T. (2013). Flourishing across Europe: Application of a new conceptual framework for defining well-being. *Social Indicators Research, 110*(3), 837–861. https://doi.org/10.1007/s11205-011-9966-7

Hutz, C. S., Midgett, A., Pacico, J. C., Bastianello, M. R., & Zanon, C. (2014). The relationship of hope, optimism, self-esteem, subjective well-being, and personality in Brazilians and Americans. *Psychology, 5*(6), 514–522. https://doi.org/10.4236/psych.2014.56061

IndexMundi. (2020). *South Africa ethnic groups*. Retrieved May 17, 2021, from https://www.indexmundi.com/south_africa/ethnic_groups.html

Joshanloo, M., Wissing, M. P., Khumalo, I. P., & Lamers, S. M. (2013). Measurement invariance of the mental health continuum-short form (MHC-SF) across three cultural groups. *Personality and Individual Differences, 55*(7), 755–759. https://doi.org/10.1016/j.paid.2013.06.002

Kern, M. L., Waters, L. E., Adler, A., & White, M. E. (2014). A multidimensional approach to measuring well-being in students: Application of the PERMA framework. *The Journal of Positive Psychology, 10*(3), 262–271. https://doi.org/10.1080/17439760.2014.936962

Keyes, C. L. M. (2002). The mental health continuum: From languishing to flourishing in life. *Journal of Health and Social Research, 43*, 207–222. https://doi.org/10.2307/3090197

Keyes, C. L. (2004). The nexus of cardiovascular disease and depression revisited: The complete mental health perspective and the moderating role of age and gender. *Aging & Mental Health, 8* (3), 266–274. https://doi.org/10.1080/13607860410001669804

Keyes, C. L. M. (2005). Mental illness and/or mental health? Investigating axioms of the complete state model of health. *Journal of Consulting and Clinical Psychology, 73*, 539–548. https://doi.org/10.1037/0022-006X.73.3.539

Keyes, C. L. M. (2007). Promoting and protecting mental health as flourishing: A complementary strategy for improving national mental health. *American Psychologist, 62*(2), 95–108. https://doi.org/10.1037/0003-066X.62.2.95

Khodarahimi, S. (2013). Hope and flourishing in an Iranian adult sample: Their contributions to the positive and negative emotions. *Applied Research in Quality of Life, 8*(3), 361–372. https://doi.org/10.1007/s11482-012-9192-8

Kollamparambil, U. (2020). Happiness, happiness inequality and income dynamics in South Africa. *Journal of Happiness Studies, 21*(1), 201–222. https://doi.org/10.1007/s10902-019-00075-0

Krafft, A. M., & Choubisa, R. (2018). Hope in the Indian psychology context: Philosophical foundations and empirical findings. In A. M. Krafft, P. Perrig-Chiello, & A. M. Walker (Eds.), *Hope for a good life. Results of the Hope-Barometer international research program* (pp. 131–163). Springer. https://doi.org/10.1007/978-3-319-78470-0_7

Krafft, A. M., & Walker, A. M. (2018a). Exploring the concept and experience of Hope – Theoretical and methodological foundations. In A. M. Krafft, P. Perrig-Chiello, & A. M. Walker (Eds.), *Hope for a good life. Results of the Hope-Barometer international research program* (pp. 3–19). Springer. https://doi.org/10.1007/978-3-319-78470-0_1

Krafft, A. M., & Walker, A. M. (2018b). Exploring the concept and experience of Hope – Empirical findings and the virtuous circle of Hope. In A. M. Krafft, P. Perrig-Chiello, & A. M. Walker (Eds.), *Hope for a good life. Results of the Hope-Barometer international research program* (pp. 21–60). Springer. https://doi.org/10.1007/978-3-319-78470-0_2

Krafft, A. M., Martin-Krumm, C., & Fenouillet, F. (2019). Adaptation, further elaboration, and validation of a scale to measure hope as perceived by people: Discriminant value and predictive utility vis-à-vis dispositional hope. *Assessment, 26*(8), 1594–1609. https://doi.org/10.1177/1073191117700724

Krafft, A. M., Guse, T., & Maree, D. (2021). Distinguishing perceived hope and dispositional optimism: Theoretical foundations and empirical findings beyond future expectancies and cognition. *Journal of Well-being Assessment, 4*, 217–243. https://doi.org/10.1007/s41543-020-00030-4

Levin, J. (2020). Human flourishing and population health: Meaning, measurement, and implications. *Perspectives in Biology and Medicine, 63*(3), 401–419. https://doi.org/10.1353/pbm.2020.0029

Li, Z., Mao, X., He, Z., Zhang, B., & Yin, X. (2018). Measure invariance of Snyder's dispositional Hope scale in American and Chinese college students. *Asian Journal of Social Psychology, 21*, 263–270. https://doi.org/10.1111/ajsp.12332

Ling, Y., Huebner, E. S., Fu, P., Zeng, Y., & He, Y. (2016). A person-oriented analysis of hope in Chinese adolescents. *Personality and Individual Differences, 101*, 446–450. https://doi.org/10.1016/j.paid.2016.06.048

Lopez, S. J., Snyder, C. R., & Pedrotti, J. T. (2003). Hope: Many definitions, many measures. In S. J. Lopez & C. R. Snyder (Eds.), *Positive psychological assessment: A handbook of models and measures* (pp. 91–106). American Psychological Association. https://doi.org/10.1037/10612-006

Loubser, R., & Kotzé, H. (2017). Religiosity in South Africa among the public and elites. *Scriptura: Journal for Contextual Hermeneutics in Southern Africa, 116*(1), 1–12.

Marujo, H. Á., Velez, M. J., Gonçalves, S. P., Neto, L. M., Krafft, A. M., & Casais, M. (2021). The value of hope: Validation of the perceived hope scale in the Portuguese population. *Current Psychology, 2021*. https://doi.org/10.1007/s12144-021-02115-6

Mason, H. D. (2019). Gratitude, well-being and psychological distress among South African university students. *Journal of Psychology in Africa, 29*(4), 354–360. https://doi.org/10.1080/14330237.2019.1647492

Matsuoka, A. K. (2015). Ethnic/racial minority older adults and recovery: Integrating stories of resilience and hope in social work. *British Journal of Social Work, 45*(Suppl 1), 135–152. https://doi.org/10.1093/bjsw/bcv120

Mattingly, C. (2010). *The paradox of hope: Journeys through a clinical borderland*. University of California Press.

Minkov, M., Dutt, P., Schachner, M., Morales, O., Sanchez, C., Jandosova, J., Khassenbekov, Y., & Mudd, B. (2017). A revision of Hofstede's individualism-collectivism dimension: A new national index from a 56-country study. *Cross Cultural & Strategic Management, 24*, 386–404. https://doi.org/10.1108/CCSM-11-2016-0197

Munoz, R. T., Hanks, H., & Hellman, C. M. (2020). Hope and resilience as distinct contributors to psychological flourishing among childhood trauma survivors. *Traumatology, 26*(2), 177. https://doi.org/10.1037/trm0000224

My life elsewhere. (n.d.). *Country size comparison*. Retrieved June 22, 2021, from https://www.mylifeelsewhere.com/country-size-comparison/spain/south-africa.

National Statistics Institute (INE). (2020a). *Indicadores de calidad de vida. Tasas de paro*. Retrieved February 1, 2022, from https://www.ine.es/uc/so9TTJ9F

National Statistics Institute (INE). (2020b). *Educación. Nivel de formación de la población adulta*. Retrieved February 1, 2022, from https://www.ine.es/uc/ppiKlgCu

Nel, E. C. (2019). The impact of workplace bullying on flourishing: The moderating role of emotional intelligence. *SA Journal of Industrial Psychology, 45*(1), 1–9. https://doi.org/10.4102/sajip.v45i0.1603

Oishi, S., & Gilbert, E. A. (2016). Current and future directions in culture and happiness research. *Current Opinion in Psychology, 8*, 54–58. https://doi.org/10.1016/j.copsyc.2015.10.005

Permanent Immigration Observatory (Observatorio permanente para la inmigración). (2020). Catálogo de publicaciones de la Administración General del Estado. Ministerio de Inclusión, Seguridad Social y Migraciones. NIPO: 121–20–014-0. https://www.ine.es/prensa/cp_e2020_p.pdf.

Peterson, C., Ruch, W., Beermann, U., Park, N., & Seligman, M. E. P. (2007). Strengths of character, orientations to happiness, and life satisfaction. *The Journal of Positive Psychology, 2*(3), 149–156. https://doi.org/10.1080/17439760701228938

Rand, K. L., Martin, A. D., & Shea, A. M. (2011). Hope, but not optimism, predicts academic performance of law students beyond previous academic achievement. *Journal of Research in Personality, 45*(6), 683–686. https://doi.org/10.1016/j.jrp.2011.08.004

Robles-Bello, M. A., Sánchez-Teruel, D., & Valencia-Naranjo, N. (2020). Variables protecting mental health in the Spanish population affected by the COVID-19 pandemic. *Current Psychology, 41*, 5640–5651. https://doi.org/10.1007/s12144-020-01132-1

Ryan, R. M., & Deci, E. L. (2001). On happiness and human potentials: A review of research on hedonic and eudaimonic well-being. *Annual Review of Psychology, 52*(1), 141–166. https://doi.org/10.1146/annurev.psych.52.1.14

Ryff, C. D. (1995). Psychological well-being in adult life. *Current Directions in Psychological Science, 4*(4), 99–104. https://doi.org/10.1111/1467-8721.ep10772395

Sachs, J. D., Layard, R., & Helliwell, J. F. (2018). *World happiness report 2018* (No. id: 12761).

Sancam, H., Deveci, M., & Ahmetoglu, E. (2020). The examination of hope, intolerance of uncertainty and resilience levels in parents having disabled children. *Global Journal of Psychology Research: New Trends and Issues, 10*(1), 118–131. https://doi.org/10.18844/gjpr.v10i1.4398

Santini, Z. I., Torres-Sahli, M., Hinrichsen, C., Meilstrup, C., Madsen, K. R., Rayce, S. B., Baker, M. M., Have, M. T., Schotanus-Dijkstra, M., & Koushede, V. (2020). Measuring positive mental health and flourishing in Denmark: Validation of the mental health continuum-short form (MHC-SF) and cross-cultural comparison across three countries. *Health and Quality of Life Outcomes, 18*(1), 1–15. https://doi.org/10.1186/s12955-020-01546-2

Scioli, A., Ricci, M., Nyugen, T., & Scioli, E. R. (2011). Hope: Its nature and measurement. *Psychology of Religion and Spirituality, 3*(2), 78–97. https://doi.org/10.1037/a0020903

Scioli, A., Scioli-Salter, E. R., Sykes, K., Anderson, C., & Fedele, M. (2016). The positive contributions of hope to maintaining and restoring health: An integrative, mixed-method approach. *The Journal of Positive Psychology, 11*(2), 135–148. https://doi.org/10.1080/17439760.2015.1037858

Seligman, M. E. P. (2011). *Flourish: A visionary new understanding of happiness and well-being*. Free Press.

Slezackova, A., Cefai, C., & Prosek, T. (2018). Psychosocial correlates and predictors of perceived Hope across cultures: A study of Czech and Maltese contexts. In A. M. Krafft, P. Perrig-Chiello, & A. M. Walker (Eds.), *Hope for a good life. Social indicators research series* (Vol. 72, pp. 165–197). Springer. https://doi.org/10.1007/978-3-319-78470-0_8

Slezackova, A., Guse, T., & Prosek, T. (2021). The role of perceived hope in harmony in life among Czech and South African adults. In R. K. Pradhan & U. Kumar (Eds.), *International handbook of advances in emotion, wellbeing, and resilience: Theoretical perspectives and practical applications* (pp. 77–94). Apple Academic Press.

Snyder, C. R. (1994). *The psychology of hope*. The Free Press.

Snyder, C. R. (2000). *Handbook of hope: Theory, measures, and applications*. Academic.

Snyder, C. R. (2002). Hope theory: Rainbows in the mind. *Psychological Inquiry, 24*(4), 249–275. https://doi.org/10.1207/S15327965PLI1304_01

Snyder, C. R., Harris, C., Anderson, J. R., Holleran, S. A., Irving, L. M., Sigmon, S. T., & Harney, P. (1991). The will and the ways: Development and validation of an individual-differences measure of hope. *Journal of Personality and Social Psychology, 60*(4), 570–585. https://doi.org/10.1037/0022-3514.60.4.570

Statistics South Africa. (2018, May). *Youth unemployment still high*. Retrieved September 2021, from http://www.statssa.gov.za/?p=11129

Statistics South Africa (2020, September). *SA economy sheds 2,2 million jobs in Q2 but unemployment levels drop*. Retrieved from http://www.statssa.gov.za/?p=13633.

Tang, L. (2019). Recovery, hope and agency: The meaning of hope amongst Chinese users of mental health services in the UK. *The British Journal of Social Work, 49*(2), 282–299. https://doi.org/10.1093/bjsw/bcy033
UNDP. (2020). *The 2020 human development report*. United Nations Development Programme.
Walton, E., Bowman, B., & Osman, R. (2015). Promoting access to higher education in an unequal society. *South African Journal of Higher Education, 29*, 262–269.
Węziak-Białowolska, D., McNeely, E., & VanderWeele, T. J. (2019). Human flourishing in cross cultural settings. Evidence from the United States, China, Sri Lanka, Cambodia, and Mexico. *Frontiers in Psychology, 10*, 1269. https://doi.org/10.3389/fpsyg.2019.01269

Valle Flores-Lucas is Associate Professor at Valladolid University, in the psychology department. She obtained her PHD (Psychology) from University Autónoma of Madrid in 2001. She led the Postgraduate course on Positive Psychology and Humour sense at Valladolid University. She Her research work has been centred on two main research lines: developmental language and communication disorders, and in the last years, she started another research line in the field of Positive Psychology mainly in the study of hope and its relations with other positive strengths and its applications on education. She is member of the Spanish Positive Psychology Society.

Raquel Martínez-Sinovas is an assistant professor University and sports psychologist. She has an international Ph.D. "Cum Laude" in Psychology by Valladolid University. She has a postgraduate formation as specialist in Positive Psychology and Sense of Humor from the University of Valladolid. Her research has been focussed in hope in educative fields.

Raúl López-Benítez is an Associate professor in the Department of Psychology at Valladolid University, Spain. He has a Ph. D. in Psychology by Granada University and his research examines how humor is related to psychological processes, as emotion or cognition in adults, and he is starting to research in other strengths like hope.

Tharina Guse is a counselling psychologist and obtained an MA (Counselling Psychology) degree from the Potchefstroom University (now North-West University) in 1989. She was in full-time private practice for the next 15 years providing psychotherapy for children, adolescents and adults. In 2003 she obtained her PhD (Psychology) from Potchefstroom University. She returned to academia in 2005 and joined the University of Johannesburg. Since April 2018 she is a professor and Head of the Department of Psychology at the University of Pretoria. Currently she serves on the Professional Board for Psychology of the Health Professions Council of South Africa (HPCSA). She is also President of the recently founded South African Positive Psychology Association (SAPPA). Her research focuses are on positive psychology in general and in particular on psycho-social well-being, positive psychology interventions and psychological strengths such as hope and gratitude. Closely aligned with this broad focus she also conducts research on the application of hypnosis for the promotion of mental health and well-being.

Chapter 9
Mastering the COVID-19 Pandemic Crisis: From Anxiety to Hope

Andreas M. Krafft, JohnBosco Chika Chukwuorji, Rajneesh Choubisa, Stella Comte, Fabien Fenouillet, Valle Flores-Lucas, Tharina Guse, Elżbieta Kasprzak, Charles Martin-Krumm, Helena Agueda Marujo, Chitra Nair, Mark Sinclair, Alena Slezackova, Patryk Stecz, and Olga Varsos

A. M. Krafft (✉)
Institute of Systemic Management and Public Governance, University of St. Gallen, St. Gallen, Switzerland
e-mail: andreas.krafft@unisg.ch

J. C. Chukwuorji
Department of Psychology, University of Nigeria, Nsukka, Nigeria

R. Choubisa
Department of Humanities and Social Sciences, Birla Institute of Technology and Science, (BITS) Pilani, Pilani, India

S. Comte
Department of Psychology, University of Cagliari, Cagliari, Italy

F. Fenouillet
Interdisciplinary Laboratory in Neuroscience, Physiology and Psychology: Learning, Physical Activity and Health, Université Paris Nanterre, Nanterre, France

V. Flores-Lucas
Department of Psychology, University of Valladolid, Valladolid, Spain

T. Guse
Department of Psychology, University of Pretoria, Pretoria, South Africa

E. Kasprzak
Department of Work and Organisational Psychology, Institute of Psychology, Kazimierz Wielki University of Bydgoszcz, Bydgoszcz, Poland

C. Martin-Krumm
Vulnerability, Capability, and Recovery Laboratory, Ecole de Psychologues Praticiens de Paris, Paris, France

H. A. Marujo
Instituto Superior de Ciências Sociais e Politicas, University of Lisbon, Lisbon, Portugal

C. Nair
K. N. M. Government Arts and Science College Kanjiramkulam, University of Kerala, Thiruvananthapuram, India

A. M. Krafft et al. (eds.), *Hope across cultures*, Cross-Cultural Advancements in Positive Psychology 14, https://doi.org/10.1007/978-3-031-24412-4_9

Abstract This chapter presents selected results of the Hope Barometer survey during the pandemic years of 2020 and 2021. Against the background of the intense feelings of stress and anxiety in these times of crisis, we first review current theories on psychological stress and coping, present results of our empirical studies during the pandemic and then focus on the role and importance of hope in relation to positive coping styles, well-being, and stress-related personal growth. A central aim of our research is to investigate the role of culture in the perception of stress and hope (as the counterpart of anxiety) and in the choice of different coping strategies, as evident in their relationship to experiences of well-being and personal growth. We compared the results of 11 countries with cross-sectional data collected in November 2019 ($N = 9092$), November 2020 ($N = 9536$) and November 2021 ($N = 9093$). After reporting general findings, we engage in an analysis of the most striking differences between the countries. Our results revealed that a majority of the participants experienced moderate stress levels, but with significant differences between the samples and notable changes between 2020 and 2021. Most people, especially in more collectivistic countries such as Nigeria, South Africa, India, and Portugal, remained hopeful, applied positive coping strategies, and enjoyed moderate to high levels of well-being and personal growth. Our findings highlight the importance of emotion-focused, social, and religious coping sources, besides problem-focused coping, for mastering the crisis, which are predominant in collectivistic societies.

9.1 Introduction

During the years 2020 and 2021, the worldwide COVID-19 pandemic has transformed many aspects of society resulting not only in a global health but also in an economic, social, and political crisis with profound implications for people's lives. In order to reduce the number of infections, governments around the globe have implemented several measures, such as general lockdowns, reducing economic and social activities to a minimum, temporary closing of education and cultural institutions, restricting mobility, confining people to stay at home and to work remotely, imposing social distancing to avoid close contact and determining other

M. Sinclair
Mentor Education, Windsor, VIC, Australia

A. Slezackova
Department of Medical Psychology and Psychosomatics, Faculty of Medicine, Masaryk University, Brno, Czech Republic

P. Stecz
Department of Clinical Psychology and Psychopathology, Institute of Psychology, University of Łódź, Łódź, Poland

O. Varsos
Centre for Positive Change, Melbourne, VIC, Australia

far-reaching safety procedures and limitations to public life. The threat to one's physical health combined with experiences of social isolation, economic hardships and uncertainty about the future have provoked many kinds of fears as well as feelings of anxiety and helplessness but have also inspired new energies and hopes.

Many studies in several countries have already investigated the negative and in some cases traumatic consequences of the pandemic crisis on the mental health of the population such as psychological distress, fear, anxiety, depression, burn-out, and further stress-related disorders (Alshehri et al., 2020; Boyraz & Legros, 2020; Bridgland et al., 2021; Brooks et al., 2020; Cooke et al., 2020; Horn et al., 2020; Husky et al., 2020; Lakhan et al., 2020; Maia & Dias, 2020; Rehman et al., 2021; Roy et al., 2020; Taylor et al., 2020a, 2020b; Torales et al., 2020; Tsamakis et al., 2020; Usher et al., 2020; Wu et al., 2020). Beyond the obvious burdens on the physical and mental health of the population, one main question has been how people reacted to the threats, challenges and uncertainties and what they did in order to cope with stressful situations and mitigate their negative effects (Agha, 2021; Ahuja, 2021; Bhattacharjee & Ghosh, 2021; Budimir et al., 2021; Engelbrecht et al., 2021; Garbóczy et al., 2021; Guszkowska & Dąbrowska-Zimakowska, 2022; Kar et al., 2021; Minahan et al., 2021; Morales-Rodríguez, 2021; Polizzi et al., 2020; Rogowska et al., 2021; Szkody et al., 2021).

From another line of research, several authors have highlighted the importance of hope in seemingly hopeless situations, especially when uncertainty regarding the future is high and perceived personal control is low (Averill et al., 1990; Bruininks & Malle, 2005; Scioli & Biller, 2009; Tennen et al., 2002; Tong et al., 2010). Erikson (1959) has recognized that hope emerges out of fear and anxiety, and understood it as the first and fundamental human virtue necessary for our psychosocial development. Hope is not only the counterpart of fear and anxiety but also of despair, cynicism, apathy, helplessness, and dejection (Govier, 2011; Marcel, 1951).

Several authors have underlined the role of (individualistic and collectivistic) cultures in the perception of stress and in the appraisal and choice of diverse coping strategies (Aldwin, 2004; Chun et al., 2006; Heppner et al., 2006; Hu et al., 2018). Furthermore, Averill et al. (1990) as well as Averill and Sundararajan (2005) investigated the nature and role of hope across individualistic and collectivistic cultures, concluding that people in different countries differ not only with regard to the kind of targets they hope for, but also with regard to the actions performed in order to fulfill them.

Most of the current psychological research during the pandemic was centered on the study of stress, anxiety, coping strategies, and their positive and negative outcomes related to mental disorders. The focus of the Hope Barometer during these crisis years was to investigate the phenomenon of hope in relation to perceived stress, coping styles, stress-related growth, and well-being across countries. Based on Lazarus' (1966, 1990) transactional and dynamic theory of stress and coping as well as contemporary research findings demonstrating the predominance of posttraumatic growth after stressful experiences (Armeli et al., 2001; Linley et al., 2008; Tedeschi & Calhoun, 2004), the aim of this chapter is to explore the role of hope in mastering stressful situations and the way people in different countries not only coped with, but also experienced personal growth as a consequence of the COVID-19 pandemic. In our study we therefore assessed the levels and changes of people's perceived stress, hope, and well-being in relation to specific coping strategies and their association with areas of personal growth.

9.2 Theoretical Background

9.2.1 Psychological Stress: Between Anxiety and Hope

Recent studies during the COVID-19-pandemic in several countries revealed that the sources and levels of stress varied significantly between different population groups. The most important sources of stress were the fear of becoming infected, worries related to the financial and economic consequences of the lockdowns, being isolated from family and friends, the daily bad and fake news in the mass media, and the general uncertainty about the future (Agha, 2021; Taylor et al., 2020a). Most studies showed that the levels of stress were more pronounced among young people and individuals with lower financial and social resources (Bhattacharjee & Ghosh, 2021; Kar et al., 2021; Maia & Dias, 2020; Rehman et al., 2021). Some studies also found substantial changes between the first and the second waves of COVID-19. Not only did levels of perceived stress increase and levels of life-satisfaction decrease, but significant changes in coping styles also occurred (Rogowska et al., 2021).

The effect of the COVID-19 pandemic on people's well-being can be understood using Lazarus' theory of stress and coping (Lazarus, 1966; Lazarus & Folkman, 1984). Basically, psychological stress is conceptualized as a prominently subjective phenomenon. Lazarus' transactional model is focused on the relationship between the person and the environment. A person starts to feel stressed once he or she perceives that external or even internal demands exceed personal resources to manage them. The subjective appraisal of the stressors and the available resources and strategies to cope with them are key elements. This means that psychological stress relates to the significance of a certain stressor as appraised by the individual.

People can differ greatly in the perception of stressors depending on their life situation, social relationships, character traits, and past experiences. Moreover, stress is not a simple phenomenon, but it is a complex and multifaceted one. Psychologically speaking, individual perception of stress is linked to three essential experiences (Cohen et al., 1983):

1. Unpredictability: The less one can assess and predict future events, the more uncertain and subsequently stressed one will feel.
2. Uncontrollability: When situations get out of control or people have the impression that they cannot sufficiently handle essential aspects in life, this in turn increases the feeling of stress because one feels at the mercy of external conditions.
3. Overload: Increasing demands as well as new and constantly changing situations can result in personal overload.

The appraisal process of the relationship between the individual and the environment is by and large influenced by basic beliefs as well as by positive and negative emotions and consists of two interrelated phases called primary and secondary appraisal (Lazarus, 1990, 1993). During the primary appraisal the individual can perceive the stressor as harming, threatening, or challenging, depending not only on the objective facts but also on his or her personal beliefs, attitudes, and characteristics. Whereas harm refers to the perception of damage or loss, threat is the anticipation of a possible future harm. Experiencing a stressor as harming or threatening is associated with negative emotions such as anxiety, sadness, anger, or frustration that may block mental processes, impairing well-being and possibly creating psychological problems.

Interpreting stressors as challenges, instead, is associated with feelings of hope, defined as "fearing the worst but wanting better" (Lazarus, 1993, p. 13). A hopeful attitude is motivating, mobilizing, and expansive and it is the central attitude to overcoming obstacles. Whether a stressor is interpreted as threatening or challenging is also influenced by secondary appraisal, which is the process of assessing what can be done to manage the situation based on one's resources to cope with the stressors. This secondary appraisal has an impact on the primary appraisal of the stressors and determines the concrete reactions to it.

The perception of stress and the reaction to it are basically a dynamic process. The interplay between first and secondary appraisal and the subsequent coping activities are constantly changing (Lazarus, 1990). The way people cope with a stressful situation will affect the way they appraise it and vice-versa. Changes take place in people's emotions, beliefs, motivation, coping responses, and outcomes. For example, at the beginning of the pandemic in 2020 many people felt vulnerable and overwhelmed. After several months, people learned to adapt to the circumstances and rearranged their lives. Original fears could be converted in manageable challenges and hopes. Other people, instead, might have downplayed the severity of the pandemic, believing everything would be fine again after few weeks or months. After a year these people could have felt disappointed and frustrated. Furthermore, the quick availability of vaccines changed the appraisal of the situation, but the appearance of new variants of the virus aggravated the conditions again (Bhattacharjee & Ghosh, 2021; Guszkowska & Dąbrowska-Zimakowska, 2022; Rogowska et al., 2021).

All these experiences and responses are part of a constantly changing appraisal and coping process that is very subjective and emotional in nature and gives rise to a back and forth between anxiety and hope. Therefore, Lazarus (1993, p. 10) comes to the following conclusion: "Knowing, for example, that in a given encounter (or as a consistent pattern across encounters) the individual feels angry, anxious, guilty, sad, happy, or hopeful tells us much more than knowing merely that he/she is harmed, threatened, or challenged." Most people are able to learn new strategies to manage a stressful situation and to modify their behavior to deal with changing conditions. Whereas almost all research during 2020 and 2021 focused on stress and related negative emotions such as anxiety, fear, anger, and depression, only a few studies (e.g., Gallagher et al., 2021; Hu et al., 2021) investigated the role of hope and positive growth during the pandemic.

9.2.2 Coping Strategies and the Experience of Hope

Whether a stressful situation is assessed as threatening or challenging and therefore faced with fear or hope can be determined by the kind of coping activities and strategies people choose to master it. Based on the work of Lazarus and Folkman (1984), coping activities have been classified into three categories: problem-focused, emotion-focused, and dysfunctional coping. People are either able to influence the circumstances which they are confronting or they can alter the way in which they interpret these circumstances. This means that coping can and must take place not only in deeds but also (and primarily) in thoughts and feelings (Lazarus, 1966),

In many situations, people can do something to improve the current conditions, for themselves, for their families, at work, etc. Problem-focused coping is about confronting a stressful situation, taking it as a challenge and changing something for the better (solving problems, finding new solutions, etc.). However, in order to be able to understand unfavorable circumstances as challenges instead of as threats, we firstly have to change the way we interpret what is happening. This secondary appraisal based on an emotion-focused coping approach makes external conditions look much more benign and tractable in the first place and reduce their frightening character (Lazarus, 1993). This makes it possible to convert apparently insurmountable threats into manageable challenges by simultaneously engaging in an emotional shift from anxiety to hope. The unfavorable alternative, characterized by help- and hopelessness, is to feel overwhelmed by the threats, which usually leads people to deal with them in an inappropriate way, such as denying or distancing oneself from reality, refraining from any constructive response, or even engaging in harmful reactions like substance abuse and aggressive behavior (Carver et al., 1989).

Carver and his colleagues identified and defined four problem-focused, five emotion-focused, and five dysfunctional coping strategies (Carver, 1997; Carver et al., 1989), which can be associated with the perception of hope:

Category I: Problem-focused coping strategies

1. *Active coping*: Concrete measures are taken to change the situation or mitigate the negative effects of a situation. Active coping contains the hope for improvement.
2. *Planning*: As long as no concrete measures can be taken, possible strategies for action and future steps can be envisioned and planned. Planning is an expression of hope in terms of engagement and patience.
3. *Self-direction*: Focusing on things that one can influence (e.g., one's own tasks in the family or at work). This does not solve the problem immediately, but the focus is directed to what is currently feasible to do. Self-direction demonstrates the will to refrain from giving up and to remain hopeful, waiting for future opportunities.

4. *Instrumental support*: Seeking specific support from other people. This can be of a material nature (e.g., receiving financial aid) or relate to active help in accomplishing concrete tasks (e.g., caring for children). Instrumental support is a source of hope.

Category II: Emotion-focused coping strategies

1. *Acceptance*: Reality is accepted as it is but without capitulating to it. This could be a precondition for active and constructive coping. The opposite of acceptance is denial. Hope always recognizes reality, instead of escaping from it.
2. *Positive reframing*: A positive reassessment of the situation takes place without denying the negative aspects. For example, not only the problems but also the opportunities are seen in the situation. Positive reframing turns anxiety into hope.
3. *Emotional support*: The other form of social support is aimed at personal moral and emotional encouragement. In difficult situations people need a sympathetic ear, understanding and human closeness. Emotional support is an extraordinary hope booster.
4. *Religion*: For many people, belief in God or a Higher Power and involvement in a religious community are valuable resources for coping with a crisis. Thus, for many individuals, religious faith is a foundation of hope.
5. *Humor*: One takes the situation with a pinch of cheerful serenity. However, the humor must be healthy and not fatalistic. Humor can be an expression of hopeful serenity and calm.

Category III: Dysfunctional coping strategies

1. *Denial*: Sometimes looking away can have a positive effect, for example, by making one worry less about the future. However, denying a reality often only creates additional problems, especially if nothing is done to improve the situation. Denial is based on fear rather than on hope.
2. *Venting*: Negative feelings are allowed and expressed openly. Such a reaction can be temporarily useful if it leads to feeling relieved. In the longer term, however, the negative consequences are usually greater. Venting is associated with negative feelings instead with hope.
3. *Disengagement*: Disengagement is exactly the opposite of commitment and an expression of a lack of courage and help. This occurs when individuals refrain from any attempt to change something or to achieve certain goals. Disengagement is a manifestation of help- and hopelessness.
4. *Self-blame*: In some situations, people may tend to look for the causes of their problems only within themselves and therefore feel guilty. Especially when self-esteem is low, people tend to blame themselves ("If only I hadn't . . .", etc.). Self-blame impairs self-confidence and hope.
5. *Substance abuse*: In the event of anxiety, worry, loss of control, and excessive demands, people sometimes resort to excessive consumption of alcohol and harmful substances. This only worsens the situation (their own health, social relationships, etc.). Substance abuse is a consequence of overwhelming help- and hopelessness.

Several studies during the pandemic have shown the predominance of emotion- and problem-focused coping strategies to overcome anxiety and to re-establish well-being as well as the negative effects of dysfunctional coping styles (Agha, 2021; Ahuja, 2021; Bhattacharjee & Ghosh, 2021; Budimir et al., 2021; Garbóczy et al., 2021; Guszkowska & Dąbrowska-Zimakowska, 2022; Kar et al., 2021; Mahamid & Bdier, 2021; Minahan et al., 2021; Morales-Rodríguez, 2021; Rogowska et al., 2021). In a study among participants from 20 countries, Kar et al. (2021) reported that "hoping for the best" was the most frequently adopted strategy to cope with anxiety and that dysfunctional reactions such as "avoiding thinking about it" and "struggling to cope" were related to significantly higher levels of anxiety and depression. Similarly, in a representative study in Austria, the authors disclosed that positive thinking, active stress coping, and social support were positively related to psychological life quality, well-being, and negatively predicted perceived stress, depression, and anxiety (Budimir et al., 2021). The combination of emotion- and problem-focused coping styles reveal that hope and a positive attitude must not be confounded with wishful thinking. Garbóczy et al. (2021) similarly indicated that whereas a positive attitude was associated with lower levels of psychological stress, wishful thinking, to the contrary, was related with higher levels of stress and anxiety. Furthermore, in line with Lazarus' transactional model of stress, some studies have evidenced a shift in coping styles during 2020 and 2021. In Poland for example, Rogowska et al. (2021) observed that during this period problem-oriented strategies decreased and emotion-focused behaviors slightly increased.

9.2.3 The Role of Culture

The role of culture as a significant factor in relation to the perception of stress and the adoption of different coping styles has received increased attention among researchers. Tseng (2001), for example, has highlighted that culture has a broad impact on stress in multiple dimensions, since "... culture influences the occurrence of stress, modifies the perception or appraisal of the stress, is involved in the selection of a coping style, and has an impact on the supporting resources available to the subject" (p. 125). Culturally anchored values, beliefs, norms, and habits can influence how people deal with stressful situations, but certain social expectations and norms can also be reasons causing distress in the individual. The prescription of roles and duties together with the pressure to perform or the expectation to behave in a certain manner could increase the demands on the individual, exacerbating instead of alleviating the perception of stress (Chun et al., 2006; Moos, 1984, 2002).

On the other hand, people socialized within a certain culture could have the propensity to appraise a stressful situation in a specific way by attributing the same meaning to it and to choose similar coping patterns, which consist of generally accepted and expected attitudes and behaviors in dealing with the stressors (Tseng, 2001). Cross-cultural literature on stress and coping has identified several cultural factors that seem to influence the appraisal and the coping styles in different societies and social groups such as the type of self-construal, the kinds of control, attribution styles as well as coping goals, and motivations (Aldwin, 2004; Chun et al., 2006; Heppner et al., 2006; Hu et al., 2018; Kuo et al., 2006). Basically, all these authors recognize fundamental differences in how people growing up and living in individualistic and collectivistic cultures perceive and cope with stress. However, it is important to be aware of both the more generalizable psychological universals at an individual level as well as culture specific patterns at the social level (Heppner et al., 2006).

According to Markus and Kitayama (1991, 2003), Shulruf et al. (2007, 2011) as well as Triandis (1996, 2001), people from individualistic and collectivistic cultures differ with regard to their independent vs. interdependent self-construals, the internal or external control locus, a primary vs. a secondary control target (on the environment or on oneself), as well as regarding the type of individual or social goals they engage in. Reverting to the person-environment transactional stress model of Lazarus and Folkman (1984), sociocultural groups can develop different beliefs regarding the origin and meaning of stressors and the appropriate means to cope with them (Aldwin, 2004). For example, whereas people from individualistic cultures may attribute causes of events to themselves or to other individuals (i.e., looking for and blaming the culprit), individuals from collectivistic cultures may have the tendency to attribute the origin of events to general and impersonal circumstances (such as fate, destiny, providence, etc.). Furthermore, Chun et al. (2006) hypothesized that individualistic cultures would be more prone to interpret stressful situations as challenges, and that collectivistic cultures would tend to understand them as threats in order to avoid possible harm and losses. This would imply that, based on primary appraisal and assuming all other parameters are equal, people from collectivistic cultures would display higher levels of stress than people from individualistic cultures.

However, people also differ with regard to the secondary appraisal which takes into account the resources available in order to cope with the stressors. Individuals from individualistic cultures seem to have a stronger focus on the internal locus of control such as self-confidence, individual capabilities, etc., developing coping strategies centering on one's own needs and directed to change the external environment to promote positive outcomes (especially for oneself). Alternately, people from collectivistic cultures prefer to focus on external coping sources like social support and religious faith, by simultaneously emphasizing the secondary control of their internal cognitive and emotional states in order to adapt to the external circumstances and avoid harm to themselves and others (Chun et al., 2006; Yeh et al., 2006). Consequently, in individualistic cultures people would be more oriented to engage in problem-focused coping activities (e.g., active coping and striving), and in collectivistic cultures individuals would favor more passive and emotion-focused coping strategies (e.g., family support, emotional backing, and religious practices) with the goal to preserve social cohesion and harmony (Hu et al., 2018). However, we must keep in mind that at the level of the individual person, individualistic and collectivistic characteristics may coexist and vary in degree due to different socialization and acculturation experiences and personality traits (Kuo et al., 2006).

In summary, cultural values, beliefs, norms and habits can influence levels of stress, anxiety, hope, and well-being of the population in several ways: Specifically, this can occur by posing certain stressors on the individual (pressures and expectations), by influencing the appraisal of a given stressful situation (as threat or challenge), by focusing on the available (individual or social) resources, and by motivating the adoption of certain (problem- or emotion-focused) coping strategies. Beyond these socio-psychological mechanisms, we also have to be aware of the role and impact of institutions such as the economic, the political, the education, and the health system, charity organizations, neighborhood associations, and social groups, etc. (Aldwin, 2004), which can provide resources to alleviate existing burdens or vice-versa make a sad situation even worse (due to mismanagement, corruption, lack of funds, etc.).

9.2.4 Posttraumatic Growth and Hope

The pandemic has occasioned widespread emotional distress in almost all people, sectors, and communities of society. Most psychological studies performed during the pandemic have centered on mental health risks and the appearance of posttraumatic stress disorders such as long-lasting anxiety, sadness, depression, and related physical dysfunctions such as fatigue, headaches, and insomnia, which have been well documented (e.g., Boyraz & Legros, 2020; Casagrande et al., 2020; Kar et al., 2021; Liu et al., 2020; Minahan et al., 2021).

From a positive psychological perspective, one major question is how people could find new meaning out of this crisis situation and possibly experience positive changes and personal growth (Linley & Joseph, 2011). For example, beyond the uncertainty due to changes at work and the worries about the future, many people reported positive experiences such as having enjoyed spending more time with their family and children, having had more time to pursue other activities or hobbies, and having performed more physical activity during the lockdowns (de Quervain et al., 2020). The Swiss Household Panel reported shifts in people's mindsets during and after the pandemic (Tillmann et al., 2021). For many people, the world after the pandemic is no longer the same. Other things became much more important than before. Many people desire a different life and do not want to go back to the previous ways of living. Some people have rearranged their lives, changing their jobs, or even starting their own businesses, and others have become more spiritual. Especially people who were negatively affected by the pandemic and lost their jobs have developed a different idea of a good life.

All these experiences show that life crises can offer new possibilities for positive personal change and growth. Psychological research has referred to these phenomena using different terms such as stress-related or posttraumatic growth (Armeli et al., 2001). The most common term coined by Calhoun and Tedeschi is that of posttraumatic growth (PTG), which is defined as the "experience of positive change that occurs as a result of the struggle with highly challenging life crises" (Tedeschi & Calhoun, 2004, p. 1). This means that "posttraumatic growth describes the experience of individuals whose development, at least in some areas, has surpassed what was present before the struggle with crises occurred. The individual has not only survived, but has experienced changes that are viewed as important, and that go beyond what was the previous status quo. Posttraumatic growth is not simply a return to baseline—it is an experience of improvement that for some persons is deeply profound" (p. 4).

Tedeschi and Calhoun (1995) identified five main areas of growth after a stressful or traumatic situation:

1. *Appreciation of life and new life philosophy*: People look at life with different eyes. They develop a new mindfulness and perceive each day more consciously. They realize how precious life is, feeling gratitude for many small and big things in life. Life is taken with greater ease and they enjoy every moment appreciating what they have.
2. *Personal strength and self-awareness*: People feel stronger and more confident because they know they can handle difficult situations. They feel more experienced and may also feel that they have grown personally and became better persons.
3. *New possibilities and priorities*: People realize what is really important and valuable to them. They develop new interests and set new priorities. Sometimes, life takes on a new direction. New paths and perspectives open up and people want to do more good in life and change things in a positive way.
4. *Relationships with other people*: Individuals recognize how important and valuable social relationships are. Relationships with family members and friends become deeper and more intimate. The person is able to form closer and more empathetic relationships with others. He or she feels more sensitivity and compassion for others and is increasingly willing to give and accept help.
5. *Religiosity and Spirituality*: People's religious faith and spirituality are strengthened. They develop more interest in and understanding of spiritual matters and a greater engagement with existential questions take place.

Previous research on stress-related and posttraumatic growth revealed that the experiences of positive effects after traumatic experiences are by far more numerous than the cases of post-traumatic stress disorders (Tedeschi & Calhoun, 2004). However, the negative and positive effects after a crisis experience coexist and are emotional in nature. The direct impact of a negative life event is primarily negative, leading to uncertainty, distress, and anxiety. The secondary effect is related to a person's response to the event (Armeli et al., 2001). How the individual assesses and copes with the initial negative experience is crucial in determining whether a positive turn may occur or not. Positive reframing, the support of others, and an active engagement in dealing with the negative situation have proven to be particularly effective in fostering personal development and growth (Collins et al., 1990).

Considering that PTG has a strong emotional component, one central aim in our research was to assess the relationship between PTG and hope. Fredrickson (2013) highlighted the transformative character of hope as one of the ten most frequently experienced positive emotions in daily life, which has the effect of fostering personal growth. Hope, as a positive emotion broadens the mindset, the scope of attention, and the thought and action repertoire, nurturing psychological, social, and even physical resources to cope with adversity. The second important effect of hope as a positive emotion is that it transforms the individual for the better. While certain emotions such as experiencing a good mood and pleasure nourish hedonic happiness, hope can be considered part of the eudaimonic domain of flourishing, connected to inner personal growth, meaning in life, and relations with others (Cohn & Fredrickson, 2009). Similarly, Joseph and Linley (2005) also claimed that posttraumatic growth can be related to an increase in eudaimonic instead of hedonic well-being, since eudaimonic or psychological well-being is strongly connected with existential life challenges. Furthermore, because of the broadening and growth effect, hopeful people tend to display more altruistic and generative behavior by helping others, taking a long-term view of things, instead of satisfying short-term needs, thinking beyond the struggles of the present moment, and adopting moral values such as friendship, gratitude, generativity, selflessness, kindness, and inclusiveness towards strangers (Cohn & Fredrickson, 2006).

Tedeschi and Calhoun (2004) have explicitly pointed out that traumatic events such as an earthquake or a financial crisis can also affect entire countries and societies and that these collective experiences can trigger social change for the better or the worse. Crises can generate a cultural, political, and economic shift with far reaching social consequences. Existing values and behaviors (e.g., travel and consumption habits) can be questioned and transformed by creating new ideas about what is good for society and which measures have to be taken in order to improve the general quality of life and the natural environment.

Whether the pandemic has generated a positive effect on the population, changing or developing a society for the better has not been examined yet and has still to be investigated. Furthermore, previous research has shown that the relationship between posttraumatic growth, perceived distress, and well-being is not always clear. PTG is sometimes, but not always, related to lower perceived stress and higher levels of well-being (Tedeschi & Calhoun, 2004). In our study, based on data collected in November 2021 and including samples from 11 countries, we assessed the degree of growth experienced by people in the five domains of PTG and examined the results in relation with reported levels of perceived hope, stress, as well as hedonic, psychological, and social well-being.

9.3 The Current Study

9.3.1 General Aim

The general aim of our study was to investigate the levels of perceived stress and hope during the pandemic years of 2020 and 2021 reported by participants in 11 countries. We also examined how they coped with the stressful situations, to what extent they experienced personal growth until the end of 2021, and how these phenomena relate to each other and with levels of well-being. Doing so, we intended to assess three novel aspects related to the phenomena of stress, coping, personal growth, hope, and well-being in the context of a global crisis situation: (1) The role of hope in relation to the appraisal of stress, coping strategies, and possible positive outcomes in terms of stress-related growth; (2) The temporal development of these psychological states across the two years of the pandemic (from the end of 2019 until the end of 2021); and (3) The similarities and differences between samples from 11 countries with very different cultural backgrounds.

9.3.2 Objectives

Our study had six objectives:

1. To compare levels of hope and hedonic psychological and social well-being for the eleven samples at three time points (at the end of 2019, 2020, and 2021) as well as levels of perceived stress at the end of 2020 and 2021 to find general trends and differences between samples.
2. To assess levels of problem-focused, emotion-focused, and dysfunctional coping styles across the samples both in 2020 and in 2021 and to identify similarities and individual patterns between the samples.
3. To examine associations between coping styles and levels of hope, perceived stress, and general well-being across countries in 2020 and 2021.
4. To investigate levels of posttraumatic growth in five areas at the end of 2021 and distinguish universal from sample specific patterns.
5. To evaluate associations between the five areas of posttraumatic growth and coping strategies employed in 2021 in the different samples.
6. To explore the relationships between posttraumatic growth, perceived hope, perceived stress, and hedonic, psychological, and social well-being across the eleven investigated countries at the end of 2021.

Basically, we expected the following:

1. Countries with higher levels of hope will display significant lower levels of distress and higher levels of well-being.
2. Problem-focused and emotion-focused coping strategies will be predominant vis-á-vis dysfunctional coping activities but significant differences between

samples, especially with regard to the intensity of emotion-focused coping activities, will emerge (e.g., emotional support and religious practices).
3. In more collectivistic countries emotion-focused strategies such as social support and religious practices will be more strongly associated with hope, stress, and well-being than in individualistic countries.
4. Because of its strong emotional basis, post-traumatic growth will be stronger in collectivistic countries than in individualistic countries.
5. Socially and religious oriented coping strategies will have positive effects on the social and religious dimensions of growth and be more pronounced in predominantly collectivistic countries.
6. Dimensions of posttraumatic growth will be more positively associated with psychological and social well-being than with hedonic well-being.

9.3.3 Procedure and Participant Samples

Data collection took place through announcements in online newspapers, social media, and e-mails in three cross-sectional waves in November 2019 ($N = 9092$), November 2020 ($N = 9536$) and November 2021 ($N = 9093$). No incentives were offered. We selected 11 countries which participated to the Hope Barometer survey during all three years, resulting in a total of 33 samples. People younger than 18 were excluded from the analysis. The questionnaire was delivered in English (Australia, Northern and Southern India, Nigeria, and South Africa), Spanish (Spain), Czech (Czech Republic), Italian (Italy and Southern Switzerland), Polish (Poland), Portuguese (Portugal), Malayalam (Southern India), French (France and West Switzerland), and German (Center and East Switzerland). The demographic structure of the samples is exhibited in Appendix 9.1.

According to the ranking delivered by Hofstede, Portugal, and Nigeria, and to a large extent also India, are the three countries amongst our samples with the highest levels of collectivistic values. These countries are characterized by interdependence, strong bonds to family members and extended relationships, and a strong commitment and responsibility towards social groups. Australia, Italy, France, and Switzerland are characterized as individualistic, where predominant values are independence and individual performance with the prevalence of an internal locus of control vis-à-vis an external locus of control. In these countries people look after themselves and their immediate families. South Africa, Spain, Czechia, and Poland have an intermediate position between individualism and collectivism. South Africa has unique features due to multi-ethnic constitution of its society. Research studies which assessed the level of individualism-collectivism in South Africa revealed that Black, native language speaking people and individuals with lower education tend to be more collectivistic than White, English-speaking people and persons with a higher education, who are more individualistic (Chipp et al., 2013; Eaton & Louw, 2000). Our samples of 2019 and 2020 contain around two thirds of white and one third of black, Colored and Indian people. The sample of 2021 is more balanced including around 50% White and 50% Black, Colored, and Indian people.

9.3.4 *Measures*

Perceived Hope
The general level of perceived hope was assessed with the Perceived Hope Scale (PHS) (Krafft et al., 2019, 2021; Marujo et al., 2021; Slezackova et al., 2020). The PHS consists of six items to measure the level of hope as perceived by people, free from any preconceptions regarding the nature and quality of hope. The PHS is especially suitable to assess the level of general hope in different cultures since it avoids any bias regarding potential sources, roots, dimensions, and elements of hope. The items of the PHS evaluate the degree of hope in general ("I feel hopeful"), in one's life ("I am hopeful with regard to my life") and especially in difficult situations ("Even in difficult times I am able to remain hopeful"). Further items assess the belief in the possibility of fulfillment of one's hopes ("My hopes are usually fulfilled"), the quality of hope with regard to one's quality of life ("Hope improves the quality of my life"), and the intensity of hope vis-à-vis the feeling of anxiety ("In my life hope outweighs anxiety"). The six positively worded items were rated on a 6-point Likert scale from 0 (strongly disagree) to 5 (strongly agree). In the current study the six items achieved a high internal consistency in all 33 samples (3 x 11) with Cronbach alpha values between $\alpha = 0.80$ and 0.92.

Perceived Stress
The level of distress was evaluated using the Perceived Stress Scale (PSS) (Cohen et al., 1983). The PSS measures the extent to which critical life situations are rated as more or less stressful, unpredictable, uncontrollable, and overloading. The six negatively and four positively expressed items are formulated in such a way that they are of a general nature and therefore relatively free of specific life situations. The PSS is particularly well suited for determining chronic stress under long-lasting life circumstances as well as subjective expectations regarding future events or developments. The ten questions of the PSS, rated on a five-point-scale from 0 (never) to 4 (often), were focused on the respondents' feelings and thoughts during the current year (2020 and 2021 respectively). The scale revealed good reliability coefficients throughout all 33 samples between $\alpha = 0.76$ and 0.91.

Hedonic, Psychological and Social Well-being
Well-being was assessed with the Mental Health Continuum Short Form (MHC-SF) developed by Keyes (2002). The MHC-SF consists of 14 positively worded items, with three items representing hedonic well-being (happy, interested in life, and satisfied), six items evaluating psychological well-being (functioning well in one's personal life) and five items describing social well-being (the relationship between oneself and the larger community/society). Participants were asked to rate how often in the past month they felt in a specific manner. Items were rated on a six-point scale

from 1 (never) to 6 (every day). Reliability coefficients were good, achieving levels between $\alpha = 0.86$ and 0.95 for the general score, between $\alpha = 0.78$ and 0.92 for hedonic well-being, between $\alpha = 0.79$ and 0.90 for psychological well-being, and between $\alpha = 0.74$ and 0.89 for social well-being.

Coping Strategies

To measure coping strategies, we used the Brief COPE (Carver, 1997) which comprises 28 items to assess 14 different coping styles represented by two items each. Four coping styles describe problem-focused strategies, five are defined as emotion-focused strategies, and the other five describe dysfunctional strategies (see the descriptions of the 14 coping styles in a previous section). Participants rated how often in the current year they used each strategy in dealing with stressful situations occasioned by the pandemic on a 4-point scale (1 = not at all to 4 = a lot). Most Cronbach alpha reliability scores were acceptable to good at around 0.70.

Posttraumatic Growth

In November 2021 we implemented the short form of the Posttraumatic Growth Inventory (PTGI-SF) (Cann et al., 2010) which comprises 10 items with two items associated to each of the five sub-scales respectively (see the descriptions of the five domains in a previous section). The items were rated on a scale from 0 (*I did not experience this change as a result of the pandemic*) to 5 (*I experienced this change to a very great degree as a result of the pandemic*). The instruction given was "*Please indicate for each of the statements below the degree to which your life has changed as a result of the COVID-19 pandemic*". Cronbach alpha reliability scores were good to high with a mean level of 0.76.

9.3.5 *Data Analysis*

Using multi-group confirmatory factor analysis (MGCFA) we first wanted to demonstrate measurement invariance of the Perceived Hope Scale across all 3 x 11 samples in 2019, 2020, and 2021 respectively. The fit of the general model by means of maximum likelihood estimation was evaluated using the comparative fit index (CFI), the Tucker-Lewis index (TLI) (study criterion ≥ 0.95 as ideal and ≥ 0.90 as the minimum acceptable level), the root mean square error of approximation (RMSEA) and the standardized root mean residual SRMR (study criterion ≤ 0.08) (Hu & Bentler, 1999). The test for measurement invariance was performed in four steps, from configurational invariance (equal form), to metric invariance (equal loadings), to scalar invariance (equal intercepts), and finally to strict invariance (equal residuals). The recommended criteria to demonstrate invariance are changes in CFI and TLI between comparison and nested models of ≥ -0.010, a change in RMSEA of ≤ 0.015 and a variation in SRMR of ≤ 0.030 (for loading invariance) and ≤ 0.010 (for intercept invariance) (Chen, 2007).

In accordance with the six above mentioned objectives, we computed mean values and standard deviations for all variables and performed analyses of variance

(ANOVA) across all samples. Afterwards, partial bivariate Pearson correlations controlled for gender, age, marital status, education, main activity, and professional status, were calculated for every sample between the following variables: (1) the 14 coping strategies and hope, stress, and well-being in 2020 and 2021, (2) the 14 coping styles and the five domains of posttraumatic growth in 2021, and (3) the five domains of posttraumatic growth and hope, stress, and well-being in 2021. All statistical analyses were performed with IBM SPSS and AMOS version 27.0.

9.3.6 *Results*

9.3.6.1 Group Invariance of the PHS

In order to be able to compare mean values of the PHS and relate them to the other variables, we tested group invariance using all the investigated samples in 2019, 2020, and 2021. Table 9.1 contains the results of all three MGCFA including the fit indices for the general samples followed by the four models to test different types of invariance. The overall fit indices for the total samples revealed that the one-factor model achieved good model fit (CFI and TLI > 0.95 in 2019, 2020 and CFI > 0.90

Table 9.1 Multigroup Confirmatory Factor Analysis and Group Invariance for the Perceived Hope Scale 2019–2021

	X^2	df	CFI	TLI	RMSEA	SRMR
Total sample 2019 (11 groups, $N = 9092$)	402.20	9	0.986	0.977	0.070	0.020
Country invariance						
Configurational Invariance (equal form)	4200.54	261	0.856	0.909	0.041	0.057
Metric Invariance (equal loadings)	4210.66	266	0.856	0.910	0.040	0.057
Scalar Invariance (equal intercepts)	4233.58	272	0.855	0.912	0.040	0.057
Full uniqueness (measurement residuals)	4251.93	279	0.855	0.914	0.040	0.057
Total sample 2020 (11 groups, $N = 9536$)	386.07	9	0.987	0.978	0.066	0.020
Country invariance						
Configurational Invariance (equal form)	1976.53	261	0.940	0.962	0.026	0.087
Metric Invariance (equal loadings)	1992.89	266	0.940	0.963	0.026	0.086
Scalar Invariance (equal intercepts)	2075.57	272	0.937	0.962	0.026	0.086
Full uniqueness (measurement residuals)	2082.99	279	0.937	0.963	0.026	0.085
Total sample 2021 (11 groups, $N = 9093$)	323.09	9	0.989	0.982	0.063	0.017
Country invariance						
Configurational Invariance (equal form)	2297.56	261	0.932	0.957	0.029	0.046
Metric Invariance (equal loadings)	2311.47	266	0.932	0.958	0.029	0.046
Scalar Invariance (equal intercepts)	2391.85	272	0.930	0.957	0.029	0.046
Full uniqueness (measurement residuals)	2412.46	279	0.929	0.958	0.029	0.046

Note: CFI Comparative fit index, TLI Tucker-Lewis index, RMSEA Root mean square error of approximation, SRMR Standardized root mean residual

and TLI > 0.95 in 2021, RMSEA and SRMR ≤ 0.08) (Hu & Bentler, 1999). Furthermore, the model fit of the individual samples also revealed adequate results. The equal form used as baseline model provided a good fit to the data, suggesting reasonable support for configurational invariance across the groups, with exception of the CFI in 2019. According to Marsh (1994) and Marsh et al. (1996) the TLI could be considered as more appropriate than the CFI, because it also takes into account the model complexity. Furthermore, all indices comparing the nested models with the baseline model were under the threshold values recommended by the literature (Chen, 2007, CFI and TLI > −0.01, RMSEA and SRMR < 0.015) (Marsh, 1994). This means that the PHS demonstrated strong measurement invariance and that it is possible to compare the PHS scores between the national samples. The perceived hope construct measured with the PHS seemed to be conceptualized in a similar way across cultures and was suitable to be examined in relationship to other constructs.

9.3.6.2 Perceived Hope, Perceived Stress, and Well-being 2019-2021

We started our analysis by comparing mean values of perceived hope, perceived stress, and well-being between 2019 and 2021 and between all country samples (see Table 9.2).

Perceived Hope 2019-2021

The first remarkable result is that in 2020 and 2021 people in all countries experienced moderate to high levels of hope clearly above the center of the scale ($M > 3.0$). This means that during the pandemic, and despite the cumbersome times, most people could remain hopeful for the future.

The highest levels of hope during all three years were reported by people in Nigeria, Australia, and South Africa. Participants in India reported high levels of hope in 2019 and 2020, but moderate levels of hope in 2021. In Portugal, people showed higher levels of hope in 2019 and 2021 but moderate levels of hope in 2020. The lowest levels of perceived hope were reported by participants in Spain, Poland, France, and Switzerland (especially in the French and Italian regions). Participants from Italy and Czechia were in between and displayed moderate levels of hope.

Regarding the development of the levels of hope between 2019 and 2020, people in Czechia, France, Poland, Switzerland, and South Africa recorded an increase or constant level of hope in 2020 but a clear decline in 2021. In contrast, people in Portugal and Spain reported a marked drop of hope in 2020 but an upsurge in 2021. Whereas in Australia and Italy the levels of hope remained almost constant from 2019 to 2021, people in Nigeria and India demonstrated a negative trend.

Perceived Stress 2020-2021

The slight but evident ups and downs in levels of hope could be related to the experience and appraisal of distress. Based on previous studies, stress levels can be divided into three ranges (Cohen et al., 1997): (1) low stress levels are expressed by mean values between 0 and 1.3 with "normal" levels around 1.3-1.4; (2) moderate

Table 9.2 Mean values, standard deviations and ANOVA for Perceived Hope, Well-being and Perceived Stress

		Perceived Hope		Well-being		Perceived Stress	
		M	*SD*	*M*	*SD*	*M*	*SD*
Australia	2021	3.66	0.91	4.24	1.11	1.80	0.63
	2020	3.72	0.91	4.40	0.96	1.69	0.62
	2019	3.71	0.88	4.42	1.01		
Czech Republic	2021	3.31	0.97	3.68	1.07	1.86	0.60
	2020	3.47	0.99	3.86	0.93	2.05	0.64
	2019	3.41	0.97	3.82	0.97		
France	2021	3.07	1.10	3.75	0.95	1.99	0.67
	2020	3.43	1.05	3.91	0.87	1.94	0.68
	2019	3.22	1.00	3.96	0.78		
India	2021	3.39	0.87	4.17	1.05	2.03	0.50
	2020	3.54	0.81	3.95	0.99	2.13	0.54
	2019	3.69	0.82	4.16	1.01		
Italy	2021	3.53	0.99	3.99	1.00	1.95	0.60
	2020	3.49	0.98	3.86	0.96	1.98	0.56
	2019	3.43	1.11	3.93	0.91		
Nigeria	2021	4.13	0.63	4.56	0.84	1.90	0.59
	2020	4.20	0.61	4.48	0.72	1.87	0.48
	2019	4.21	0.61	4.51	0.80		
Poland	2021	3.17	1.03	3.50	1.16	2.00	0.76
	2020	3.39	1.04	3.64	1.08	1.98	0.72
	2019	3.26	0.99	3.67	1.07		
Portugal	2021	3.63	0.94	4.04	0.97	1.92	0.62
	2020	3.43	0.95	3.88	0.90	2.08	0.64
	2019	3.50	1.00	4.19	0.96		
South Africa	2021	3.58	0.99	4.16	1.13	1.94	0.48
	2020	3.70	0.86	4.24	0.81	1.97	0.60
	2019	3.65	0.98	4.21	1.07		
Spain	2021	3.32	0.93	3.98	1.03	2.03	0.67
	2020	3.10	0.96	4.17	0.90	2.28	0.58
	2019	3.28	0.95	4.12	0.96		
Switzerland	2021	3.28	1.09	3.80	1.04	1.93	0.70
	2020	3.39	1.00	3.84	1.00	1.91	0.66
	2019	3.24	1.08	3.88	1.05		
ANOVA *F*/Eta^2	2021	36.77*	0.052	22.83*	0.028	3.96*	0.006
	2020	15.03*	0.016	17.02*	0.018	14.11*	0.015
	2019	74.40*	0.076	44.48*	0.047		

Notes. *$P < 0.001$

stress levels are characterized by mean values between 1.4 and 2.6, slightly impairing satisfaction and well-being; (3) high stress levels are revealed by values between 2.7 and 4.0. In this case, the perception of stress might have a strong impact on satisfaction and personal well-being.

The first key finding in Table 9.2 is that stress levels in all samples appear to be within the moderate range but with significant differences between samples especially in 2021. During 2020 and 2021, the vast majority of people experienced a level of stress that was significantly above the "normal" level. In 2020 people in Spain, Portugal, India, and Czechia reported the highest and people in Australia, Nigeria, and Switzerland the lowest levels of stress, with people in Poland, South Africa, Italy, and France in the middle between both extremes. From 2020 to 2021, the levels of stress remained almost constant in Italy, Nigeria, Poland, and South Africa. People in Australia, France, and Switzerland experienced a slight increase and people in Spain, Portugal, Czechia, and India a slight reduction in the perception of stress.

Well-being 2019-2020

The levels of well-being are moderate to high in all samples, in some samples close to and in others clearly above the center or the scale ($M > 3.5$). In general terms, people in Nigeria, Australia, South Africa, India, and Portugal reported the highest levels of well-being and people in Poland and Czechia the lowest. A negative trend in the levels of well-being especially during 2021 could be observed in Australia, Czechia, France, Poland, Spain, and Switzerland. Participants in India, Italy, Nigeria, and Portugal experienced a decline in well-being decline during 2020 but an upturn in 2021, almost regaining the levels of 2019. Therefore, at the end of 2021, people in Nigeria, Australia, India, South Africa, and Portugal reported significant higher levels of well-being than people in Poland, Italy, Czechia, Switzerland, and France.

9.3.6.3 Coping Styles 2020-2021

The next analysis examined the coping styles that participants in the various countries employed in order to deal with the stressful experiences in 2020 and 2021. Tables 9.3, 9.4 and 9.5. present the levels of coping styles in 2020 and 2021, classified in the three categories emotion-focused (Table 9.3), problem-focused (Table 9.4), and dysfunctional coping (Table 9.5). Across all countries, the positive coping styles received much more adherence than the dysfunctional reactions. In general terms, the principal coping styles were acceptance, positive reframing, active coping, self-direction, and planning. In comparison to the other countries, participants in South Africa, Czechia, Poland, India, and Spain asked for more emotional support in 2020, and people in Poland, South Africa, and India also in 2021. The lowest levels of emotional support were reported in Australia, Switzerland, and France, and also in Spain in 2021 (mainly individualistic countries). Instrumental social support was especially important for people in India, Nigeria,

Table 9.3 Mean values and Standard Deviations of Emotion-Focused Coping Styles 2020–2021

		Acceptance		Positive Reframing		Emotional Support		Religion		Humor	
	Years	*M*	*SD*	*M*	*SD*	*M*	*SD*	*M*	*SD*	*M*	*SD*
Australia	2021	3.18	0.82	2.68	0.94	2.20	0.90	1.94	1.05	2.28	0.95
	2020	3.26	0.69	2.69	0.84	2.19	0.88	1.83	0.97	2.04	0.85
Czech Republic	2021	2.94	0.77	2.55	0.81	2.37	0.86	1.60	0.85	2.37	0.93
	2020	3.33	0.64	2.72	0.85	2.65	0.86	1.78	0.90	2.65	0.93
France	2021	3.12	0.70	2.82	0.80	2.29	0.82	1.69	0.88	2.02	0.80
	2020	3.12	0.76	2.93	0.77	2.27	0.84	1.83	0.93	2.17	0.84
India	2021	2.87	0.79	2.68	0.79	2.49	0.83	2.27	0.94	2.13	0.85
	2020	3.01	0.74	2.82	0.76	2.55	0.77	2.25	0.99	2.32	0.96
Israel	2021	3.23	0.62	3.03	0.70	2.57	0.83	1.82	0.90	2.73	0.89
	2020	3.17	0.59	3.05	0.69	2.55	0.84	1.81	0.93	2.87	0.88
Italy	2021	3.26	0.63	2.73	0.71	2.26	0.82	1.95	0.86	2.24	0.99
	2020	3.16	0.64	2.67	0.79	2.31	0.80	1.85	0.91	2.32	0.90
Nigeria	2021	2.77	0.84	2.75	0.82	2.33	0.90	2.81	0.93	1.90	0.86
	2020	2.84	0.76	2.72	0.81	2.34	0.82	2.98	0.91	1.85	0.85
Poland	2021	3.38	0.59	2.68	0.84	2.71	0.87	1.56	0.83	2.06	0.66
	2020	3.28	0.62	2.75	0.80	2.56	0.84	1.72	0.88	1.98	0.61
Portugal	2021	3.25	0.69	2.98	0.81	2.33	0.95	2.22	1.10	2.46	0.92
	2020	3.26	0.71	2.78	0.84	2.38	0.92	1.93	1.01	2.45	0.96
South Africa	2021	3.13	0.74	2.89	0.81	2.45	0.95	2.86	1.06	2.19	0.95
	2020	3.43	0.55	2.87	0.73	2.77	0.91	2.56	1.20	2.04	0.90
Spain	2021	3.18	0.66	2.31	0.70	2.21	0.87	1.59	0.79	2.07	0.92
	2020	3.17	0.61	2.83	0.72	2.50	0.86	1.46	0.68	2.08	1.00
Switzerland	2021	2.94	0.88	2.61	0.88	1.88	0.77	1.60	0.88	2.14	0.89
	2020	2.94	0.82	2.69	0.83	2.01	0.82	1.60	0.88	2.08	0.86

(continued)

Table 9.3 (continued)

	Years	Acceptance		Positive Reframing		Emotional Support		Religion		Humor	
		M	*SD*	*M*	*SD*	*M*	*SD*	*M*	*SD*	*M*	*SD*
ANOVA *F*/Eta^2	2021	19.44*	0.022	23.04*	.027	85.03*	.091	135.09*	.138	18.82*	0.022
	2020	26.77*	0.027	4.15*	.040	57.10*	.057	67.99*	.067	25.61*	0.026

Notes. *$P < 0.001$

Table 9.4 Mean values and Standard Deviations of Problem-Focused Coping Styles 2020–2021

		Active Coping		Self-direction		Planning		Instrumental Support	
	Years	M	SD	M	SD	M	SD	M	SD
Australia	2021	3.05	0.82	2.46	0.92	2.86	0.82	2.01	0.83
	2020	2.97	0.77	2.43	0.82	2.79	0.92	2.01	0.83
Czech Republic	2021	2.52	0.75	2.62	0.86	2.54	0.82	2.15	0.76
	2020	2.46	0.74	2.81	0.86	2.48	0.82	2.23	0.82
France	2021	2.37	0.82	2.61	0.75	2.36	0.83	2.18	0.78
	2020	2.52	0.78	2.66	0.77	2.49	0.88	2.22	0.79
India	2021	2.76	0.69	2.66	0.74	2.76	0.73	2.48	0.78
	2020	2.73	0.72	2.74	0.72	2.93	0.75	2.51	0.79
Israel	2021	2.97	0.61	2.90	0.74	2.96	0.65	2.43	0.77
	2020	2.64	0.75	2.93	0.69	2.82	0.75	2.33	0.83
Italy	2021	2.78	0.66	2.46	0.77	2.99	0.70	2.18	0.78
	2020	2.70	0.66	2.50	0.73	2.88	0.69	2.18	0.75
Nigeria	2021	2.95	0.88	2.48	0.86	2.89	0.88	2.42	0.90
	2020	3.00	0.85	2.49	0.82	2.99	0.84	2.48	0.82
Poland	2021	2.44	0.86	2.57	0.90	2.73	0.89	2.51	0.89
	2020	2.40	0.85	2.48	0.83	2.77	0.84	2.36	0.79
Portugal	2021	2.85	0.81	2.66	0.89	2.98	0.71	2.20	0.90
	2020	2.69	0.77	2.68	0.85	2.91	0.76	2.14	0.89
South Africa	2021	3.11	0.75	2.81	0.81	3.09	0.78	2.39	0.96
	2020	2.98	0.76	2.72	0.71	2.90	0.74	2.42	0.93
Spain	2021	2.70	0.68	2.42	0.82	2.42	0.72	2.08	0.84
	2020	2.75	0.70	2.83	0.72	2.31	0.75	2.33	0.84
Switzerland	2021	2.45	0.82	2.41	0.85	2.51	0.83	1.69	0.75
	2020	2.47	0.80	2.51	0.80	2.50	0.81	1.75	0.75
ANOVA *F*/ Eta^2	2021	58.52*	0.065	23.45*	0.027	53.29*	0.059	123.80*	0.128
	2020	28.00*	0.029	10.82*	0.011	38.19*	0.039	89.42*	0.086

Notes. *$P < 0.001$

South Africa, and Poland (mainly collectivistic countries) and the least important for people in Australia and Switzerland (mainly individualistic countries). Religious coping was particularly high in Nigeria, South Africa, India, and Portugal (mainly collectivistic countries), and the least important in Switzerland and Spain (mainly individualistic countries).

Comparing changes in coping styles by country between 2020 and 2021, the following patterns were the most remarkable: Levels of disengagement rose in Australia, Czechia, France, Italy, South Africa, and Switzerland, probably denoting a certain fatigue with the burdens imposed by the longer than expected lasting pandemic. At the same time, the levels of acceptance declined in Australia, Czechia, India, Nigeria, and South Africa, and a further decline took place in positive reframing in Czechia, France, India, Poland, Spain, and Switzerland. Emotional and instrumental social support declined in Czechia, Spain, and Switzerland but

Table 9.5 Mean Values and Standard Deviations of Dysfunctional Coping Styles 2020–2021

		Denial		Venting		Disengagement		Self-blame		Substance Abuse	
	Years	M	SD	M	SD	M	SD	M	SD	M	SD
Australia	2021	1.44	0.69	1.97	0.80	1.52	0.68	1.64	0.82	1.47	0.78
	2020	1.34	0.62	1.90	0.73	1.39	0.65	1.63	0.80	1.45	0.72
Czech Republic	2021	2.10	0.69	2.21	0.78	1.82	0.67	2.16	0.77	1.39	0.69
	2020	1.68	0.70	2.33	0.77	1.57	0.61	2.06	0.76	1.31	0.57
France	2021	1.37	0.58	2.51	0.78	1.78	0.71	1.63	0.72	1.36	0.67
	2020	1.43	0.64	2.52	0.72	1.67	0.67	1.57	0.67	1.39	0.66
India	2021	1.86	0.83	2.16	0.76	1.78	0.78	2.12	0.84	1.33	0.70
	2020	1.85	0.88	2.23	0.74	2.01	0.87	2.19	0.95	1.31	0.69
Israel	2021	1.51	0.66	2.52	0.68	1.59	0.65	1.86	0.70	1.18	0.53
	2020	1.51	0.63	2.50	0.69	1.73	0.64	1.81	0.72	1.34	0.71
Italy	2021	1.38	0.65	2.38	0.65	1.32	0.50	1.69	0.63	1.17	0.45
	2020	1.35	0.62	2.36	0.65	1.25	0.50	1.63	0.64	1.20	0.50
Nigeria	2021	2.03	1.00	2.15	0.80	1.60	0.77	1.69	0.88	1.48	0.90
	2020	1.91	0.91	2.17	0.75	1.66	0.73	1.72	0.83	1.35	0.69
Poland	2021	1.31	0.53	2.40	0.72	1.66	0.63	1.74	0.84	1.36	0.66
	2020	1.40	0.63	2.40	0.66	1.60	0.64	1.61	0.67	1.44	0.73
Portugal	2021	1.33	0.58	2.42	0.84	1.37	0.65	1.67	0.72	1.19	0.53
	2020	1.27	0.56	2.37	0.82	1.42	0.66	1.56	0.69	1.18	0.51
South Africa	2021	1.92	0.95	2.32	0.82	1.74	0.84	2.08	0.98	1.61	0.94
	2020	1.35	0.64	2.22	0.67	1.33	0.54	1.78	0.78	1.39	0.73
Spain	2021	1.56	0.72	2.28	0.73	1.62	0.59	1.74	0.83	1.23	0.54
	2020	1.71	0.82	2.21	0.70	1.66	0.59	1.85	0.85	1.28	0.59

Switzerland	2021	1.53	0.76	1.97	0.76	1.83	0.78	1.42	0.65	1.35	0.70
	2020	1.54	0.73	2.02	0.76	1.71	0.72	1.45	0.65	1.35	0.67
ANOVA *F*/Eta^2	2021	64.57*	0.071	51.34*	0.057	26.66*	0.031	121.24*	0.125	13.42*	0.016
	2020	24.77*	0.025	36.60*	0.037	37.64*	0.038	58.52*	0.058	7.06*	0.007

Notes. $^*P < 0.001$

increased in Poland. Moreover, the levels of religious coping intensified in Italy, Portugal, South Africa, and Spain and slightly diminished in Czechia, France, Nigeria, and Poland.

9.3.6.4 Correlations Between Coping Styles and Perceived Hope, Perceived Stress, and Well-being

In this section we evaluate the partial bivariate Pearson correlation coefficients of each individual sample in 2020 and 2021 between the 14 coping styles, on the one hand, and the levels of perceived hope, perceived stress, and well-being, on the other. Our aim is to highlight the most striking results, identifying similarities, and differences between samples.

Correlations between Coping Styles and Perceived Hope 2020-2021
A central question of our study concerns the extent to which the different coping styles are associated with the general level of perceived hope (see Table 9.6). In almost all samples the highest correlation coefficients with perceived hope were, first, positive reframing, second, acceptance, active coping, and religious coping, and third, planning. Negative correlation coefficients were found for the relationships between perceived hope and the dysfunctional coping styles of disengagement and self-blame. Furthermore, perceived hope was barely or even not at all associated with humor, self-direction, denial, and venting.

Emotional and instrumental social support displayed low to moderate correlation coefficients with perceived hope, particularly in Poland, South Africa, Czechia, India, and Italy (in 2020). Interestingly, in the Portuguese sample the association between hope and social support was not significant. In a separate analysis, not reported here, we detected that this is due to the significant associations between hope and the demographic variables, especially with age and the main activity participants were involved in. Correlation coefficients between perceived hope and religious coping were notably strong in samples from South Africa, Portugal, Poland, Nigeria, France, and Australia, of moderate size also in India, Italy, and Switzerland and not significant at all in Spain.

Interestingly, in some cases the results varied from one year to the other. The reason may be grounded in individual differences between the samples of 2020 and 2021, but could also correspond to changes in general conditions and experiences. For example, in Czechia, India, and Italy, the association between social support (emotional and instrumental) and hope was stronger in 2020 than in 2021, but in South Africa and Nigeria the coefficient was stronger in 2021 than in 2020. In some countries, like Czechia, France, India, Italy, South Africa, and Spain, the negative relationship between self-blame and perceived hope was more accentuated in 2020 than in 2021, but in other countries like Australia, Poland, and Portugal, it was the other way around.

Table 9.6 Partial Bivariate Pearson Correlations of Coping Styles with Perceived Hope 2020–2021

	Australia		Czech Republic		France		India		Italy	
Years	2020	2021	2020	2021	2020	2021	2020	2021	2020	2021
Acceptance	0.152*	0.025	0.082	0.197**	0.374**	0.226**	0.131*	0.275**	0.231**	0.154*
Positive Reframing	0.295**	0.449**	0.420**	0.405**	0.506**	0.369**	0.301**	0.274**	0.447**	0.302**
Emotional Support	0.071	0.164	0.254**	0.156**	0.101	0.060	0.209**	0.115*	0.192**	0.142
Religion	0.218**	0.286**	0.224**	0.077	0.328**	0.241**	0.142*	0.160**	0.215**	0.158*
Humor	0.175*	0.121	0.100	0.147**	0.249**	0.175**	−0.142*	0.057	0.042	0.225**
Active Coping	0.177*	0.351**	0.284**	0.210**	0.403**	0.261**	0.258**	0.304**	0.298**	0.373**
Self-direction	0.056	0.010	−0.008	0.001	0.081	0.050	0.111	0.173**	0.037	−0.041
Planning	0.049	0.124	0.126*	0.052	0.355**	0.302**	0.243**	0.271**	0.333**	0.297**
Instrumental Support	−0.054	0.207*	0.175**	0.095*	0.113	0.116*	0.187**	0.093*	0.204**	0.118
Denial	0.080	0.135	−0.159*	−0.171**	−0.036	−0.005	−0.086	−0.015	−0.021	0.016
Venting	−0.098	0.078	0.086	0.022	0.154*	0.200**	0.022	−0.021	0.179**	0.075
Disengagement	−0.169*	−0.210*	−0.202**	−0.237**	−0.212**	−0.236**	−0.112	−0.201**	−0.169**	−0.218**
Selfblame	−0.279**	−0.336**	−0.329**	−0.272**	−0.240**	−0.191**	−0.198**	−0.068	−0.181**	−0.124
Substance Abuse	−0.166*	−0.190*	−0.111	−0.189**	−0.231**	−0.167**	−0.131*	−0.045	−0.104*	−0.176*

(continued)

Table 9.6 (continued)

	Australia		Czech Republic		France		India		Italy	
Years	2020	2021	2020	2021	2020	2021	2020	2021	2020	2021

	Nigeria		Poland		Portugal		South Africa		Spain		Switzerland	
Years	2020	2021	2020	2021	2020	2021	2020	2021	2020	2021	2020	2021
Acceptance	0.233**	0.029	0.252**	0.135	0.292**	0.235**	0.279**	0.309**	0.111	0.236**	0.268**	0.217**
Positive Reframing	0.345**	0.237*	0.407**	0.459**	0.393**	0.424**	0.369**	0.432**	0.338**	0.364**	0.439**	0.390**
Emotional Support	0.104	0.184*	0.305**	0.352**	0.035	0.028	0.169	0.308**	−0.054	0.041	0.068**	0.136**
Religion	0.300**	0.207*	0.242**	0.322**	0.309**	0.326**	0.499**	0.398**	0.179	0.094	0.170**	0.167**
Humor	−0.035	0.101	0.057	0.071	0.008	0.115*	0.036	0.090*	0.102	0.029	0.202**	0.188**
Active Coping	0.179*	0.119	0.163*	0.201*	0.238**	0.218**	0.189*	0.412**	0.098	0.237**	0.219**	0.223**
Self-direction	0.143	0.040	−0.042	−0.082	−0.039	0.098*	−0.144	0.075	0.047	0.009	0.082**	0.089**
Planning	0.230**	0.019	0.209**	0.369**	0.238**	0.269**	−0.018	0.266**	0.088	0.221**	0.183**	0.152**
Instrumental Support	0.090	0.254**	0.263**	0.284**	0.107	0.042	−0.023	0.248**	−0.062	−0.016	0.004	0.067**
Denial	−0.012	0.071	−0.082	−0.075	−0.048	0.002	0.060	−0.018	−0.031	−0.115*	−0.091**	−0.084**
Venting	0.057	0.056	−0.022	−0.071	−0.038	0.037	−0.185*	−0.037	−0.143	0.032	−0.054**	−0.031*
Disengagement	−0.152	−0.188*	−0.423**	−0.547**	−0.195*	−0.291**	−0.228**	−0.256**	−0.123	−0.135*	−0.157**	−0.159**
Selfblame	−0.144	−0.123	−0.205**	−0.276**	−0.253**	−0.319**	−0.429**	−0.269**	−0.476**	−0.279**	−0.199**	−0.171**
Substance Abuse	−0.206*	0.048	−0.177**	−0.152	−0.168*	−0.158**	−0.215*	−0.178**	−0.337**	−0.115*	−0.182**	−0.203**

Notes. **Correlation is significant at 0.01 level, *Correlation is significant at 0.05 level. Control variables: Gender, age, marital status, education, main activity, professional status

Correlations Between Coping Styles and Perceived Stress 2020-2021
According to Lazarus' (1990, 1993) stress theory, the availability of coping resources might affect the secondary appraisal of the stressful situation. Emotion- and problem focused coping styles might have a favorable effect in reducing the level of distress, while dysfunctional coping strategies would have a detrimental effect in exacerbating the level of stress even more. Over almost all investigated samples, the strongest positive associations with perceived stress emerged with dysfunctional reactions, especially with disengagement, self-blame, and in some countries, also substance abuse, denial, and venting (see Table 9.7). Furthermore, whereas the emotion-focused coping styles of acceptance and positive reframing displayed moderate associations with perceived stress in most countries, problem-focused coping activities were only slightly or not at all associated with stress.

Social support (emotional and instrumental) and religiosity showed almost no association with perceived stress. Religious coping was significantly related to lower levels of perceived stress only in South Africa. In Portugal and Spain, emotional and instrumental support were even associated with higher levels of perceived stress, which could simply mean that people with higher levels of stress reached out to obtain more social support. Similarly, in some countries (e.g., Spain), self-direction was associated with higher levels of stress. A noteworthy case is that of Nigeria, where emotion- and problem-focused coping styles did not correspond with a reduction of stress in 2020 and even showed positive correlation with stress in 2021. Nigerian people with higher levels of stress used different coping styles, but these attitudes and activities apparently did not help in appraising the stressor more positively and in reducing the level of stress.

Correlations Between Coping Styles and Well-being 2020-2021
Beyond the question of whether the awareness regarding the availability of different coping styles can reduce the levels of stress, a further enquiry concerns the association of coping styles with the general level of well-being (see Table 9.8). It is worth mentioning, that the correlation coefficients between perceived hope and well-being yielded moderate to high values of between $r = 0.40$ and $r = 0.60$ ($p < 0.001$). Similarly to hope, well-being correlated most strongly with positive reframing, active coping, acceptance, and planning, but in some countries also with emotional and instrumental support and religious coping. Again, self-blame and disengagement showed the most negative associations with well-being. The strongest association between emotional and instrumental support and well-being could be found in samples from Poland, South Africa, India, Italy, and Czechia. Correlation coefficients in samples from Australia, Spain, Switzerland, Nigeria, Portugal, and France were less pronounced. The association of religious coping with well-being was especially strong in South Africa, Portugal, Poland, India, France, and Nigeria and the lowest in Spain, Czechia, Italy, and Switzerland. Humor and self-direction only displayed low or no association with well-being. One interesting result was that even though instrumental support had little association with perceived hope and stress, it was positively associated with well-being in Czechia, France, India, Italy, Poland, Portugal, and South Africa.

Table 9.7 Partial Bivariate Pearson Correlations of Coping Styles with Well-being 2020–2021

	Australia		Czech Republic.		France		India		Italy	
Years	2020	2021	2020	2021	2020	2021	2020	2021	2020	2021
Acceptance	0.245**	0.134	0.105	0.132**	0.389**	0.235**	0.186**	0.241**	0.262**	0.186*
Positive Reframing	0.252**	0.400**	0.355**	0.352**	0.486**	0.378**	0.329**	0.293**	0.358**	0.262**
Emotional Support	0.134	0.184*	0.248**	0.264**	0.143*	0.171**	0.291**	0.279**	0.276**	0.242**
Religion	0.106	0.257**	0.166**	0.092*	0.252**	0.219**	0.225**	0.221**	0.159**	0.128
Humor	0.165*	0.168	0.019	0.104*	0.213**	0.263**	0.051	0.043	0.090	0.127
Active Coping	0.275**	0.452**	0.261**	0.281**	0.428**	0.249**	0.311**	0.322**	0.329**	0.277**
Self-direction	0.071	−0.103	−0.041	−0.010	0.065	0.107*	0.159**	0.130**	−0.030	−0.023
Planning	0.082	0.180*	0.146*	0.155**	0.427**	0.271**	0.157*	0.274**	0.343**	0.283**
Instrumental Support	0.034	0.211*	0.283**	0.189**	0.209**	0.202**	0.273**	0.282**	0.264**	0.210**
Denial	−0.030	0.079	−0.080	−0.109*	−0.090	−0.037	0.048	0.034	−0.087	−0.061
Venting	−0.120	−0.063	0.060	0.035	0.166*	0.274**	0.057	0.022	0.157**	0.113
Disengagement	−0.185**	−0.344**	−0.237**	−0.154**	−0.199**	−0.197**	−0.056	−0.171**	−0.119*	−0.168*
Selfblame	−0.298**	−0.419**	−0.256**	−0.182**	−0.293**	−0.242**	−0.210**	−0.220**	−0.184**	−0.185*
Substance Abuse	−0.136	−0.242**	−0.112	−0.114*	−0.119	−0.180**	0.036	0.060	−0.163**	−0.201**

	Nigeria		Poland		Portugal		South Africa		Spain		Switzerland	
Years	2020	2021	2020	2021	2020	2021	2020	2021	2020	2021	2020	2021
Acceptance	0.032	0.012	0.277**	0.181*	0.453**	0.238**	0.358**	0.251**	0.126	0.317**	0.269**	0.229**
Positive Reframing	0.291**	0.243**	0.355**	0.514**	0.374**	0.444**	0.427**	0.379**	0.153	0.414**	0.404**	0.397**
Emotional Support	0.116	0.181*	0.303**	0.381**	0.092	0.055	0.212*	0.320**	−0.165	0.113*	0.131**	0.177**
Religion	0.210*	0.169*	0.195**	0.216**	0.246**	0.257**	0.339**	0.328**	0.103	0.076	0.132**	0.133**
Humor	0.001	0.104	0.210**	0.137	0.094	0.170**	0.016	0.103*	−0.051	0.087	0.191**	0.210**
Active Coping	0.195*	0.048	0.286**	0.308**	0.285**	0.273**	0.376**	0.367**	0.218*	0.250**	0.251**	0.258**
Self-direction	0.127	0.006	−0.004	−0.137	0.112	0.123**	−0.190*	0.007	−0.009	0.035	0.096**	0.087**
Planning	0.101	−0.006	0.344**	0.422**	0.377**	0.314**	0.145	0.196**	0.155	0.311**	0.200**	0.181**
Instrumental Support	0.093	0.204*	0.229**	0.300**	0.196*	0.097*	0.159	0.244**	−0.166	0.100	0.068**	0.103**
Denial	0.070	0.006	−0.142*	−0.113	−0.047	−0.046	0.023	0.030	−0.067	−0.072	−0.114**	−0.088**
Venting	−0.176*	−0.013	0.010	−0.046	0.031	0.090*	−0.162	−0.067	−0.113	−0.004	−0.028*	0.018
Disengagement	−0.238**	−0.003	−0.321**	−0.445**	−0.150	−0.252**	−0.308**	−0.257**	−0.212*	−0.090	−0.188**	−0.184**
Selfblame	−0.404**	−0.275**	−0.164*	−0.206*	−0.164*	−0.352**	−0.399**	−0.319**	−0.514**	−0.220**	−0.205**	−0.183**
Substance Abuse	−0.125	−0.021	−0.112	−0.092	−0.185*	−0.193**	−0.168	−0.164**	−0.364**	−0.070	−0.198**	−0.213**

Notes. **Correlation is significant at 0.01 level, *Correlation is significant at 0.05 level. Control variables: Gender, age, marital status, education, main activity, professional status

Table 9.8 Partial Bivariate Pearson Correlations of Coping Styles with Perceived Stress 2020–2021

	Australia		Czech Republic		France		India		Italy	
Years	2020	2021	2020	2021	2020	2021	2020	2021	2020	2021
Acceptance	-0.172^{*}	-0.012	-0.185^{**}	-0.190^{**}	-0.320^{**}	-0.230^{**}	0.079	-0.046	-0.315^{**}	-0.341^{**}
Positive Reframing	-0.083	-0.226^{**}	-0.288^{**}	-0.296^{**}	-0.403^{**}	-0.225^{**}	-0.176^{**}	-0.145^{**}	-0.312^{**}	-0.251^{**}
Emotional Support	0.175^{*}	0.106	0.017	-0.053	0.073	0.057	0.012	-0.010	-0.110^{*}	0.028
Religion	0.020	-0.031	-0.086	0.070	-0.154^{*}	-0.063	-0.053	-0.023	0.005	0.027
Humor	-0.064	-0.141	-0.001	-0.124^{**}	-0.219^{**}	-0.184^{**}	0.100	0.084	-0.026	-0.139
Active Coping	-0.074	-0.335^{**}	-0.055	-0.093^{*}	-0.254^{**}	-0.100^{*}	-0.081	-0.188^{**}	-0.252^{**}	-0.164^{*}
Self-direction	0.091	0.239^{**}	0.196^{**}	0.115^{*}	0.080	-0.020	0.059	0.228^{**}	0.097	0.175^{*}
Planning	0.121	-0.039	0.115	0.023	-0.228^{**}	-0.104^{*}	0.042	-0.071	-0.253^{**}	-0.204^{**}
Instrumental Support	0.272^{**}	0.161	0.000	0.038	0.036	0.024	-0.090	0.036	-0.037	0.082
Denial	0.173^{*}	0.123	0.242^{**}	0.312^{**}	0.177^{**}	0.160^{**}	0.073	0.196^{**}	0.155^{**}	0.247^{**}
Venting	0.402^{**}	0.260^{**}	0.192^{**}	0.127^{**}	-0.029	-0.098^{*}	0.199^{**}	0.232^{**}	0.060	0.176^{*}
Disengagement	0.285^{**}	0.485^{**}	0.201^{**}	0.293^{**}	0.290^{**}	0.224^{**}	0.226^{**}	0.281^{**}	0.253^{**}	0.280^{**}
Selfblame	0.380^{**}	0.490^{**}	0.358^{**}	0.343^{**}	0.368^{**}	0.331^{**}	0.341^{**}	0.408^{**}	0.287^{**}	0.368^{**}
Substance Abuse	0.219^{**}	0.351^{**}	0.217^{**}	0.209^{**}	0.288^{**}	0.241^{**}	-0.011	0.125^{**}	0.167^{**}	0.211^{**}

	Nigeria		Poland		Portugal		South Africa		Spain		Switzerland	
Years	2020	2021	2020	2021	2020	2021	2020	2021	2020	2021	2020	2021
Acceptance	0.045	0.187^{*}	-0.334^{**}	-0.271^{**}	-0.251^{**}	-0.192^{**}	-0.235^{**}	-0.200^{**}	0.015	-0.305^{**}	-0.338^{**}	-0.297^{**}
Positive Reframing	-0.199^{*}	0.166^{*}	-0.249^{**}	-0.368^{**}	-0.255^{**}	-0.320^{**}	-0.193^{*}	-0.273^{**}	−0.022	-0.201^{**}	-0.357^{**}	-0.325^{**}
Emotional Support	0.057	0.061	−0.007	-0.271^{**}	0.186^{*}	0.189^{**}	0.091	-0.132^{**}	0.274^{**}	0.182^{**}	0.142^{**}	0.100^{**}
Religion	−0.077	0.092	−0.074	−0.112	0.002	−0.042	-0.200^{*}	-0.169^{**}	−0.157	0.049	0.018	0.048^{**}
Humor	0.021	0.028	−0.030	−0.052	0.045	−0.067	−0.029	0.040	−0.001	−0.075	-0.181^{**}	-0.223^{**}
Active Coping	−0.091	0.209^{*}	−0.040	-0.224^{**}	−0.012	−0.085	−0.084	-0.236^{**}	0.023	−0.092	-0.092^{**}	-0.073^{**}
Self-direction	0.105	0.433^{**}	0.217^{**}	0.068	0.099	0.012	0.143	0.218^{**}	0.238^{*}	0.245^{**}	0.098^{**}	0.111^{**}
Planning	0.068	0.234^{*}	-0.221^{**}	-0.332^{**}	−0.087	-0.101^{*}	0.245^{**}	−0.080	−0.036	-0.126^{*}	−0.004	0.058^{**}
Instrumental Support	0.089	0.007	−0.045	-0.180^{*}	0.116	0.175^{**}	0.241^{**}	−0.029	0.252^{**}	0.218^{**}	0.153^{**}	0.121^{**}
Denial	0.056	0.174	0.268^{**}	0.165	0.291^{**}	0.170^{**}	0.209^{*}	0.164^{**}	0.184	0.254^{**}	0.281^{**}	0.261^{**}
Venting	0.264^{**}	0.321^{**}	0.295^{**}	0.142	0.242^{**}	0.147^{**}	0.365^{**}	0.229^{**}	0.343^{**}	0.130^{*}	0.186^{**}	0.189^{**}
Disengagement	0.225^{**}	0.261^{**}	0.445^{**}	0.460^{**}	0.215^{**}	0.350^{**}	0.377^{**}	0.385^{**}	0.279^{**}	0.257^{**}	0.232^{**}	0.221^{**}
Selfblame	0.416^{**}	0.325^{**}	0.292^{**}	0.303^{**}	0.405^{**}	0.452^{**}	0.534^{**}	0.449^{**}	0.521^{**}	0.455^{**}	0.312^{**}	0.288^{**}
Substance Abuse	0.146	0.111	0.172^{**}	0.001	0.293^{**}	0.259^{**}	0.335^{**}	0.321^{**}	0.099	0.155^{**}	0.278^{**}	0.262^{**}

Notes. **Correlation is significant at 0.01 level, *Correlation is significant at 0.05 level. Control variables: Gender, age, marital status, education, main activity, professional status

9.3.6.5 Posttraumatic Growth 2021

One of the objectives of the current study was to investigate possible fields of personal growth as a positive consequence of having dealt successfully with the pandemic crisis. Table 9.9 presents the mean values and standard deviations of the five areas of posttraumatic growth at the end of 2021 per country. In almost all samples, the most pronounced growth was reported in the areas of appreciation of life and personal strength and the least in the field of spiritual change (with exception of Nigeria).

Comparing the countries with each other yielded interesting results. Whereas participants in Nigeria, South Africa, Portugal, and in some areas, also India, registered the highest scores in almost all categories (above the center of the scale $M = 2.5$), participants in Switzerland and Poland achieved the lowest results (below $M = 2.5$). Spiritual change was especially pronounced in Nigeria, South Africa, and (to a lesser extent) Portugal and extremely low in Poland, Switzerland, France, Czechia, and Spain, with India, Australia, and Italy in between. People in Nigeria, South Africa, Portugal, and India reported significantly greater growth in the domain of interpersonal relationships than participants in Switzerland, Poland, France, and Czechia. Moreover, people in Nigeria, South Africa, Portugal, and Australia more often experienced the appearance of new possibilities than people in Switzerland, Poland, Czechia, and France.

9.3.6.6 Correlations between Coping Styles and Posttraumatic Growth

In this section we examine which coping styles displayed a significant correlation with the level of personal growth in the five domains and whether there are certain common and some country specific findings worth to be highlighted (see Appendix 9.2). Generally, positive reframing and active coping were the two coping strategies exhibiting significant correlation coefficients with nearly all growth domains in almost all countries. This was followed by social support (emotional and instrumental) and planning. Acceptance, humor, self-direction, and the dysfunctional coping activities were the least associated with personal growth.

Religious coping showed a positive relationship with many domains of personal growth, especially in Australia, Italy, Nigeria, Portugal, South Africa, and to a lesser degree also in Switzerland. In all countries, people who were high in religious coping did also experience high levels of positive spiritual change. Receiving emotional and instrumental support displayed strong positive correlations with most areas of growth in Nigeria and South Africa and in many other countries it was especially related to enhanced interpersonal relationships. Interestingly, in some countries denial and venting displayed significant positive associations with some or even many areas of personal growth (e.g., denial in Australia). This could be interpreted as a sign of relief at the end of 2021 as some countries returned to a certain normality.

Table 9.9 Mean Values and Standard Deviations of Posttraumatic Growth Domains

	Appreciation of Life		Personal Strength		New Possibilities		Relating to others		Spiritual Change	
	M	*SD*	*M*	*SD*	*M*	*SD*	*M*	*SD*	*M*	*SD*
Australia	2.85	1.52	2.66	1.60	2.47	1.61	2.41	1.62	1.62	1.70
Czech Republic	2.55	1.43	2.34	1.43	1.92	1.33	2.00	1.30	1.02	1.32
France	2.49	1.34	2.25	1.38	2.02	1.38	1.84	1.37	0.96	1.24
India	2.50	1.50	2.64	1.57	2.33	1.50	2.62	1.50	1.78	1.51
Italy	2.77	1.34	3.15	1.15	2.26	1.26	2.41	1.38	1.57	1.42
Nigeria	3.33	1.17	3.93	0.91	3.61	1.04	3.50	1.12	3.61	1.32
Poland	1.98	1.54	1.83	1.58	1.58	1.46	1.66	1.57	0.86	1.24
Portugal	2.94	1.35	2.88	1.39	2.65	1.43	2.64	1.41	1.91	1.61
South Africa	3.29	1.43	3.32	1.54	2.95	1.54	2.96	1.57	2.79	1.81
Spain	3.01	1.36	2.67	1.36	2.36	1.31	2.47	1.40	1.08	1.19
Switzerland	2.40	1.47	2.36	1.51	1.64	1.39	1.67	1.43	0.92	1.30
ANOVA										
F	28.17		40.36		75.95		73.74		125.36	
Sig.	$p < 0.001$		$p < 0.001$		$p < 0.001$		$p < 0.001$		$p < 0.001$	
Eta^2	0.040		0.056		0.101		0.098		0.156	

9.3.6.7 Correlations between Posttraumatic Growth and Perceived Hope, Stress, and Well-being

An unresolved issue discussed in the literature is whether posttraumatic growth is associated with lower levels of stress and higher levels of well-being (hedonic or psychological) (Tedeschi & Calhoun, 2004). Our final analysis in this chapter aimed to assess the relationships between the five areas of posttraumatic growth, on the one hand, and perceived hope, stress, and the three domains of hedonic, psychological, and social well-being, on the other, among the 11 samples (see Appendix 9.3). We will report the most general and noteworthy findings.

In most countries, the areas of personal growth were positively related to perceived hope, hedonic, psychological, and social well-being but slightly or moderately negatively correlated with perceived stress. This means that, at least in our samples, until the end of 2021, people with higher levels of stress experienced lower degrees of personal growth. Another noteworthy finding was that in many countries, appreciation of life was only slightly, or not at all, associated with hope and well-being. Spiritual change and changes in interpersonal relationships were mainly positively associated with hope and social well-being. In South Africa, spiritual change was moderately correlated not only with perceived hope and social well-being, but also with psychological and hedonic well-being. The Indian sample displayed the lowest correlation coefficients and in the Italian sample personal strengths were strongly related to hope and well-being.

9.4 Findings and Discussion

Many psychological studies between 2020 and 2021 focused on studying the negative effects of the worldwide COVID-19 pandemic crisis on mental health, with special emphasis on the perceived levels of distress, uncertainty, fear, anxiety, and depression. Furthermore, several studies have shown the importance of cultural characteristics in the perception of stress and the coping styles chosen to deal with it. From a positive psychological standpoint, the aim of the Hope Barometer survey of 2020 and 2021 was to investigate the levels of perceived stress in relation to a hopeful attitude towards the future as reported by people in 11 countries. Hope has been characterized as a positive emotion that helps people to cope with stressful situations, enhancing well-being and fostering personal growth.

This section commences with the presentation of the general findings of our study with regard to common patterns about the levels of perceived hope, stress, well-being, coping styles and personal growth, and the associations between them. Afterwards we analyze the sample specific results in order to find individual patterns that could reveal meaningful differences between countries. One main research question was whether people in collectivistic countries experienced and dealt with the pandemic crisis differently than people in more individualistic countries.

9.4.1 General Findings

During 2020 and 2021 most people in our study reported moderate to high levels of hope and at the same time moderate but clearly above the "normal" perceived levels of stress characterized by feelings of unpredictability, uncontrollability, and overload. Moreover, despite the burdens of the crisis, people reported moderate to high levels of well-being, in some countries below the levels of 2019, but in other countries with a loss in 2020 and a clear recovery in 2021. In general, over-all samples, people were able to display positive coping styles such as accepting the new reality by simultaneously adopting a positive stance and actively coping with the challenging situation.

Hope and well-being of the participants in our study were primarily related to the possibility of reframing the negative events in a positive way, to the capacity of accepting and actively coping with everyday challenges, but also to finding relief and comfort in religious faith and practices. In some countries, levels of well-being were positively related to the availability of social support. To the contrary, disengaging from any effort to positively deal with the current situation and blaming oneself were the reactions most negatively related with hope and well-being.

Higher levels of perceived stress were primarily related to dysfunctional coping styles such as disengagement, self-blame, and denial. Acceptance and positive reframing showed a much stronger association with lower levels of perceived stress than the problem-focused styles, revealing the importance of emotion-focused coping styles. However, social support and religious coping, were either weakly or even not significantly related to lower levels of perceived stress, although showing significant positive associations with perceived hope and well-being.

Most of the participants in our samples reported moderate levels of posttraumatic growth, especially with regard to the appreciation of life and the awareness of personal strengths, but much less in relation to the spiritual dimension. Personal growth correlated positively with positive reframing and active coping and also with social support. In some countries, personal growth was also related to religious coping. Furthermore, personal growth was positively associated with perceived hope and well-being, but not or only marginally with a reduction of perceived stress. Positive changes in spiritual awareness and relating to others were significantly associated with higher levels of perceived hope and social well-being. Besides these outcomes, we did not find any further clear pattern regarding the association of personal growth and the individual dimensions of hedonic, psychological, and social well-being.

To summarize, the results of our study confirm the findings of other authors and reveal new aspects that have not been investigated before. The COVID-19 pandemic intensified the level of stress as already reported in other studies (e.g., Alshehri et al., 2020; Bridgland et al., 2021; Horn et al., 2020; Maia & Dias, 2020) affecting the mental health of the population. However, most people could remain hopeful and face the threats and challenges in a positive way. In line with previous research and our own assumptions, emotion-focused coping styles such as acceptance and

Table 9.10 Relative Levels of Hope, Well-being, and Stress across Countries

	Hope	Well-being	Stress
Higher	Nigeria, Australia, South Africa, India, Portugal	Nigeria, Australia, South Africa, India, Portugal	Spain, Portugal, India, Czechia
Moderate	Czechia, Italy	Italy, France, Spain	South Africa, Italy, France
Lower	Spain, Poland, France, Switzerland	Poland, Czechia, Switzerland	Nigeria, Australia, Poland, Switzerland
Increase 2020-21	Italy, Portugal		Switzerland, Australia, France
Decrease 2020-21	France, India, Czechia	Australia, Czechia, France, Poland, Spain and Switzerland	Spain, Portugal, Czechia, India

positive reframing and religious faith were especially important in order to remain hopeful and preserve well-being (see also Agha, 2021; Guszkowska & Dąbrowska-Zimakowska, 2022; Kar et al., 2021; Rogowska et al., 2021). Supporting the results of Ahuja (2021) and Szkody et al. (2021), the value of social support and religious coping seems to be less related to reducing the levels of stress as to fostering the feelings of hope and well-being. Furthermore, personal growth occurred across the samples of our study, and was especially related to hope and well-being but not with a reduction of perceived stress. However, our findings could not confirm that posttraumatic growth would be associated with an increase in psychological well-being as opposed to subjective well-being, proposed by claims of Joseph and Linley (2005).

9.4.2 *Country Specific Findings*

Beyond these general findings, some noteworthy results specific to individual countries emerged from our study, confirming the importance of cultural values and norms with regard to the perception of stress and hope and the choice of particular coping styles.

An overview of the levels of hope, well-being, and perceived stress across countries are presented in Table 9.10. The first remarkable results are that participants in Nigeria, Australia, South Africa, India, and Portugal reported the highest levels of hope and well-being. On the other hand, people in Spain, Poland, France, and Switzerland displayed the lowest hope scores and samples from in Poland and Czechia the lowest levels of well-being. Furthermore, people in Australia, Czechia, France, Poland, Spain, and Switzerland experienced a clear decline in well-being during 2020-2021. With regard to the perceived burdens of the pandemic, people in Spain, Portugal, India, and Czechia experienced high levels of stress, while those from Nigeria, Australia and Switzerland reported lower levels of stress. However, whereas in Switzerland, Australia and France levels of stress increased from 2020 to 2021, in Spain, Portugal, Czech, and India, it decreased.

Portugal and Switzerland are two exemplary cases showing opposite characteristics. Compared to the other countries, participants in Portugal demonstrated high levels of hope and well-being but also experienced high levels of stress. Interestingly, levels of hope increased during this period and the level of stress decreased. On the other hand, people in Switzerland perceived relatively lower levels of stress but also reported lower levels of hope and well-being. Additionally, levels of stress increased and well-being declined.

Theoretically, we assumed that people in countries with higher levels of hope will display lower levels of distress and higher levels of well-being. This assumption was only partly supported. Participants in Australia and Nigeria reported higher levels of hope and well-being and lower levels of distress. However, those in Portugal and India reported higher levels of hope and well-being but also higher levels of stress. This suggests that people can remain hopeful despite higher levels of stress, but also that lower levels of stress do not always result in higher levels of hope and well-being.

We then examined possible differences in coping styles preferred by participants from different countries. Beyond the common patterns presented in the previous section, noteworthy differences appeared regarding social support, religious coping, and some individual trends also emerged. People in Poland, South Africa, India, and to a lesser extent also in Czechia and Spain, reported higher levels of emotional and instrumental support and people in Nigeria only instrumental support. Similarly, the association of social support and hope and well-being was the highest in the South African, Polish, Czech, and Indian samples. On the other hand, levels of social support and also the association of social support with well-being were the lowest in Australia, Switzerland, France, and Spain. Interestingly, in 2021 people in Czechia and Switzerland reported lower levels of social support and also declining levels of positive reframing (as in Australia, Poland, and Spain), and a rise in disengagement (as in Australia, France, and Italy).

Higher levels of religious coping were expressed by participants from Nigeria, South Africa, India, and Portugal and lower levels by those from Spain, Switzerland, Poland, and France. Furthermore, religious coping showed stronger correlations with hope and well-being in South Africa, Nigeria, Portugal, Poland, and India. In South Africa, higher levels of religious coping were even significantly associated with lower levels of perceived stress. In Spain, Czechia, and Switzerland, the correlation coefficients between religious coping and hope and well-being were the lowest. Thus, our theoretical assumption that people from more collectivistic countries would demonstrate higher levels of social support and religious coping, as proposed by authors such as Chun et al. (2006) and Hu et al. (2018), was largely confirmed, especially regarding to the importance of religious coping. However, social support and religious coping were barely associated with lower levels of stress. To the contrary, in Spain, Portugal, and Nigeria, higher levels of social support were associated with higher levels of stress.

Finally, we assessed the differences in the levels of posttraumatic growth between the 11 investigated samples as a secondary effect of successfully dealing with the pandemic. Because of its strong emotional basis, we expected that posttraumatic growth would be more pronounced in collectivistic countries, compared to individualistic countries. This assumption was largely confirmed. Participants from Nigeria, South Africa, Portugal, and India reported significantly higher levels of personal growth, especially in the social and spiritual domains, than those from Switzerland, Poland, France, and Czechia. Moreover, people in Nigeria, South Africa and Portugal scored much higher in the specific domain of the appearance of new possibilities than people in Switzerland, Poland, Czechia, and France. Remarkably, in the Nigerian and South African samples, all posttraumatic growth domains were positively associated with social and religious coping styles, supporting our assumption.

To summarize, levels of hope and well-being during 2020-2021 were moderate to high despite the moderately high levels of distress, especially among people in more collectivistic countries such as Nigeria, South Africa, India, and Portugal, but also in the largely individualistic Australia. People in the collectivistic countries of Nigeria, South Africa, India, and Portugal exposed much more emotional coping strategies such as religious coping and social support than people in individualistic countries such as Australia, Switzerland, France, Spain, and Czechia. Furthermore, in most of the collectivistic countries, social support and religious coping presented stronger positive correlations with hope and well-being than the samples from the individualistic countries. Moreover, people in Nigeria, South Africa, Portugal, and India reported the highest levels of personal growth, especially in the social and religious dimension. In Nigeria and South Africa, higher levels of social support and religious coping corresponded with higher levels in almost all dimensions of personal growth.

9.5 Limitations

Due to the cross-sectional design of our study and the convenient collection of data from people active in online platforms and social media, a number of limitations need to be addressed. First of all, our samples are not representative of the demographic structure of the investigated countries and show significant differences in the number and the demographic characteristics of their participants. Moreover, the online survey makes the participation of socio-economic groups with limited or no internet access, especially in economically less developed regions, difficult or even impossible. Therefore, the comparison of results from one year to the other must be interpreted with care, since the effects could be attributed, at least in part, to differences in the composition of the samples. Furthermore, we are not able to infer causal relationships and assume that the diverse variables are reciprocally interrelated. For example, questions of whether hopeful people were able to cope with stress more effectively, or whether the level of hope was a consequence of successfully coping with stress must be answered using a longitudinal study design.

We are moreover aware that the point of time to assess the long-term effects of the pandemic in terms of PTG may be too early, that the positive effects reported by people could be to a certain extent of illusory nature and that the self-report measures along with the cross-sectional design of our study could be important limitations that have to be taken into account when interpreting the results. We know and understand the concerns addressed by authors that consider self-report measures of personal growth to be, to a certain extent, misleading (Boals & Schuler, 2018; Jayawickreme & Blackie, 2014; Maercker & Zoellner, 2004; Nolen-Hoeksema & Davis, 2004). On the one hand we used a scale which only assesses positive changes, and on the other hand people tend to answer growth questions tinted by their own desires and illusions.

9.6 Conclusions

Our study during 2020 and 2021 was centered on the question of how people in different countries perceived and dealt with the COVID-19 pandemic crisis. The focus was not to investigate the negative effects of the crisis, such as anxiety and depression, but on positive coping strategies, hope for the future, well-being, and personal growth. Besides the stress and burdens to physical and mental health resulting from the pandemic, our study demonstrates that most people around the world were able to remain hopeful, to positively cope with the emerging challenges and that they furthermore experienced personal growth in some areas. Particularly, people from more collectivistic countries have benefited from social support and religious coping strategies, also showing higher levels of hope, well-being, and personal growth, despite experiencing higher levels of stress in some cases.

Our findings contribute to support the argument that in every crisis there are as many opportunities as threats, and that we can face such crises either with anxiety or hope. The question is not whether the crisis is good or bad. What is important is our personal attitude towards what is happening and the way we behave in the face of it. We always have a choice: we can make a difficult situation even worse by adopting a negative attitude, or we can look the unpleasant facts in the eyes and let something good come out of them. It depends on the individual to see the situation from a new perspective and, within the scope of one's own possibilities, to change something for the better. Crises can be understood as life tests that can trigger positive turns and lead to personal growth.

However, this does not mean that we always have to master life crises alone and by our own efforts. Events often take us to the limits of our own possibilities and capabilities. They teach us to turn to other people and even to a transcendent Higher Power, to trust them, and to accept help from them. This is the great power of hope. By being aware of the problems and difficulties of our times and accepting them as a challenge, we can believe in a good future. Simultaneously, we can have trust that due to our own personal strengths, in conjunction with other people, we will be able to solve the problems and overcome the difficulties so that our most ardent wishes and desires can be fulfilled. The current study has shown that people all over the world are capable of doing so.

Appendices

Appendix 9.1

Appendix 9.1.1: Demographic Structure of the Samples 2019

Number of participants, mean age and standard deviation and GDP per capita

	Australia	Czechia	France	India	Italy	Nigeria	Poland	Portugal	South Africa	Spain	Switzerland
N	474	469	94	1092	272	665	481	507	574	529	3935
%	5.2%	5.2%	1.0%	12.0%	3.0%	7.3%	5.3%	5.6%	6.3%	5.8%	43.3%
M_{age}	47.53	32.75	28.22	31.15	41.86	32.26	31.58	36.45	39.27	35.19	15.22
SD_{age}	13.05	15.54	13.61	12.60	13.78	8.47	10.82	14.74	14.85	46.82	15.67

Gender

		Australia	Czechia	France	India	Italy	Nigeria	Poland	Portugal	South Africa	Spain	Switzerland
Male	n	232	132	15	529	75	434	140	124	*252*	116	1797
	%	48.9%	28.1%	15.0%	48.4%	27.6%	65.3%	29.1%	24.5%	*43.9%*	21.9%	45.7%
Female	n	242	337	79	563	197	231	341	383	*322*	413	2138
	%	51.1%	71.9%	84.0%	51.6%	72.4%	34.7%	70.9%	75.5%	*56.1%*	78.1%	54.3%

Marital Status

		Australia	Czechia	France	India	Italy	Nigeria	Poland	Portugal	South Africa	Spain	Switzerland
Still living with my parents	n	20	136	37	469	45	112	85	142	106	206	231
	%	4.2%	29.0%	39.4%	42.9%	16.5%	16.8%	17.7%	28.0%	18.5%	38.9%	5.9%
Single, unmarried	n	41	67	21	140	36	295	71	84	82	67	589

(continued)

		Australia	Czechia	France	India	Italy	Nigeria	Poland	Portugal	South Africa	Spain	Switzerland
	%	8.6%	14.3%	22.3%	12.8%	13.2%	44.4%	14.8%	16.6%	14.3%	12.7%	15.0%
Living in a partnership but in separate households	n	16	44	9	9	33	11	43	17	14	26	314
	%	3.4%	9.4%	9.6%	0.8%	12.1%	1.7%	8.9%	3.4%	2.4%	4.9%	8.0%
Living together in a partnership	n	54	70	8	18	60	4	101	65	92	58	719
	%	11.4%	14.9%	8.5%	1.6%	22.1%	0.6%	21.0%	12.8%	16.0%	11.0%	18.3%
Married	n	298	117	16	428	79	228	166	150	224	150	1531
	%	62.9%	24.9%	17.0%	39.2%	29.0%	34.3%	34.5%	29.6%	39.0%	28.4%	38.9%
Divorced / separated	n	42	27	3	16	16	11	14	46	43	21	459
	%	8.9%	5.8%	3.2%	1.5%	5.9%	1.7%	2.9%	9.1%	7.5%	4.0%	11.7%
Widowed	n	3	8	0	12	3	4	1	3	13	1	92
	%	0.6%	1.7%	0.0%	1.1%	1.1%	0.6%	0.2%	0.6%	2.3%	0.2%	2.3%

Education

		Australia	Czechia	France	India	Italia	Nigeria	Poland	Portugal	South Africa	Spain	Switzerland
Did not finish school	n	4	0	18	4	0	1	0	0	6	12	41
	%	0.8%	0.0%	19.1%	0.4%	0.0%	0.2%	0.0%	0.0%	1.0%	1.1%	1.0%
Primary school	n	0	16	1	36	18	0	4	1	4	61	190
	%	0.0%	3.4%	1.1%	3.3%	6.6%	0.0%	0.8%	0.2%	0.7%	5.9%	4.8%
Secondary school	n	54	287	6	214	54	23	185	147	211	361	1111
	%	11.4%	61.2%	6.4%	19.6%	19.9%	3.5%	38.5%	29.0%	32.1%	34.5%	28.2%
Professional training/Diploma	n	126	0	5	526	69	22	64	226	140	271	2146
	%	40.0%	0.0%	5.3%	48.2%	52.7%	3.3%	13.3%	44.6%	24.4%	25.9%	54.5%
University	n	131	166	64	312	131	619	228	124	212	349	447
	%	41.6%	35.4%	68.1%	28.6%	48.2%	93.1%	47.4%	24.5%	37.1%	66.0%	11.4%

Main activity

		Australia	Czechia	France	India	Italy	Nigeria	Poland	Portugal	South Africa	Spain	Switzerland
In education or training (student)	n	23	236	62	504	62	171	144	171	83	216	197
	%	4.9%	50.3%	66.0%	46.2%	22.8%	25.7%	29.9%	33.7%	14.5%	40.8%	5.0%
Household/raising children	n	16	15	2	118	13	7	18	2	16	12	181
	%	3.4%	3.2%	2.1%	10.8%	4.8%	1.1%	3.7%	0.4%	2.8%	2.3%	4.6%
Part-time job	n	77	33	5	57	41	102	33	45	73	62	830
	%	16.2%	7.0%	5.3%	5.2%	15.1%	15.3%	6.9%	8.9%	12.7%	11.7%	21.1%
Fulltime job	n	312	155	21	352	126	276	269	260	293	202	1777
	%	65.8%	33.0%	22.3%	32.2%	46.3%	41.5%	55.9%	51.3%	51.0%	38.2%	45.2%
Unemployed	n	22	0	2	46	16	103	7	17	68	13	212
	%	4.6%	0.0%	2.1%	4.2%	5.9%	15.5%	1.5%	3.4%	11.8%	2.5%	5.4%
Retired	n	24	30	2	15	14	6	10	12	41	24	738
	%	5.1%	6.4%	2.1%	1.4%	5.1%	0.9%	2.1%	2.4%	7.1%	4.5%	18.8%

Professional status

		Australia	Czechia	France	India	Italy	Nigeria	Poland	Portugal	South Africa	Spain	Switzerland
No position in an organization (e.g., at school, housekeeping, unemployed, retired)	n	47	154	24	224	69	101	32	111	127	136	657
	%	9.9%	32.8%	25.5%	20.5%	25.4%	15.2%	6.7%	21.9%	22.1%	25.7%	16.7%
In education / training	n	23	91	43	499	34	159	147	68	90	98	168
	%	4.9%	19.4%	45.7%	45.7%	12.5%	23.9%	30.6%	13.4%	15.7%	18.5%	4.3%
Employee	n	150	155	12	242	55	162	195	199	138	196	1705
	%	31.6%	33.0%	12.8%	22.2%	20.2%	24.4%	40.5%	39.3%	24.0%	37.1%	43.3%
Junior / Middle management	n	64	32	0	70	16	79	49	71	102	42	729

(continued)

		Australia	Czechia	France	India	Italy	Nigeria	Poland	Portugal	South Africa	Spain	Switzerland
	%	13.5%	6.8%	0.0%	6.4%	5.9%	11.9%	10.2%	14.0%	17.8%	7.9%	18.5%
Senior management / Board of directors	n	49	6	8	18	21	47	9	22	37	37	275
	%	10.3%	1.3%	8.5%	1.6%	7.7%	7.1%	1.9%	4.3%	6.4%	7.0%	7.0%
Entrepreneur / Business owner	n	141	31	7	39	77	117	49	36	80	20	401
	%	29.7%	6.6%	7.4%	3.6%	28.3%	17.6%	10.2%	7.1%	13.9%	3.8%	10.2%

Religion

		Australia	Czechia	France	India	Italy	Nigeria	Poland	Portugal	South Africa	Spain	Switzerland
Catholic	n	80	101	33	224	130	326	308	244	41	288	1100
	%	16.9%	21.5%	35.1%	20.5%	47.8%	49.0%	64.0%	48.1%	7.1%	54.4%	28.0%
Protestant	n	43	11	2	14	0	131	4	10	69	2	796
	%	9.1%	2.3%	2.1%	1.3%	0.0%	19.7%	0.8%	2.0%	12.0%	0.4%	20.2%
Another Christian church or community	n	66	26	0	25	2	155	11	5	265	1	138
	%	13.9%	5.5%	0.0%	2.3%	0.7%	23.3%	2.3%	1.0%	46.2%	0.2%	3.5%
Muslim	n	5	0	1	215	1	14	0	2	16	2	71
	%	1.1%	0.0%	1.1%	19.7%	0.4%	2.1%	0.0%	0.4%	2.8%	0.4%	1.8%
Jewish	n	17	1	3	0	1	0	0	0	5	0	11
	%	3.6%	0.2%	3.2%	0.0%	0.4%	0.0%	0.0%	0.0%	0.9%	0.0%	0.3%
Hindu	n	14	0	0	533	1	0	0	0	8	0	1
	%	3.0%	0.0%	0.0%	48.8%	0.4%	0.0%	0.0%	0.0%	1.4%	0.0%	0.0%
Buddhist	n	9	5	1	0	9	0	2	3	1	0	27
	%	1.9%	1.1%	1.1%	0.0%	3.3%	0.0%	0.4%	0.6%	0.2%	0.0%	0.7%
	n	95	156	15	37	32	28	50	96	92	35	340

(continued)

		Australia	Czechia	France	India	Italy	Nigeria	Poland	Portugal	South Africa	Spain	Switzerland
I am a spiritual person outside the traditional world religions	%	20.0%	33.3%	16.0%	3.4%	11.8%	4.2%	10.4%	18.9%	16.0%	6.6%	8.6%
Without religion or confession	n	121	137	38	24	86	4	96	120	48	170	1352
	%	25.5%	29.2%	40.4%	2.2%	31.6%	0.6%	20.0%	23.7%	8.4%	32.1%	34.4%
Something different	n	24	32	1	20	10	7	10	27	29	31	99
	%	5.1%	6.8%	1.1%	1.8%	3.7%	1.1%	2.1%	5.3%	5.1%	5.9%	2.5%

Appendix 9.1.2: Demographic Structure of the Samples 2020

Number of participants, mean age and standard deviation and GDP per capita

	Australia	Czechia	France	India	Italy	Nigeria	Poland	Portugal	South Africa	Spain	Switzerland
N	210	257	235	272	406	149	227	567	133	112	6968
%	2.2%	2.7%	2.5%	2.9%	4.3%	1.6%	2.4%	5.9%	1.4%	1.2%	73.1%
M_{age}	50.24	26.60	44.46	22.63	43.53	31.86	39.45	33.09	44.62	19.96	48.37
SD_{age}	13.23	10.33	13.48	8.87	13.82	7.82	11.61	14.97	16.62	3.51	21.20

Gender

		Australia	Czechia	France	India	Italy	Nigeria	Poland	Portugal	South Africa	Spain	Switzerland
Male	n	125	57	45	163	106	87	50	139	34	16	2636
	%	59.5%	22.2%	19.1%	59.9%	26.1%	58.4%	22.0%	24.5%	25.6%	14.3%	37.8%
Female	n	85	200	190	109	300	62	177	428	99	96	4332
	%	40.5%	77.8%	80.9%	40.1%	73.9%	41.6%	78.0%	75.5%	74.4%	85.7%	62.2%

Marital Status

		Australia	Czechia	France	India	Italy	Nigeria	Poland	Portugal	South Africa	Spain	Switzerland
Still living with my parents	n	8	92	10	214	82	28	21	242	21	100	278
	%	3.8%	35.8%	4.3%	78.7%	20.2%	18.8%	9.3%	42.7%	15.8%	89.3%	4.0%
Single, unmarried	n	28	51	35	26	39	60	20	73	25	7	945
	%	13.3%	19.8%	14.9%	9.6%	9.6%	40.3%	8.8%	12.9%	18.8%	6.3%	13.6%
Living in a partnership but in separate households	n	6	31	21	0	41	3	13	16	4	2	471
	%	2.9%	12.1%	8.9%	0.0%	10.1%	2.0%	5.7%	2.8%	3.0%	1.8%	6.8%
Living together in a partnership	n	26	50	62	2	77	0	32	68	5	2	1358
	%	12.4%	19.5%	26.4%	0.7%	19.0%	0.0%	14.1%	12.0%	3.8%	1.8%	19.5%
Married	n	119	27	68	28	139	57	123	132	71	1	3118
	%	56.7%	10.5%	28.9%	10.3%	34.2%	38.3%	54.2%	23.3%	53.4%	0.9%	44.7%
Divorced / separated	n	20	5	33	0	24	0	16	31	4	0	626
	%	9.5%	1.9%	14.0%	0.0%	5.9%	0.0%	7.0%	5.5%	3.0%	0.0%	9.0%
Widowed	n	3	1	6	2	4	1	2	5	3	0	172
	%	1.4%	0.4%	2.6%	0.7%	1.0%	0.7%	0.9%	0.9%	2.3%	0.0%	2.5%

Education

		Australia	Czechia	France	India	Italia	Nigeria	Poland	Portugal	South Africa	Spain	Switzerland
Did not finish school	n	4	0	2	2	1	1	1	0	0	0	48
	%	1.9%	0.0%	0.9%	0.7%	0.2%	0.7%	0.4%	0.0%	0.0%	0.0%	0.7%
Primary school	n	1	1	1	0	15	0	2	0	0	0	251
	%	0.5%	0.4%	0.4%	0.0%	3.7%	0.0%	0.9%	0.0%	0.0%	0.0%	3.6%
Secondary school	n	12	147	6	95	91	3	37	192	15	51	1819
	%	5.7%	57.2%	2.6%	34.8%	22.2%	2.0%	16.1%	33.7%	11.3%	45.5%	26.1%
Professional training/Diploma	n	38	0	73	8	0	6	20	18	10	6	3885

(continued)

		Australia	Czechia	France	India	Italia	Nigeria	Poland	Portugal	South Africa	Spain	Switzerland
	%	18.1%	0.0%	31.0%	2.9%	0.0%	4.0%	8.7%	3.2%	7.5%	5.4%	55.8%
University	n	155	109	153	168	302	139	170	359	108	55	965
	%	73.8%	42.4%	65.1%	61.5%	73.8%	93.3%	73.9%	63.1%	81.2%	49.1%	13.8%

Main activity

		Australia	Czechia	France	India	Italy	Nigeria	Poland	Portugal	South Africa	Spain	Switzerland
In education or training (student)	n	13	182	28	243	95	44	26	11	30	112	253
	%	6.2%	70.8%	11.9%	89.3%	23.4%	29.5%	11.5%	6.7%	22.6%	100.0%	3.6%
Household/raising children	n	5	5	3	1	12	2	17	1	4	0	355
	%	2.4%	1.9%	1.3%	0.4%	3.0%	1.3%	7.5%	0.6%	3.0%	0.0%	5.1%
Part-time job	n	19	14	44	2	51	16	15	18	12	0	1722
	%	9.1%	5.4%	18.7%	0.7%	12.6%	10.7%	6.6%	10.9%	9.0%	0.0%	24.7%
Fulltime job	n	142	47	130	15	203	57	151	114	72	0	3174
	%	67.9%	18.3%	55.3%	5.5%	50.0%	38.3%	66.5%	69.1%	54.1%	0.0%	45.6%
Unemployed	n	18	6	15	7	26	28	7	7	1	0	306
	%	8.6%	2.3%	6.4%	2.6%	6.4%	18.8%	3.1%	4.2%	0.8%	0.0%	4.4%
Retired	n	12	3	15	4	19	2	11	14	14	0	1158
	%	5.7%	1.2%	6.4%	1.5%	4.7%	1.3%	4.8%	8.5%	10.5%	0.0%	16.6%

Professional status

		Australia	Czechia	France	India	Italy	Nigeria	Poland	Portugal	South Africa	Spain	Switzerland
No position in an organization (e.g. at school, housekeeping, unemployed, retired)	n	26	108	30	68	110	28	22	27	20	44	1182
	%	12.4%	42.0%	12.8%	25.0%	27.1%	18.8%	9.7%	16.4%	15.0%	39.3%	17.0%
In education/training	n	8	69	28	185	57	39	31	11	34	59	266

(continued)

		Australia	Czechia	France	India	Italy	Nigeria	Poland	Portugal	South Africa	Spain	Switzerland
	%	3.8%	26.8%	11.9%	68.0%	14.0%	26.2%	13.7%	6.7%	25.6%	52.7%	3.8%
Employee	n	54	58	49	8	89	36	83	79	28	8	2952
	%	25.8%	22.6%	20.9%	2.9%	21.9%	24.2%	36.6%	47.9%	21.1%	7.1%	42.4%
Junior / Middle management	n	32	9	62	6	18	14	36	22	19	1	1361
	%	15.3%	3.5%	26.4%	2.2%	4.4%	9.4%	15.9%	13.3%	14.3%	0.9%	19.5%
Senior management / Board of directors	n	28	1	33	5	31	7	15	8	13	0	439
	%	13.4%	0.4%	14.0%	1.8%	7.6%	4.7%	6.6%	4.8%	9.8%	0.0%	6.3%
Entrepreneur / Business owner	n	61	12	33	0	101	25	40	18	19	0	768
	%	29.2%	4.7%	14.0%	0.0%	24.9%	16.8%	17.6%	10.9%	14.3%	0.0%	11.0%

Religion

		Australia	Czechia	France	India	Italy	Nigeria	Poland	Portugal	South Africa	Spain	Switzerland
Catholic	n	23	58	74	7	222	82	121	244	1	59	2025
	%	13.3%	22.6%	31.5%	2.6%	54.7%	55.0%	53.3%	43.0%	0.8%	52.7%	29.1%
Protestant	n	21	8	4	6	1	34	3	11	29	0	1373
	%	10.0%	3.1%	1.7%	2.2%	0.2%	22.8%	1.3%	1.9%	21.8%	0.0%	19.7%
Another Christian church or community	n	27	9	0	6	2	25	3	14	42	0	247
	%	12.9%	3.5%	0.0%	2.2%	0.5%	16.8%	1.3%	2.5%	31.6%	0.0%	3.5%
Muslim	n	2	0	4	10	0	1	0	1	2	0	104
	%	1.0%	0.0%	1.7%	3.7%	0.0%	0.7%	0.0%	0.2%	1.5%	0.0%	1.5%
Jewish	n	6	0	1	0	0	0	0	1	2	0	21
	%	2.9%	0.0%	0.4%	0.0%	0.0%	0.0%	0.0%	0.2%	1.5%	0.0%	0.3%

(continued)

		Australia	Czechia	France	India	Italy	Nigeria	Poland	Portugal	South Africa	Spain	Switzerland
Hindu	n	12	0	2	198	0	1	0	0	3	0	9
	%	5.7%	0.0%	0.9%	72.8%	0.0%	0.7%	0.0%	0.0%	2.3%	0.0%	0.1%
Buddhist	n	4	3	0	0	10	0	2	3	3	0	42
	%	1.9%	1.2%	0.0%	0.0%	2.5%	0.0%	0.9%	0.5%	2.3%	0.0%	0.6%
I am a spiritual person outside the traditional world religions	n	36	89	28	18	41	2	31	122	26	5	527
	%	17.1%	34.6%	11.9%	6.6%	10.1%	1.3%	13.7%	21.5%	19.5%	4.5%	7.6%
Without religion or confession	n	65	76	110	17	104	1	60	171	15	43	2422
	%	31.0%	29.6%	46.8%	6.3%	25.6%	0.7%	26.4%	30.2%	11.3%	38.4%	34.8%
Something different	n	9	14	12	10	26	3	7	0	10	5	198
	%	4.3%	5.4%	5.1%	3.7%	6.4%	2.0%	3.1%	0.0%	7.5%	4.5%	2.8%

Appendix 9.1.3: Demographic Structure of the Samples 2021

Number of participants, mean age and standard deviation and GDP per capita

	Australia	Czechia	France	India	Italy	Nigeria	Poland	Portugal	South Africa	Spain	Switzerland
N	138	692	406	485	188	121	148	494	563	312	5546
%	1.5	7.4	4.4	5.2	2.0	1.3	1.6	5.3	6.0	3.4	59.6
M_{age}	49.30	45.24	37.96	22.12	47.73	33.07	31.16	43.68	38.87	42.24	48.75
SD_{age}	11.45	16.75	15.44	21.99	12.34	8.08	12.46	15.63	14.52	16.87	14.52

Gender

		Australia	Czechia	France	India	Italy	Nigeria	Poland	Portugal	South Africa	Spain	Switzerland
Male	n	75	59	69	283	43	67	28	108	260	96	2391

(continued)

		Australia	Czechia	France	India	Italy	Nigeria	Poland	Portugal	South Africa	Spain	Switzerland
	%	54.3%	30.6%	17.0%	58.4%	22.9%	55.4%	18.9%	21.9%	46.2%	30.8%	43.4%
Female	n	63	134	335	200	145	54	118	386	303	214	3118
	%	45.7%	69.4%	82.5%	41.2%	77.1%	44.6%	79.7%	78.1%	53.8%	68.6%	56.6%

Marital Status

		Australia	Czechia	France	India	Italy	Nigeria	Poland	Portugal	South Africa	Spain	Switzerland
Still living with my parents	n	4	33	63	388	25	18	43	96	97	72	195
	%	2.9%	17.1%	15.5%	80.0%	13.3%	14.9%	29.1%	19.4%	17.2%	23.1%	3.5%
Single, unmarried	n	14	25	59	66	20	54	21	67	130	29	873
	%	10.1%	13.0%	14.5%	13.6%	10.6%	44.6%	14.2%	13.6%	23.1%	9.3%	15.7%
Living in a partnership but in separate households	n	1	17	46	3	13	0	6	12	15	14	371
	%	0.7%	8.8%	11.3%	0.6%	6.9%	0.0%	4.1%	2.4%	2.7%	4.5%	6.7%
Living together in a partnership	n	26	36	75	7	34	1	25	75	78	50	1103
	%	18.8%	18.7%	18.5%	1.4%	18.1%	0.8%	16.9%	15.2%	13.9%	16.0%	19.9%
Married	n	80	70	133	20	78	47	45	176	196	119	2313
	%	58.0%	36.3%	32.8%	4.1%	41.5%	38.8%	30.4%	35.6%	34.8%	38.1%	41.7%
Divorced / separated	n	13	9	28	1	15	1	7	60	39	21	543
	%	9.4%	4.7%	6.9%	0.2%	8.0%	0.8%	4.7%	12.1%	6.9%	6.7%	9.8%
Widowed	n	0	3	2	0	3	0	1	8	8	7	148
	%	0.0%	1.6%	0.5%	0.0%	1.6%	0.0%	0.7%	1.6%	1.4%	2.2%	2.7%

Education

		Australia	Czechia	France	India	Italia	Nigeria	Poland	Portugal	South Africa	Spain	Switzerland
Did not finish school	n	1	1	1	0	1	0	0	1	3	0	32
	%	0.7%	0.1%	0.2%	0.0%	0.5%	0.0%	0.0%	0.2%	0.5%	0.0%	0.6%

(continued)

		Australia	Czechia	France	India	Italia	Nigeria	Poland	Portugal	South Africa	Spain	Switzerland
Primary school	n	0	18	1	1	3	1	0	6	1	9	183
	%	0.0%	2.6%	0.2%	0.2%	1.6%	0.8%	0.0%	1.2%	0.2%	2.9%	3.3%
Secondary school	n	21	221	15	147	45	5	75	114	166	60	1219
	%	15.2%	31.9%	3.7%	35.5%	23.9%	4.2%	50.7%	23.1%	29.5%	19.2%	22.0%
Professional training / Diploma	n	38	262	84	3	6	4	9	25	138	41	3224
	%	27.5%	37.9%	20.7%	0.7%	3.2%	3.3%	6.1%	5.1%	24.5%	13.2%	58.1%
University	n	78	190	305	264	133	111	64	348	255	202	888
	%	56.5%	27.5%	75.1%	63.77%	70.7%	91.7%	43.2%	70.4%	45.3%	64.7%	16.0%

Main activity

		Australia	Czechia	France	India	Italy	Nigeria	Poland	Portugal	South Africa	Spain	Switzerland
In education or training (student)	n	8	64	133	438	20	34	72	108	75	82	158
	%	5.8%	33.2%	32.8%	90.3%	10.6%	28.1%	48.6%	21.9%	13.3%	26.3%	2.8%
Household / raising children	n	3	8	7	4	7	4	3	0	11	7	260
	%	2.2%	4.1%	1.7%	0.8%	3.7%	3.3%	2.0%	0.0%	2.0%	2.2%	4.7%
Part-time job	n	24	11	57	8	22	16	11	44	69	21	1222
	%	17.4%	5.7%	14.0%	1.6%	11.7%	13.2%	7.4%	8.9%	12.3%	6.7%	22.0%
Fulltime job	n	87	98	177	18	109	53	58	284	314	151	2654
	%	63.0%	50.8%	43.6%	3.7%	58.0%	43.8%	39.2%	57.5%	55.8%	48.4%	47.9%
Unemployed	n	10	2	9	14	15	14	3	17	50	11	219
	%	7.2%	1.0%	2.2%	2.9%	8.0%	11.6%	2.0%	3.4%	8.9%	3.5%	3.9%
Retired	n	6	10	23	3	15	0	1	41	44	40	1033
	%	4.3%	5.2%	5.7%	0.6%	8.0%	0.0%	0.7%	8.3%	7.8%	12.8%	18.6%

Professional status

		Australia	Czechia	France	India	Italy	Nigeria	Poland	Portugal	South Africa	Spain	Switzerland
No position in an organization (e.g., at school, housekeeping, unemployed, retired)	n	17	47	58	86	30	11	2	118	120	88	918
	%	12.3%	24.4%	14.3%	17.7%	16.0%	9.1%	1.4%	23.9%	21.3%	28.2%	16.6%
In education / training	n	10	53	88	375	22	34	72	39	73	41	177
	%	7.2%	27.5%	21.7%	77.3%	11.7%	28.1%	48.6%	7.9%	13.0%	13.1%	3.2%
Employee	n	37	9	66	11	50	28	34	184	144	117	2185
	%	26.8%	4.7%	16.3%	2.3%	26.6%	23.1%	23.0%	37.2%	25.6%	37.5%	39.4%
Junior / Middle management	n	15	30	94	6	16	20	15	56	103	27	1225
	%	10.9%	15.5%	23.2%	1.2%	8.5%	16.5%	10.1%	11.3%	18.3%	8.7%	22.1%
Senior management / Board of directors	n	25	34	57	3	22	10	6	19	49	24	387
	%	18.1%	17.6%	14.0%	0.6%	11.7%	8.3%	4.1%	3.8%	8.7%	7.7%	7.0%
Entrepreneur / Business owner	n	34	20	43	4	48	18	19	78	74	15	654
	%	24.6%	10.4%	10.6%	0.8%	25.5%	14.9%	12.8%	15.8%	13.1%	4.8%	11.8%

Religion

		Australia	Czechia	France	India	Italy	Nigeria	Poland	Portugal	South Africa	Spain	Switzerland
Catholic	n	20	37	123	29	96	73	58	207	49	153	1512
	%	14.5%	19.2%	30.3%	6.0%	51.1%	60.3%	39.2%	41.9%	8.7%	49.0%	27.3%
Protestant	n	14	2	10	13	0	26	0	4	67	0	1093
	%	10.1%	1.0%	2.5%	2.7%	0.0%	21.5%	0.0%	0.8%	11.9%	0.0%	19.7%
Another Christian church or community	n	15	3	2	20	2	17	2	11	272	1	206
	%	10.9%	1.6%	0.5%	4.1%	1.1%	14.0%	1.4%	2.2%	48.3%	0.3%	3.7%
Muslim	n	1	0	8	18	0	0	0	1	11	0	63
	%	0.7%	0.0%	2.0%	3.7%	0.0%	0.0%	0.0%	0.2%	2.0%	0.0%	1.1%
Jewish	n	1	0	5	1	0	1	0	1	5	1	13

(continued)

		Australia	Czechia	France	India	Italy	Nigeria	Poland	Portugal	South Africa	Spain	Switzerland
	%	0.7%	0.0%	1.2%	0.2%	0.0%	0.8%	0.0%	0.2%	0.9%	0.3%	0.2%
Hindu	n	3	0	1	340	0	0	0	0	3	0	5
	%	2.2%	0.0%	0.2%	70.1%	0.0%	0.0%	0.0%	0.0%	0.5%	0.0%	0.1%
Buddhist	n	6	3	3	2	6	0	1	6	5	3	35
	%	4.3%	1.6%	0.7%	0.4%	3.2%	0.0%	0.7%	1.2%	0.9%	1.0%	0.6%
I am a spiritual person outside the traditional world religions	n	26	71	54	24	24	1	27	143	76	33	397
	%	18.8%	36.8%	13.3%	4.9%	12.8%	0.8%	18.2%	28.9%	13.5%	10.6%	7.2%
Without religion or confession	n	40	72	186	19	38	0	54	121	48	109	2035
	%	29.0%	37.3%	45.8%	3.9%	20.2%	0.0%	36.5%	24.5%	8.5%	34.9%	36.7%
Something different	n	12	5	14	19	22	3	6	0	27	12	187
	%	8.7%	2.6%	3.4%	3.9%	11.7%	2.5%	4.1%	0.0%	4.8%	3.8%	3.4%

Appendix 9.2

Appendix 9.2.1

Australia: Partial Bivariate Pearson Correlations of Coping Styles with Posttraumatic Growth Domains

	Appreciation of Life	Personal Strength	New Possibilities	Relating to others	Spiritual Change
Acceptance	0.073	0.292**	0.145	0.333**	0.049
Positive Reframing	0.312**	0.449**	0.441**	0.515**	0.468**
Emotional Support	0.115	0.231**	0.136	0.339**	0.099
Religion	0.334**	0.471**	0.443**	0.405**	0.729**
Humor	−0.044	0.091	0.032	0.048	−0.046

(continued)

	Appreciation of Life	Personal Strength	New Possibilities	Relating to others	Spiritual Change
Active Coping	0.210*	0.278**	0.345**	0.300**	0.275**
Self-direction	0.039	0.071	0.034	0.153	0.124
Planning	0.289**	0.401**	0.368**	0.292**	0.325**
Instrumental Support	0.232**	0.361**	0.276**	0.456**	0.361**
Denial	0.285**	0.294**	0.290**	0.193*	0.425**
Venting	0.053	0.143	0.116	0.174*	0.173*
Disengagement	0.014	0.077	0.037	−0.041	0.143
Self-blame	0.055	−0.042	−0.093	−0.033	0.106
Substance Abuse	−0.042	−0.056	−0.138	−0.036	−0.103

Notes. **Correlation is significant at 0.01 level, *Correlation is significant at 0.05 level. Control variables: Gender, age, marital status, education, main activity, professional status

Appendix 9.2.2

Czech Republic: Partial Bivariate Pearson Correlations of Coping Styles with Posttraumatic Growth Domains

	Appreciation of Life	Personal Strength	New Possibilities	Relating to others	Spiritual Change
Acceptance	0.059	0.207**	0.062	0.120**	−0.058
Positive Reframing	0.174**	0.318**	0.283**	0.326**	0.172**
Emotional Support	0.244**	0.240**	0.255**	0.311**	0.190**
Religion	0.130**	0.135**	0.235**	0.225**	0.647**
Humor	0.034	0.097*	0.112*	0.087	0.038
Active Coping	0.216**	0.311**	0.347**	0.304**	0.149**
Self-direction	0.203**	0.165**	0.209**	0.162**	0.126**
Planning	0.179**	0.229**	0.190**	0.201**	0.144**

(continued)

	Appreciation of Life	Personal Strength	New Possibilities	Relating to others	Spiritual Change
Instrumental Support	0.240**	0.273**	0.278**	0.359**	0.268**
Denial	0.150**	0.102*	0.111*	0.102*	0.091*
Venting	0.149**	0.129**	0.122**	0.110*	0.098*
Disengagement	0.125**	0.069	0.098*	0.068	0.191**
Self-blame	0.113*	0.076	0.113*	0.080	0.114*
Substance Abuse	0.085	0.030	0.065	0.050	0.135**

Notes. **Correlation is significant at 0.01 level, *Correlation is significant at 0.05 level. Control variables: Gender, age, marital status, education, main activity, professional status

Appendix 9.2.3

France: Partial Bivariate Pearson Correlations of Coping Styles with Posttraumatic Growth Domains

	Appreciation of Life	Personal Strength	New Possibilities	Relating to others	Spiritual Change
Acceptance	0.133**	0.141**	0.162**	0.098*	0.058
Positive Reframing	0.254**	0.246**	0.234**	0.225**	0.176**
Emotional Support	0.187**	0.279**	0.188**	0.302**	0.131**
Religion	0.135**	0.113*	0.225**	0.205**	0.661**
Humor	0.072	0.125*	0.085	0.201**	0.021
Active Coping	0.185**	0.233**	0.231**	0.206**	0.084
Self-direction	0.213**	0.200**	0.154**	0.163**	0.048
Planning	0.160**	0.224**	0.244**	0.183**	0.097
Instrumental Support	0.139**	0.264**	0.158**	0.272**	0.087
Denial	0.168**	0.090	0.072	0.056	0.109*
Venting	0.141**	0.261**	0.150**	0.238**	0.099*
Disengagement	0.061	−0.010	−0.039	−0.115*	0.030

(continued)

	Appreciation of Life	Personal Strength	New Possibilities	Relating to others	Spiritual Change
Self-blame	0.044	0.008	0.047	0.038	0.063
Substance Abuse	0.048	−0.097	0.045	−0.034	−0.021

Notes. **Correlation is significant at 0.01 level, *Correlation is significant at 0.05 level. Control variables: Gender, age, marital status, education, main activity, professional status

Appendix 9.2.4

India: Partial Bivariate Pearson Correlations of Coping Styles with Posttraumatic Growth Domains

	Appreciation of Life	Personal Strength	New Possibilities	Relating to others	Spiritual Change
Acceptance	0.229**	0.269**	0.210**	0.257**	0.047
Positive Reframing	0.227**	0.296**	0.320**	0.263**	0.107*
Emotional Support	0.182**	0.197**	0.119**	0.229**	0.141**
Religion	0.097*	0.130**	0.135**	0.130**	0.436**
Humor	0.083	0.117*	0.092*	0.107*	0.152**
Active Coping	0.282**	0.282**	0.295**	0.171**	0.088
Self-direction	0.282**	0.227**	0.210**	0.203**	0.153**
Planning	0.343**	0.283**	0.274**	0.228**	0.099*
Instrumental Support	0.173**	0.147**	0.143**	0.181**	0.190**
Denial	0.034	0.100*	0.167**	0.066	0.196**
Venting	0.219**	0.189**	0.246**	0.181**	0.220**
Disengagement	0.018	−0.013	0.102*	0.011	0.199**
Self-blame	0.144**	0.077	0.057	0.049	0.124**
Substance Abuse	0.054	0.092*	0.162**	0.072	0.243**

Notes. **Correlation is significant at 0.01 level, *Correlation is significant at 0.05 level. Control variables: Gender, age, marital status, education, main activity, professional status

Appendix 9.2.5

Italy: Partial Bivariate Pearson Correlations of Coping Styles with Posttraumatic Growth Domains

	Appreciation of Life	Personal Strength	New Possibilities	Relating to others	Spiritual Change
Acceptance	0.078	0.342**	0.063	0.066	0.005
Positive Reframing	0.325**	0.294**	0.331**	0.276**	0.284**
Emotional Support	0.274**	0.153*	0.318**	0.462**	0.168*
Religion	0.314**	0.146*	0.222**	0.314**	0.721**
Humor	0.127	0.164*	0.138	0.101	−0.014
Active Coping	0.194**	0.355**	0.276**	0.285**	0.175*
Self-direction	0.154*	0.070	0.117	0.068	0.038
Planning	0.157*	0.404**	0.251**	0.227**	0.131
Instrumental Support	0.281**	0.112	0.295**	0.461**	0.230**
Denial	−0.021	−0.048	0.011	−0.014	0.140
Venting	0.271**	0.176*	0.193**	0.223**	0.168*
Disengagement	0.051	−0.217**	0.030	0.021	0.145
Self-blame	0.078	−0.168*	−0.020	0.003	0.054
Substance Abuse	0.014	−0.155*	−0.057	−0.120	−0.014

Notes. **Correlation is significant at 0.01 level, *Correlation is significant at 0.05 level. Control variables: Gender, age, marital status, education, main activity, professional status

Appendix 9.2.6

Nigeria: Partial Bivariate Pearson Correlations of Coping Styles with Posttraumatic Growth Domains

	Appreciation of Life	Personal Strength	New Possibilities	Relating to others	Spiritual Change
Acceptance	0.125	0.135	0.217*	0.044	−0.040
Positive Reframing	0.280**	0.311**	0.391**	0.352**	0.310**
Emotional Support	0.239*	0.313**	0.355**	0.392**	0.330**
Religion	0.358**	0.328**	0.312**	0.378**	0.606**
Humor	0.045	−0.095	−0.005	0.038	−0.074
Active Coping	0.372**	0.331**	0.355**	0.211*	0.298**
Self-direction	0.303**	0.222*	0.359**	0.119	0.217*
Planning	0.276**	0.355**	0.295**	0.224*	0.241**
Instrumental Support	0.273**	0.293**	0.372**	0.462**	0.327**
Denial	0.084	0.020	0.030	0.163	0.174
Venting	0.239*	0.206*	0.161	0.220*	0.214*
Disengagement	0.034	−0.038	−0.001	0.087	−0.011
Self-blame	0.106	−0.008	0.004	0.033	0.071
Substance Abuse	0.041	−0.028	0.069	0.122	0.098

Notes. **Correlation is significant at 0.01 level, *Correlation is significant at 0.05 level. Control variables: Gender, age, marital status, education, main activity, professional status

Appendix 9.2.7

Poland: Partial Bivariate Pearson Correlations of Coping Styles with Posttraumatic Growth Domains

	Appreciation of Life	Personal Strength	New Possibilities	Relating to others	Spiritual Change
Acceptance	−0.007	0.100	0.084	0.045	−0.070
Positive Reframing	0.198*	0.311**	0.311**	0.225**	0.174*
Emotional Support	0.299**	0.150	0.248**	0.254**	0.122
Religion	0.162	0.115	0.199*	0.244**	0.591**
Humor	−0.005	0.167*	0.099	0.166*	0.008
Active Coping	0.225**	0.343**	0.338**	0.233**	0.226**
Self-direction	0.177*	0.183*	0.172*	0.148	−0.023
Planning	0.171*	0.281**	0.259**	0.167*	0.117
Instrumental Support	0.184*	0.101	0.115	0.168*	0.001
Denial	0.152	0.095	0.094	0.012	0.101
Venting	0.182*	0.137	0.134	0.113	0.124
Disengagement	−0.006	0.052	0.059	−0.031	−0.068
Self-blame	0.101	0.091	0.149	0.105	0.162
Substance Abuse	−0.071	−0.053	−0.028	0.015	−0.055

Notes. **Correlation is significant at 0.01 level, *Correlation is significant at 0.05 level. Control variables: Gender, age, marital status, education, main activity, professional status

Appendix 9.2.8

Portugal: Partial Bivariate Pearson Correlations of Coping Styles with Posttraumatic Growth Domains

	Appreciation of Life	Personal Strength	New Possibilities	Relating to others	Spiritual Change
Acceptance	0.063	0.121**	0.048	0.115*	0.029
Positive Reframing	0.211**	0.287**	0.274**	0.300**	0.235**
Emotional Support	0.168**	0.072	0.116*	0.190**	0.136**
Religion	0.218**	0.203**	0.238**	0.309**	0.657**
Humor	0.069	0.098*	0.041	0.126**	0.032
Active Coping	0.276**	0.273**	0.262**	0.242**	0.168**
Self-direction	0.192**	0.178**	0.191**	0.193**	0.132**
Planning	0.281**	0.284**	0.273**	0.229**	0.224**
Instrumental Support	0.228**	0.170**	0.221**	0.280**	0.195**
Denial	0.131**	0.065	0.155**	0.098*	0.196**
Venting	0.147**	0.044	0.119**	0.128**	0.079
Disengagement	0.010	−0.046	0.020	−0.003	0.086
Self-blame	0.089*	−0.023	0.045	−0.004	0.092*
Substance Abuse	−0.001	−0.041	−0.062	−0.062	0.004

Notes. **Correlation is significant at 0.01 level. *Correlation is significant at 0.05 level. Control variables: Gender, age, marital status, education, main activity, professional status

Appendix 9.2.9

South Africa: Partial Bivariate Pearson Correlations of Coping Styles with Posttraumatic Growth Domains

	Appreciation of Life	Personal Strength	New Possibilities	Relating to others	Spiritual Change
Acceptance	0.272**	0.304**	0.255**	0.257**	0.186**
Positive Reframing	0.349**	0.446**	0.455**	0.415**	0.404**
Emotional Support	0.285**	0.330**	0.294**	0.412**	0.285**
Religion	0.268**	0.346**	0.348**	0.329**	0.632**
Humor	0.103*	0.136**	0.157**	0.153**	0.073
Active Coping	0.306**	0.430**	0.403**	0.297**	0.301**
Self-direction	0.311**	0.229**	0.287**	0.230**	0.199**
Planning	0.292**	0.360**	0.335**	0.277**	0.283**
Instrumental Support	0.273**	0.257**	0.295**	0.397**	0.289**
Denial	0.095*	0.066	0.120**	0.122**	0.119**
Venting	0.085*	0.106*	0.132**	0.047	0.103*
Disengagement	−0.025	−0.108*	−0.045	−0.037	−0.012
Self-blame	−0.055	−0.097*	−0.072	−0.061	−0.050
Substance Abuse	0.008	−0.080	−0.033	−0.017	−0.022

Notes. **Correlation is significant at 0.01 level, *Correlation is significant at 0.05 level. Control variables: Gender, age, marital status, education, main activity, professional status

Appendix 9.2.10

Spain: Partial Bivariate Pearson Correlations of Coping Styles with Posttraumatic Growth Domains

	Appreciation of Life	Personal Strength	New Possibilities	Relating to others	Spiritual Change
Acceptance	0.020	0.133*	0.004	0.028	−0.035
Positive Reframing	0.276**	0.467**	0.362**	0.363**	0.249**
Emotional Support	0.212**	0.197**	0.241**	0.302**	0.178**
Religion	0.071	0.148**	0.178**	0.169**	0.696**
Humor	0.034	0.075	0.033	0.028	−0.055
Active Coping	0.140*	0.354**	0.225**	0.206**	0.137*
Self-direction	0.330**	0.258**	0.216**	0.201**	0.121*
Planning	0.210**	0.385**	0.298**	0.223**	0.203**
Instrumental Support	0.212**	0.250**	0.276**	0.325**	0.256**
Denial	0.190**	0.108	0.162**	0.170**	0.157**
Venting	0.106	0.098	0.087	0.113*	0.100
Disengagement	0.121*	0.054	0.073	0.084	0.013
Self-blame	0.017	−0.041	0.005	0.042	0.061
Substance Abuse	−0.008	−0.072	0.054	0.004	0.081

Notes. **Correlation is significant at 0.01 level. *Correlation is significant at 0.05 level. Control variables: Gender, age, marital status, education, main activity, professional status

Appendix 9.2.11

Switzerland: Partial Bivariate Pearson Correlations of Coping Styles with Posttraumatic Growth Domains

	Appreciation of Life	Personal Strength	New Possibilities	Relating to others	Spiritual Change
Acceptance	0.132**	0.196**	0.149**	0.099**	0.017
Positive Reframing	0.274**	0.312**	0.328**	0.301**	0.179**
Emotional Support	0.251**	0.228**	0.269**	0.396**	0.222**
Religion	0.188**	0.184**	0.255**	0.277**	0.760**
Humor	0.000	0.120**	0.060**	0.062**	0.022
Active Coping	0.298**	0.311**	0.336**	0.273**	0.191**
Self-direction	0.255**	0.216**	0.228**	0.203**	0.129**
Planning	0.254**	0.288**	0.268**	0.227**	0.193**
Instrumental Support	0.219**	0.197**	0.251**	0.329**	0.223**
Denial	0.034*	0.008	0.029*	0.033*	0.092**
Venting	0.146**	0.126**	0.176**	0.132**	0.141**
Disengagement	−0.057**	−0.085**	−0.065**	−0.087**	0.007
Self-blame	0.107**	0.056**	0.135**	0.085**	0.129**
Substance Abuse	−0.032*	−0.053**	−0.036**	−0.036**	−0.005

Notes. **Correlation is significant at 0.01 level, *Correlation is significant at 0.05 level. Control variables: Gender, age, marital status, education, main activity, professional status

Appendix 9.3

Appendix 9.3.1

Australia: Partial Bivariate Pearson Correlations of Posttraumatic Growth Domains, Perceived Hope, Stress and Well-being

	Appreciation of Life	Personal Strength	New Possibilities	Relating to others	Spiritual Change
Perceived Hope	0.255**	0.460**	0.397**	0.480**	0.377**
Perceived Stress	0.017	−0.150	−0.191*	−0.181*	0.007
Hedonic Well-being	0.207*	0.380**	0.430**	0.350**	0.184*
Psychological Well-being	0.134	0.353**	0.335**	0.362**	0.171*
Social Well-being	0.272**	0.511**	0.432**	0.557**	0.308**

Notes. **Correlation is significant at 0.01 level, *Correlation is significant at 0.05 level. Control variables: Gender, age, marital status, education, main activity, professional status

Appendix 9.3.2

Czech Republic: Partial Bivariate Pearson Correlations of Posttraumatic Growth Domains, Perceived Hope, Stress and Well-being

	Appreciation of Life	Personal Strength	New Possibilities	Relating to others	Spiritual Change
Perceived Hope	0.066	0.246**	0.232**	0.252**	0.144**
Perceived Stress	0.103*	−0.094*	−0.054	−0.066	0.039
Hedonic Well-being	0.071	0.192**	0.202**	0.215**	0.090*
Psychological Well-being	0.079	0.285**	0.266**	0.243**	0.147**
Social Well-being	0.160**	0.263**	0.325**	0.393**	0.296**

Notes. **Correlation is significant at 0.01 level, *Correlation is significant at 0.05 level. Control variables: Gender, age, marital status, education, main activity, professional status

Appendix 9.3.3

France: Partial Bivariate Pearson Correlations of Posttraumatic Growth Domains, Perceived Hope, Stress and Well-being

	Appreciation of Life	Personal Strength	New Possibilities	Relating to others	Spiritual Change
Perceived Hope	0.150**	0.265**	0.289**	0.326**	0.228**
Perceived Stress	0.019	−0.120*	−0.052	−0.119*	−0.051
Hedonic Well-being	0.090	0.259**	0.187**	0.214**	0.090
Psychological Well-being	0.143**	0.310**	0.255**	0.280**	0.169**
Social Wellb-eing	0.129**	0.263**	0.235**	0.406**	0.186**

Notes. **Correlation is significant at 0.01 level, *Correlation is significant at 0.05 level. Control variables: Gender, age, marital status, education, main activity, professional status

Appendix 9.3.4

India: Partial Bivariate Pearson Correlations of Posttraumatic Growth Domains, Perceived Hope, Stress and Well-being

	Appreciation of Life	Personal Strength	New Possibilities	Relating to others	Spiritual Change
Perceived Hope	0.156**	0.203**	0.194**	0.185**	0.102*
Perceived Stress	0.024	−0.075	−0.067	−0.035	0.035
Hedonic Well-being	0.069	0.113*	0.137**	0.178**	0.080
Psychological Well-being	0.114*	0.207**	0.161**	0.244**	0.115*
Social Well-being	0.146**	0.178**	0.202**	0.229**	0.180**

Notes. **Correlation is significant at 0.01 level, *Correlation is significant at 0.05 level. Control variables: Gender, age, marital status, education, main activity, professional status

Appendix 9.3.5

Italy: Partial Bivariate Pearson Correlations of Posttraumatic Growth Domains, Perceived Hope, Stress and Well-being

	Appreciation of Life	Personal Strength	New Possibilities	Relating to others	Spiritual Change
Perceived Hope	0.308^{**}	0.517^{**}	0.414^{**}	0.311^{**}	0.245^{**}
Perceived Stress	−0.082	-0.422^{**}	-0.271^{**}	-0.188^{*}	−0.089
Hedonic Well-being	0.173^{*}	0.499^{**}	0.323^{**}	0.261^{**}	0.139
Psychological Well-being	0.188^{*}	0.555^{**}	0.378^{**}	0.386^{**}	0.195^{**}
Social Well-being	0.244^{**}	0.459^{**}	0.382^{**}	0.420^{**}	0.338^{**}

Notes. **Correlation is significant at 0.01 level, *Correlation is significant at 0.05 level. Control variables: Gender, age, marital status, education, main activity, professional status

Appendix 9.3.6

Nigeria: Partial Bivariate Pearson Correlations of Posttraumatic Growth Domains, Perceived Hope, Stress and Well-being

	Appreciation of Life	Personal Strength	New Possibilities	Relating to others	Spiritual Change
Perceived Hope	0.251^{**}	0.185^{*}	0.349^{**}	0.313^{**}	0.325^{**}
Perceived Stress	0.119	−0.040	−0.096	-0.258^{**}	−0.086
Hedonic Well-being	0.145	0.156	0.306^{**}	0.134	0.116
Psychological Well-being	0.255^{**}	0.210^{*}	0.392^{**}	0.256^{**}	0.233^{*}
Social Well-being	0.122	0.249^{**}	0.298^{**}	0.418^{**}	0.324^{**}

Notes. **Correlation is significant at 0.01 level, *Correlation is significant at 0.05 level. Control variables: Gender, age, marital status, education, main activity, professional status

Appendix 9.3.7

Poland: Partial Bivariate Pearson Correlations of Posttraumatic Growth Domains, Perceived Hope, Stress and Well-being

	Appreciation of Life	Personal Strength	New Possibilities	Relating to others	Spiritual Change
Perceived Hope	0.178*	0.173*	0.161	0.289**	0.246**
Perceived Stress	−0.141	−0.177*	−0.189*	−0.175*	−0.080
Hedonic Well-being	0.236**	0.259**	0.286**	0.284**	0.249**
Psychological Well-being	0.241**	0.309**	0.236**	0.284**	0.114
Social Well-being	0.209*	0.318**	0.296**	0.353**	0.282**

Notes. **Correlation is significant at 0.01 level, *Correlation is significant at 0.05 level. Control variables: Gender, age, marital status, education, main activity, professional status

Appendix 9.3.8

Portugal: Partial Bivariate Pearson Correlations of Posttraumatic Growth Domains, Perceived Hope, Stress and Well-being

	Appreciation of Life	Personal Strength	New Possibilities	Relating to others	Spiritual Change
Perceived Hope	0.216**	0.312**	0.316**	0.286**	0.293**
Perceived Stress	0.049	−0.116*	−0.058	−0.110*	−0.010
Hedonic Well-being	0.069	0.191**	0.153**	0.230**	0.084
Psychological Well-being	0.096*	0.238**	0.220**	0.272**	0.143**
Social Well-being	0.168**	0.274**	0.233**	0.392**	0.222**

Notes. **Correlation is significant at 0.01 level, *Correlation is significant at 0.05 level. Control variables: Gender, age, marital status, education, main activity, professional status

Appendix 9.3.9

South Africa: Partial Bivariate Pearson Correlations of Posttraumatic Growth Domains, Perceived Hope, Stress and Well-being

	Appreciation of Life	Personal Strength	New Possibilities	Relating to others	Spiritual Change
Perceived Hope	0.257**	0.419**	0.394**	0.415**	0.442**
Perceived Stress	−0.041	−0.217**	−0.181**	−0.210**	−0.183**
Hedonic Wellbeing	0.144**	0.278**	0.289**	0.337**	0.295**
Psychological Wellbeing	0.183**	0.369**	0.353**	0.354**	0.328**
Social Wellbeing	0.213**	0.355**	0.369**	0.450**	0.363**

Notes. **Correlation is significant at 0.01 level. Control variables: Gender, age, marital status, education, main activity, professional status

Appendix 9.3.10

Spain: Partial Bivariate Pearson Correlations of Posttraumatic Growth Domains, Perceived Hope, Stress and Well-being

	Appreciation of Life	Personal Strength	New Possibilities	Relating to others	Spiritual Change
Perceived Hope	0.229**	0.400**	0.339**	0.317**	0.187**
Perceived Stress	0.102	−0.141*	−0.033	−0.085	−0.012
Hedonic Well-being	0.172**	0.299**	0.246**	0.241**	0.127*
Psychological Well-being	0.211**	0.391**	0.325**	0.308**	0.233**
Social Well-being	0.220**	0.370**	0.321**	0.442**	0.279**

Notes. **Correlation is significant at 0.01 level, *Correlation is significant at 0.05 level. Control variables: Gender, age, marital status, education, main activity, professional status

Appendix 9.3.11

Switzerland: Partial Bivariate Pearson Correlations of Posttraumatic Growth Domains, Perceived Hope, Stress and Well-being

	Appreciation of Life	Personal Strength	New Possibilities	Relating to others	Spiritual Change
Perceived Hope	0.218**	0.288**	0.270**	0.335**	0.202**
Perceived Stress	0.021	−0.126**	−0.059**	−0.094**	0.021
Hedonic Well-being	0.142**	0.244**	0.197**	0.249**	0.083**
Psychological Well-being	0.178**	0.301**	0.248**	0.301**	0.151**
Social Well-being	0.206**	0.274**	0.261**	0.457**	0.200**

Notes. **Correlation is significant at 0.01 level. Control variables: Gender, age, marital status, education, main activity, professional status

References

Agha, S. (2021). Mental well-being and association of the four factors coping structure model: A perspective of people living in lockdown during COVID-19. *Ethics, Medicine and Public Health, 16*, 1–8. https://doi.org/10.1016/j.jemep.2020.100605

Ahuja, K. K. (2021). Scanning the VIRUS: A study of dimensions of stress and coping with COVID-19. *Current Psychology, 41*, 1–11. https://doi.org/10.1007/s12144-021-01369-4

Aldwin, C. M. (2004). *Culture, coping and resilience to stress* (pp. 563–573). Centre for Bhutan Studies.

Alshehri, F. S., Alatawi, Y., Alghamdi, B. S., Alhifany, A. A., & Alharbi, A. (2020). Prevalence of post-traumatic stress disorder during the COVID-19 pandemic in Saudi Arabia. *Saudi Pharmaceutical Journal, 28*(12), 1666–1673. https://doi.org/10.11588/xarep.00001333

Armeli, S., Gunthert, K. C., & Cohen, L. H. (2001). Stressor appraisals, coping, and post-event outcomes: The dimensionality and antecedents of stress-related growth. *Journal of Social and Clinical Psychology, 20*(3), 366–395. https://doi.org/10.1521/jscp.20.3.366.22304

Averill, J. R., Catlin, G., & Chon, K. K. (1990). *Rules of hope: Recent research in psychology*. Springer.

Averill, J. R., & Sundararajan, L. (2005). Hope as rhetoric: Cultural narratives of wishing and coping. In J. Eliott (Ed.), *Interdisciplinary perspectives on hope* (pp. 133–165). Nova Science.

Bhattacharjee, A., & Ghosh, T. (2021). COVID-19 pandemic and stress: Coping with the new normal. *Journal of Prevention and Health Promotion, 3*, 30–52. https://doi.org/10.1177/26320770211050058

Boals, A., & Schuler, K. L. (2018). Reducing reports of illusory posttraumatic growth: A revised version of the Stress-Related Growth Scale (SRGS-R). *Psychological Trauma: Theory, Research, Practice, and Policy, 10*(2), 190–198.

Boyraz, G., & Legros, D. N. (2020). Coronavirus disease (COVID-19) and traumatic stress: probable risk factors and correlates of posttraumatic stress disorder. *Journal of Loss and Trauma, 25*(6-7), 503–522. https://doi.org/10.1080/15325024.2020.1763556

Bridgland, V. M. E., Moeck, E. K., Green, D. M., Swain, T. L., Nayda, D. M., Matson, L. A., Hutchison, N. P., & Takarangi, M. K. T. (2021). Why the COVID-19 pandemic is a traumatic stressor. *PLoS One, 16*(1), 1–15. https://doi.org/10.1371/journal.pone.0240146

Brooks, S. K., Webster, R. K., Smith, L. E., Woodland, L., Wessely, S., Greenberg, N., & Rubin, G. J. (2020). The psychological impact of quarantine and how to reduce it: Rapid review of the evidence. *Lancet, 395*(10227), 912–920. https://doi.org/10.1016/S0140-6736(20)30460-8

Bruininks, P., & Malle, B. F. (2005). Distinguishing hope from optimism and related affective states. *Motivation and Emotion, 29*(4), 324–352. https://doi.org/10.1007/s11031-006-9010-4

Budimir, S., Probst, T., & Pieh, C. (2021). Coping strategies and mental health during COVID-19 lockdown. *Journal of Mental Health, 30*(2), 156–163. https://doi.org/10.1080/09638237.2021.1875412

Cann, A., Calhoun, L. G., Tedeschi, R. G., Taku, K., Vishnevsky, T., Triplett, K. N., & Danhauer, S. C. (2010). A short form of the posttraumatic growth inventory. *Anxiety, Stress, & Coping, 23*(2), 127–137. https://doi.org/10.1080/10615800903094273

Carver, C. S. (1997). You want to measure coping but your protocol'too long: Consider the brief cope. *International Journal of Behavioral Medicine, 4*(1), 92–100. https://doi.org/10.1207/s15327558ijbm0401_6

Carver, C. S., Scheier, M. F., & Weintraub, J. K. (1989). Assessing coping strategies: a theoretically based approach. *Journal of Personality and Social Psychology, 56*(2), 267.

Casagrande, M., Favieri, F., Tambelli, R., & Forte, G. (2020). The enemy who sealed the world: effects quarantine due to the COVID-19 on sleep quality, anxiety, and psychological distress in the Italian population. *Sleep Medicine, 75*, 12–20. https://doi.org/10.1016/j.sleep.2020.05.011

Chen, F. F. (2007). Sensitivity of goodness of fit indexes to lack of measurement invariance. *Structural Equation Modeling: A Multidisciplinary Journal, 14*(3), 464–504. https://doi.org/10.1080/10705510701301834

Chipp, K., Corder, C., & Kapelianis, D. (2013). The role of collectivism in defining the South African bottom of the pyramid. *Management Dynamics: Journal of the Southern African Institute for Management Scientists, 22*(1), 2–13.

Chun, C. A., Moos, R. H., & Cronkite, R. C. (2006). Culture: A fundamental context for the stress and coping paradigm. In L. C. J. Wong & W. J. Lonner (Eds.), *Handbook of multicultural perspectives on stress and coping* (pp. 29–53). Springer. https://doi.org/10.1007/0-387-26238-5_2

Cohen, S., Kamarck, T., & Mermelstein, R. (1983). A global measure of perceived stress. *Journal of Health and Social Behavior, 24*(4), 385–396. https://doi.org/10.2307/2136404

Cohen, S., Kessler, R. C., & Gordon, L. U. (Eds.). (1997). *Measuring stress: A guide for health and social scientists*. Oxford University Press on Demand.

Cohn, M. A., & Fredrickson, B. L. (2006). Beyond the moment, beyond the self: Shared ground between selective investment theory and the broaden-and-build theory of positive emotions. *Psychological Inquiry, 17*(1), 39–44.

Cohn, M. A., & Fredrickson, B. L. (2009). Positive emotions. In S. Lopez & C. Snyder (Eds.), *Oxford handbook of positive psychology* (Vol. 2, pp. 13–24).

Collins, R., Taylor, S., & Skokan, L. (1990). A better world or a shattered vision: Changes in life perspectives following victimization. *Social Cognition, 8*, 263–265.

Cooke, J. E., Eirich, R., Racine, N., & Madigan, S. (2020). Prevalence of posttraumatic and general psychological stress during COVID-19: A rapid review and metaanalysis. *Psychiatry Research, 292*, 113347. https://doi.org/10.1016/j.psychres.2020.113347

de Quervain, D., Aerni, A., Amini, E., Bentz, D., Coynel, D., Gerhards, C., Fehlmann, B., Freytag, V., Papassotiropoulos, A., Schicktanz, N., Schlitt, T., Zimmer, A., & Zuber, P. (2020). *The Swiss Corona Stress Study*. Report of the University of Basel.

Eaton, L., & Louw, J. (2000). Culture and self in South Africa: Individualism-collectivism predictions. *The Journal of Social Psychology, 140*(2), 210–217. https://doi.org/10.1080/00224540009600461

Engelbrecht, M. C., Heunis, J. C., & Kigozi, N. G. (2021). Post-traumatic stress and coping strategies of South African nurses during the second wave of the COVID-19 pandemic. *International Journal of Environmental Research and Public Health, 18*(15), 1–14. https://doi.org/10.3390/ijerph18157919

Erikson, E. H. (1959). *Identity and the life cycle: Selected Papers*. International Universities Press.

Fredrickson, B. L. (2013). Positive emotions broaden and build. *Advances in Experimental Social Psychology, 47*(1), 1–53. https://doi.org/10.1016/B978-0-12-407236-7.00001-2

Gallagher, M. W., Smith, L. J., Richardson, A. L., D'Souza, J. M., & Long, L. J. (2021). Examining the longitudinal effects and potential mechanisms of hope on COVID-19 stress, anxiety, and well-being. *Cognitive Behaviour Therapy, 50*(3), 234–245. https://doi.org/10.1080/16506073.2021.1877341

Garbóczy, S., Szemán-Nagy, A., Ahmad, M. S., Harsányi, S., Ocsenás, D., Rekenyi, V., Al-Tammemi, A., & Kolozsvári, L. R. (2021). Health anxiety, perceived stress, and coping styles in the shadow of the COVID-19. *BMC psychology, 9*(1), 1–13. https://doi.org/10.1186/s40359-021-00560-3

Govier, T. (2011). Hope and its opposites. *Journal of Social Philosophy, 42*(3), 239–253.

Guszkowska, M., & Dąbrowska-Zimakowska, A. (2022). Coping with stress during the second wave of the COVID-19 pandemic by Polish University students: Strategies, structure, and relation to psychological well-being. *Psychology Research and Behavior Management, 15*, 339. https://doi.org/10.2147/PRBM.S345648

Heppner, P. P., Heppner, M. J., Lee, D. G., Wang, Y. W., Park, H. J., & Wang, L. F. (2006). Development and validation of a collectivist coping styles inventory. *Journal of Counseling Psychology, 53*(1), 107.

Horn, M., Wathelet, M., Fovet, T., Amad, A., Vuotto, F., Faure, K., Astier, T., Noël, H., Henryb, M., Stéphane, S., Vaiva, G., & Fabien, D. (2020). Is COVID-19 associated with posttraumatic stress disorder? *The Journal of Clinical Psychiatry, 82*(1), 9886.

Hu, L. T., & Bentler, P. M. (1999). Cutoff criteria for fit indexes in covariance structure analysis: Conventional criteria versus new alternatives. *Structural Equation Modeling: A Multidisciplinary Journal, 6*(1), 1–55. https://doi.org/10.1080/10705519909540118

Hu, Q., Bernardo, A. B., Lam, S. W., & Cheang, P. K. (2018). Individualism-collectivism orientations and coping styles of cyberbullying victims in Chinese culture. *Current Psychology, 37*(1), 65–72. https://doi.org/10.1007/s12144-016-9490-7

Hu, Y., Ye, B., & Im, H. (2021). Hope and post-stress growth during COVID-19 pandemic: The mediating role of perceived stress and the moderating role of empathy. *Personality and Individual Differences, 178*, 110831. https://doi.org/10.1016/j.paid.2021.110831

Husky, M. M., Kovess-Masfety, V., & Swendsen, J. D. (2020). Stress and anxiety among university students in France during Covid-19 mandatory confinement. *Comprehensive Psychiatry, 102*, 152191. https://doi.org/10.1016/j.comppsych.2020.152191

Jayawickreme, E., & Blackie, L. R. (2014). Post-traumatic growth as positive personality change: Evidence, controversies and future directions. *European Journal of Personality, 28*, 312–331. https://doi.org/10.1002/per.1963

Joseph, S., & Linley, A. (2005). Positive adjustment to threatening events: An organismic valuing theory of growth through adversity. *Review of General Psychology, 9*, 262–280. https://doi.org/10.1037/1089-2680.9.3.262

Kar, N., Kar, B., & Kar, S. (2021). Stress and coping during COVID-19 pandemic: Result of an online survey. *Psychiatry Research, 295*, 113598. https://doi.org/10.1016/j.psychres.2020.113598

Keyes, C. L. (2002). The mental health continuum: From languishing to flourishing in life. *Journal of Health and Social Behavior, 43*(2), 207–222. https://doi.org/10.2307/3090197

Krafft, A. M., Guse, T., & Maree, D. (2021). Distinguishing perceived hope and dispositional optimism: Theoretical foundations and empirical findings beyond future expectancies and cognition. *Journal of Well-Being Assessment, 4*, 1–27. https://doi.org/10.1007/s41543-020-00030-4

Krafft, A. M., Martin-Krumm, C., & Fenouillet, F. (2019). Adaptation, further elaboration, and validation of a scale to measure hope as perceived by people: Discriminant value and predictive utility vis-à-vis dispositional hope. *Assessment, 26*(8), 1594–1609. https://doi.org/10.1177/1073191117700724

Kuo, B. C., Roysircar, G., & Newby-Clark, I. R. (2006). Development of the cross-cultural coping scale: Collective, avoidance, and engagement coping. *Measurement and Evaluation in Counseling and Development, 39*(3), 161–181. https://doi.org/10.1080/07481756.2006.11909796

Lakhan, R., Agrawal, A., & Sharma, M. (2020). Prevalence of depression, anxiety, and stress during COVID-19 pandemic. *Journal of Neurosciences in Rural Practice, 11*(4), 519–525. https://doi.org/10.1055/s-0040-1716442

Lazarus, R. S. (1966). *Psychological stress and the coping process*. McGraw-Hill.

Lazarus, R. S. (1990). Theory-based stress measurement. *Psychological Inquiry, 1*(1), 3–13. https://doi.org/10.1207/s15327965pli0101_1

Lazarus, R. S. (1993). From psychological stress to the emotions: A history of changing outlooks. *Annual Review of Psychology, 44*(1), 1–22.

Lazarus, R. S., & Folkman, S. (1984). *Stress, appraisal, and coping*. Springer.

Linley, P. A., & Joseph, S. (2011). Meaning in life and posttraumatic growth. *Journal of Loss and Trauma, 16*(2), 150–159. https://doi.org/10.1080/15325024.2010.519287

Linley, P. A., Joseph, S., & Goodfellow, B. (2008). Positive changes in outlook following trauma and their relationship to subsequent posttraumatic stress, depression, and anxiety. *Journal of Social and Clinical Psychology, 27*(8), 877–891. https://doi.org/10.1521/jscp.2008.27.8.877

Liu, C. H., Zhang, E., Wong, G. T. F., Hyun, S., & Hahm, H. C. (2020). Factors associated with depression, anxiety, and PTSD symptomatology during the COVID-19 pandemic: Clinical implications for U.S. young adult mental health. *Psychiatry Research, 290*, 113172. https://doi.org/10.1016/j.psychres.2020.113172

Marcel, G. (1951). *Homo viator: Introduction to a metaphysic of hope*. St. Augustines Press.

Maercker, A., & Zoellner, T. (2004). The Janus face of self-perceived growth: Toward a two-component model of posttraumatic growth. *Psychological Inquiry, 15*, 41–48.

Mahamid, F. A., & Bdier, D. (2021). The association between positive religious coping, perceived stress, and depressive symptoms during the spread of coronavirus (covid-19) among a sample of adults in Palestine: Across sectional study. *Journal of Religion and Health, 60*(1), 34–49. https://doi.org/10.1007/s10943-020-01121-5

Maia, B. R., & Dias, P. C. (2020). Anxiety, depression and stress in university students: The impact of COVID-19. *Estudos de Psicologia (Campinas), 37*, e200067. https://doi.org/10.1590/1982-0275202037e200067

Markus, H. R., & Kitayama, S. (1991). Culture and the self: Implications for cognition, emotion, and motivation. *Psychological Review, 98*(2), 224.

Markus, H. R., & Kitayama, S. (2003). Culture, self, and the reality of the social. *Psychological Inquiry, 14*(3-4), 277–283. https://doi.org/10.1080/1047840X.2003.9682893

Marsh, H. W. (1994). Confirmatory factor analysis models of factorial invariance: A multifaceted approach. *Structural Equation Modelling, 1*, 5–34. https://doi.org/10.1080/10705519409539960

Marsh, H. W., Balla, J. R., & Hau, K. (1996). An evaluation of incremental fit indices: A clarification of mathematical and empirical properties. In G. A. Marcoulides & R. E. Schumacker (Eds.), *Advanced structural equation modeling: Issues and techniques* (pp. 315–353). Lawrence Erlbaum.

Marujo, H. Á., Velez, M. J., Gonçalves, S. P., Neto, L. M., Krafft, A. M., & Casais, M. (2021). The value of hope: Validation of the perceived hope scale in the Portuguese population. *Current Psychology*, 1–9. https://doi.org/10.1007/s12144-021-02115-6

Minahan, J., Falzarano, F., Yazdani, N., & Siedlecki, K. L. (2021). The COVID-19 pandemic and psychosocial outcomes across age through the stress and coping framework. *The Gerontologist, 61*(2), 228–239. https://doi.org/10.1093/geront/gnaa205

Moos, R. H. (1984). Context and coping: Toward a unifying conceptual framework. *American Journal of Community Psychology, 12*(1), 5.

Moos, R. H. (2002). Context and coping: Toward a unifying conceptual framework. In D. Marks (Ed.), *The health psychology reader* (pp. 167–185). SAGE Publications.

Morales-Rodríguez, F. M. (2021). Fear, stress, resilience and coping strategies during COVID-19 in Spanish university students. *Sustainability, 13*(11), 5824. https://doi.org/10.3390/su13115824

Nolen-Hoeksema, S., & Davis, C. G. (2004). Theoretical and methodological issues in the assessment and interpretation of posttraumatic growth. *Psychological Inquiry, 15*, 60–64.

Polizzi, C., Lynn, S. J., & Perry, A. (2020). Stress and coping in the time of COVID-19: Pathways to resilience and recovery. *Clinical Neuropsychiatry, 17*(2), 59. https://doi.org/10.36131/CN20200204

Rehman, U., Shahnawaz, M. G., Khan, N. H., Kharshiing, K. D., Khursheed, M., Gupta, K., Kashyap, D., & Uniyal, R. (2021). Depression, anxiety and stress among Indians in times of Covid-19 lockdown. *Community Mental Health Journal, 57*(1), 42–48. https://doi.org/10.1007/s10597-020-00664-x

Rogowska, A. M., Kuśnierz, C., & Ochnik, D. (2021). Changes in stress, coping styles, and life satisfaction between the first and second waves of the COVID-19 pandemic: A longitudinal cross-lagged study in a sample of university students. *Journal of Clinical Medicine, 10*(17), 4025. https://doi.org/10.3390/jcm10174025

Roy, D., Tripathy, S., Kar, S. K., Sharma, N., Verma, S. K., & Kaushal, V. (2020). Study of knowledge, attitude, anxiety & perceived mental healthcare need in Indian population during COVID-19 pandemic. *Asian Journal of Psychiatry, 51*, 102083. https://doi.org/10.1016/j.ajp.2020.102083

Shulruf, B., Hattie, J., & Dixon, J. (2007). Development of a new measurement tool for individualism and collectivism. *Journal of Psychoeducational Assessment, 25*, 385–401. https://doi.org/10.1177/0734282906298992

Shulruf, B., Alesi, M., Ciochină, L., Faria, L., Hattie, J., Hong, F., Pepi, A. M., & Watkins, D. (2011). Measuring collectivism and individualism in the third millennium. *Social Behavior and Personality: An International Journal, 39*, 173–187. https://doi.org/10.2224/sbp.2011.39.2.173

Scioli, A., & Biller, H. (2009). *Hope in the age of anxiety*. Oxford University Press.

Slezackova, A., Prošek, T., Malatincová, T., & Krafft, A. M. (2020). Psychometrické vlastnosti české verze Škály prožívané naděje: faktorová struktura a vnitřní konzistence [Psychometric characteristics of the Czech version of The Perceived Hope Scale: Factor structure and internal consistency]. *Československá psychologie/Czechoslovak Psychology, 64*(3), 288–305.

Szkody, E., Stearns, M., Stanhope, L., & McKinney, C. (2021). Stress-buffering role of social support during COVID-19. *Family Process, 60*(3), 1002–1015. https://doi.org/10.1111/famp.12618

Taylor, S., Landry, C. A., Paluszek, M. M., Fergus, T. A., McKay, D., & Asmundson, G. J. (2020a). COVID stress syndrome: Concept, structure, and correlates. *Depression and Anxiety, 37*(8), 706–714. https://doi.org/10.1002/da.23071

Taylor, S., Landry, C. A., Paluszek, M. M., Fergus, T. A., McKay, D., & Asmundson, G. J. (2020b). Development and initial validation of the COVID stress scales. *Journal of Anxiety Disorders, 72*, 102232. https://doi.org/10.1016/j.janxdis.2020.102232

Tedeschi, R., & Calhoun, L. (1995). *Trauma and transformation: Growing in the aftermath of suffering*. Sage.

Tedeschi, R. G., & Calhoun, L. G. (2004). Posttraumatic growth: Conceptual foundations and empirical evidence. *Psychological Inquiry, 15*(1), 1–18. https://doi.org/10.1207/s15327965pli1501_01

Tennen, H., Affleck, G., & Tennen, R. (2002). Clipped feathers: The theory and measurement of hope. *Psychological Inquiry, 13*(4), 311–317.

Tillmann, R., Kuhn, U., Kühr, J., Thiévent, R., & Tabin, J. P. (2021). *Effets de la pandémie de coronavirus et du semi-confinement sur les conditions de vie: une analyse de l'enquête «COVID-19» du Panel suisse de ménages selon les catégories de revenu. Rapport final.* OFAS, FORS.

Tong, E. M., Fredrickson, B. L., Chang, W., & Lim, Z. X. (2010). Re-examining hope: The roles of agency thinking and pathways thinking. *Cognition and Emotion, 24*(7), 1207–1215. https://doi.org/10.1080/02699930903138865

Torales, J., O'Higgins, M., Castaldelli-Maia, J. M., & Ventriglio, A. (2020). The outbreak of COVID-19 coronavirus and its impact on global mental health. *International Journal of Social Psychiatry, 66*(4), 317–320. https://doi.org/10.1177/0020764020915212

Triandis, H. (1996). The psychological measurement of cultural syndromes. *American Psychologist, 51*, 407–415.

Triandis, H. C. (2001). Individualism-collectivism and personality. *Journal of Personality, 69*(6), 907–924. https://doi.org/10.1111/1467-6494.696169

Tsamakis, K., Triantafyllis, A. S., Tsiptsios, D., Spartalis, E., Mueller, C., Tsamakis, C., Chaidou, S., Spandidos, D., Fotis, L., Economou, M., & Rizos, E. (2020). COVID-19 related stress exacerbates common physical and mental pathologies and affects treatment. *Experimental and Therapeutic Medicine, 20*(1), 159–162. https://doi.org/10.3892/etm.2020.8671

Tseng, W. S. (2001). *Handbook of cultural psychiatry*. Academic.

Usher, K., Durkin, J., & Bhullar, N. (2020). The COVID-19 pandemic and mental health impacts. *International Journal of Mental Health Nursing, 29*(3), 315–318. https://doi.org/10.1111/inm.12726

Wu, D., Yu, L., Yang, T., Cottrell, R., Peng, S., Guo, W., & Jiang, S. (2020). The impacts of uncertainty stress on mental disorders of Chinese college students: Bhattacharjee and Ghosh 51 Evidence from a nationwide study. *Frontiers in Psychology, 11*, 243. https://doi.org/10.3389/fpsyg.2020.00243

Yeh, C. J., Arora, A. K., & Wu, K. A. (2006). A new theoretical model of collectivistic coping. In P. T. P. Wong, L. C. J. Wong, & W. J. Lonner (Eds.), *Handbook of multicultural perspectives on stress and coping* (pp. 55–72). Springer. https://doi.org/10.1007/0-387-26238-5_3

Andreas Krafft holds a doctoral degree in Management Sciences at the University of St. Gallen (Switzerland) with special focus on Organizational Psychology, Culture and Development. He has academic specializations in Social Psychology of Organizations, Work and Health Psychology as well as Positive Psychology from the University of Zürich. Andreas is associate researcher for Futures Studies and lecturer at the Institute of Systemic Management and Public Governance at the University of St. Gallen. Furthermore, he teaches at the University of Zürich in the field of Work and Health, at the Master of Applied Positive Psychology at the University of Lisbon, Portugal, as well as at the Master of Futures Studies from the Free University Berlin. He is co-president of swissfuture, the Swiss Society for Futures Studies, member of the executive board of SWIPPA (the Swiss Positive Psychology Association) and of the DACH-PP (German speaking Association of Positive Psychology). Since many years he leads the International Research Network of the Hope Barometer.

JohnBosco Chika Chukwuorji is a Senior Lecturer at the Department of Psychology, University of Nigeria, Nsukka. He was a Fulbright scholar and visiting researcher at Cleveland State University Cleveland, Ohio USA (2019–2020). He holds a PhD in clinical psychology obtained from the University of Nigeria Nsukka. As a research fellow in the Center for Translational and Implementation Research (CTAIR), University of Nigeria Nsukka, he is a core team member in the use of implementation science to enhance the effectiveness and quality of healthcare services in Nigeria. His research is focused on finding innovative approaches to provide quality mental healthcare for people living with challenging health conditions, forcibly displaced persons, justice-involved individuals, underserved communities and the general population. In addition to being the Editor of Nigerian Journal of Psychological Research, he is associate editor of three Journals (Fulbright Chronicles, Nigerian Journal of Psychology, Journal of International Politics & Development Studies) and editorial board member of four journals (BMC Psychology, Journal of Child and Adolescent Trauma, CPQ Women and Child Health, Journal of Psychology and Allied Disciplines).

Rajneesh Choubisa is Associate Professor of Psychology in the Department of Humanities and Social Sciences at Birla Institute of Technology and Science, (BITS) Pilani, Pilani Campus, India. He is a behavioral scientist by training and specializes in Positive Psychology from IIT Delhi. He has carried out meaningful research in the area of positive psychological measurement, positive organizational psychology and well-being promotion. He has rendered his expertise for reviewing projects at the European Commission's Institute of Advance Studies, among others. He is actively providing his expertise in the capacity of reviewer and academic editor for many top quality journals in the field. As an Indian collaborator of the Hope Barometer project, he has keen interest in exploring positive psychological variables theoretically, and also testing the practicability of these variables through customized, theory-driven, tailor-made programs and interventions.

Stella Comte is professor at the University of Cagliari, Italy. She is a member of the Italian Association of Psychology (A.I.P., Experimental Session) and of the Italian Association of Ethology. She is a referee for "Psychological Research" and "International Journal of Psychology". Her main research interest focuses on the following areas: the methodological issues of research on cognitive activity in human and animal: Vigilance and Attention, Language, Perception and Memory, as well as Cooperative Learning, Ethological studies of gulls, BFC and changes after treatment in children and adults and Theater therapy in adults and children. She has been the Scientific Responsible of a number of research projects: 2020 Creation of Help Desk for the Prevention of New Technology Addictions Foundation. She is the author of 180 scientific works, including monographies, chapters of books, scientific papers and proceedings published in national and international Journals.

Fabien Fenouillet is a professor of positive psychology of learning at the University of Paris Nanterre (UPN) and deputy director of the Interdisciplinary Laboratory in Neuroscience, Physiology and Psychology: Learning, Physical Activity and Health (LINP2-2APS). He is a specialist in motivation, particularly when this concept is applied to school, university or adult learning. He has written several books on this topic and published numerous scientific articles on the relationship between motivation and cognitive processes related to intelligence, memory, or in connection with technologies. He is committed to the optimal functioning of the human being. His research and publications apply more globally to consider different aspects of learning such as those related to well-being, interests, values but also anxiety.

Valle Flores-Lucas is Associate Professor at Valladolid University, in the psychology department. She led the Postgraduate course on Positive Psychology and Humour sense at Valladolid University. Her research work has been centred on two main research lines: developmental language and communication disorders. In the last years, she started another research line in the field of Positive Psychology mainly in the study of hope and its relations with other positive strengths and its applications on education. She is member of the Spanish Positive Psychology Society.

Tharina Guse is a counselling psychologist and obtained an MA (Counselling Psychology) degree from the Potchefstroom University (now North-West University) in 1989. She was in full-time private practice for the next 15 years providing psychotherapy for children, adolescents and adults. In 2003 she obtained her PhD (Psychology) from Potchefstroom University. She returned to academia in 2005 and joined the University of Johannesburg. Since April 2018 she is a professor and Head of the Department of Psychology at the University of Pretoria. Currently she serves on the Professional Board for Psychology of the Health Professions Council of South Africa (HPCSA). She is also President of the recently founded South African Positive Psychology Association (SAPPA). Her research focuses are on positive psychology in general and in particular on psycho-social well-being, positive psychology interventions and psychological strengths such as hope and gratitude. Closely aligned with this broad focus she also conducts research on the application of hypnosis for the promotion of mental health and well-being.

Elżbieta Kasprzak, psychologist, professor at the Kazimierz Wielki University in Bydgoszcz, Poland. Researcher of the determinants of careers and their consequences for the well-being of employees. An important area of her scientific interests are various aspects of positive functioning at work, job satisfaction, hope and passion at work, as well as the conditions and effects of job crafting and proactivity at work. Since 2015 she has been participating in the international research network of the Hope Barometer.

Charles Martin-Krumm is full Professor at the Ecole de Psychologues Praticiens de Paris (EPP). He is the director of the Vulnerability, Capability, and Recovery Laboratory at EPP. He is researcher at APEMAC UR 4360 UDL in Metz and associate at the Institut de Recherche Biomédicale des Armées (IRBA), in Brétigny. He is received the Fellow Award of the International Positive Psychology Association. Author of ten books and more than a hundred scientific publications, his research themes are related to quality of life and education in the fields of school, physical activity and sports, health and organizations.

Helena Agueda Marujo has a PhD in Psychology. She is Associate Professor at the Instituto Superior de Ciências Sociais e Politicas of the University of Lisbon, where she holds the positions of Executive Coordinator of Masters and PhDs programs in Development Human Resources

Policies; of Scientific Coordinator of the Postgraduate Degree in Applied Positive Psychology; of researcher at the Centre for Administration and Public Policy (CAPP); and of member of the Ethics Committee. She is the Coordinator of the UNESCO Chair in Education for Global Peace Sustainability at the University of Lisbon. Helena is a member of the Advisory Board of the International Positive Psychology Association and of the Board of Directors of the European Positive Psychology Network.

Chitra Nair started her career as Assistant Professor of Sociology at Government K.N.M. College, Thiruvananthapuram under University of Kerala in 2015. Her ongoing research focuses on positive psychology, improving quality of life and happiness of the marginalized, social exclusion and human rights issues, life course of centenarians and understanding the indigenous approaches to "Healthy Ageing". Her social engagements include advocacy for aged and women through local self-governments, NGOs, student level interventions, industrial partners and academic institutions. Her ongoing engagements include the Major Research Project from National Commission for Women, India to conduct research study titled 'Reproductive Rights and Choices of Fisher Women in Coastal Kerala – an Ethnographic Enquiry' and the Minor Research Project from Indian Council for Social Science Research for the research study on Intimate Partner Violence.

Mark Sinclair is an experienced educator, governance and technology professional. Dr Sinclair's career spans multi-sector education; corporate advisory at KPMG and AT Kearney and IT strategy (banking & public sectors). Dr. Sinclair has advised senior executives at over 100 organizations in a broad range of industries throughout Australia, Southeast Asia and the Middle East, helped establish a successful technology start-up and, over the last 20 years, overseen the development of an Education College that has provided education to 100,000 students.

Alena Slezackova, Ph.D., is an Associate Professor of Psychology and a Vice Head of the Dept. of Psychology and Psychosomatics, Faculty of Medicine, Masaryk University, in Brno, Czech Republic. Her scientific interests include mainly hope, mental health, and well-being. She also has a special interest in the research and practice of mindfulness. Alena is a founder and director of the Czech Positive Psychology Centre (CPPC), a member of the Advisory Council of the International Positive Psychology Association (IPPA), and a member of the Executive Board of the European Network for Positive Psychology (ENPP). She has been a member of several international research projects, and she serves on the editorial boards of five academic psychological journals. Alena is the author of the first comprehensive monograph on positive psychology in the Czech language and dozens of scientific publications in positive psychology and health psychology.

Patryk Stecz, a psychologist, is an assistant professor at the Institute of Psychology, University of Lodz, Poland. From 2014–2017 and 2021–2025, he was elected to the Executive Board of the Polish Suicidology Association. Dr Stecz completed his Ph.D. at the Medical University of Lodz. He published approx. 40 scientific works related to applied clinical psychology (attitudes towards suicide, positive suicidology, religious coping, well-being predictors in clinical and non-clinical populations, risk behavior in students with visual impairment, studies on hope). Dr Stecz has been serving psychological support at the Academic Counseling Centre (Technical University of Lodz) for students and employees with disabilities and special needs since 2008. Dr Stecz was aged 31 when he received the Medical University Rector's Scientific Award. Currently he is finishing a four-year post-graduate Clinical Psychology Specialization Program (Center of Postgraduate Medical Education).

Olga Varsos is the co-Author of the POWER Coaching and the GOAL Models, with extensive experience in executive, adult, homeless and at-risk youth coaching. These leading programs are used extensively in Australia and internationally in the not-for-profit, education, community, and indigenous youth sectors, focusing on instilling hope to establish goals to help ensure positive lasting change. Olga started her career as a social worker, firstly in the health sector before moving to project managing service delivery in the community sector. Olga has post graduate degrees in Social Work, Human Resources and is an accredited EQ Practitioner.

Chapter 10
Beacons of Hope in a Challenging World: Conclusions and Directions for Future Research and Practice

Tharina Guse, Alena Slezackova, and Andreas M. Krafft

Abstract This chapter summarizes the main tenets of our integrated hope model, followed by salient findings regarding hope in various countries and cultures, reported in this volume. We then identify challenges and future directions for research on hope across cultures and contexts.

10.1 Introduction

Now, perhaps more than ever, hope is important to human well-being (Counted et al., 2022; Gallagher et al., 2021; Yıldırım & Arslan, 2022). We find ourselves at a time in history when people across the globe are experiencing many challenges and hardships. How is it possible to remain hopeful and work towards a better future when we may feel overwhelmed by the crises of the world? This volume proposed an integrated, interdisciplinary hope model to shed light on this question and add to a more multifaceted understanding of hope. Further, we examined elements of this model in various studies across several countries.

T. Guse (✉)
Department of Psychology, University of Pretoria, Pretoria, South Africa
e-mail: tharina.guse@up.ac.za

A. Slezackova
Department of Medical Psychology and Psychosomatics, Faculty of Medicine, Masaryk University, Brno, Czech Republic

A. M. Krafft
Institute of Systemic Management and Public Governance, University of St. Gallen, St. Gallen, Switzerland

A. M. Krafft et al. (eds.), *Hope across cultures*, Cross-Cultural Advancements in Positive Psychology 14, https://doi.org/10.1007/978-3-031-24412-4_10

10.2 An Integrated Model of Hope

A key theme of this book is that hope extends beyond individual agency and includes affective, behavioural, relational, value-based, and spiritual elements. In addition, we proposed that how people hope, and what they hope for, will differ depending on the context, especially cultural context. Accordingly, we defined hope as consisting of three main elements:(1) a *wish or desire* for something that is valuable; (2) the *belief* that it may be possible for this wish to be fulfilled, although it remains uncertain or even unlikely; and (3) the *trus*t that we have the necessary internal or external resources that can facilitate the fulfillment of the wish in the face of obstacles and setbacks (see Chap. 2). These resources may be available now, or may become available in the future. The universal elements of hope, namely wish, belief, and trust, may differ across cultures and contexts based on cognitive, affective, behavioral, relational, religious, and value dimensions relevant to the context. We operationalized this understanding of hope as *perceived hope* (Krafft et al., 2019, 2021; Marujo et al., 2021; Slezackova et al., 2020).

10.3 Exploring Hope Across Cultures

Utilizing datasets from various countries obtained with the International Hope Barometer Programme from 2017–2021, we examined hope along several dimensions. First, across all samples, *levels of hope* were moderate to high and above midpoint. This suggests that, across time and context, people remained hopeful that they would attain important hoped-for goods, despite setbacks (Chap. 3). This finding underscores the importance of hope as a universal human need. However, samples from less affluent, developing countries, and to some extent those characterized as more collectivistic, seemed to display higher levels of hope than richer, more individualistic countries (Chaps. 3, 4, 8 and 9). Our findings thus seem to point to the importance of relational and affective dimensions (Braun-Lewensohn et al., 2021; Cohn & Fredrickson, 2009; Jacoby & Goldzweig, 2014) of hope.

Next, our findings indicated that *values* (Schwartz, 2012), especially values of self-transcendence (caring for the well-being of others) and of openness to change (self-mastery, looking for new challenges and novel experiences), are associated with hope. In addition, tradition, religious experiences, and achievement could also act as hope-related values. When we examined what people are hoping for (hope targets), we found that people seemed to be wishing for similar goods (Chap. 3). These were good health, a happy relationship, family or marriage, and harmony in life. Hoping for these targets aligned with domains that nurture eudaimonic well-being (Ryff, 2014) and were positively related to hope. However, wishing for hedonic and materialistic goods was unrelated to hope. These findings support the notion of hope as a transcendent virtue (Peterson & Seligman, 2004), associated with eudaimonic facets of well-being.

Third, we aimed to extend our understanding of individual hope and examined *collective hope and future expectations* across 12 countries (Chap. 4). We defined the broader concept of collective hope as a wish or desire for a better common future, the belief that the realization of a better future for all is possible (although not necessarily probable), and trust in the availability of personal, social, and other resources to deal with current challenges and to overcome obstacles and setbacks. Further, we considered people's long-term expectations concerning future quality of life as well as their outlooks regarding probable and desirable long-term future scenarios (Eckersley, 1999; Eckersley et al., 2007). While our findings pointed to a strong universal wish for a sustainable, harmonious, just, and cooperative human community, people expected the future to be characterized by crises such as environmental destruction, new diseases, and ethnic and regional conflicts. However, participants from less affluent countries such as Nigeria and Colombia held expectations of a more flourishing future scenario, expecting the world to enter a new age of sustainability, peace, and prosperity. Overall, and surprisingly, the desire for a better future had only a small impact on hope and well-being. These findings provide further evidence for context-specific manifestations of hope and future expectancies. It also points to the importance of finding ways to strengthen collective hope and positive future expectancies, as these collective resources could serve to sustain hope in challenging times (Braithwaite, 2004; Kelsey, 2016).

Since one of the central elements of our model of hope involves the belief that what we wish for might possibly (but not inevitably) be attained, it can be expected that beliefs and assumptions of the world would be related to our experiences of hope. Therefore, we further set out to examine the role of *basic beliefs and worldviews* in sustaining hope across six samples (Chap. 5). The results suggest that our basic beliefs indeed have a significant effect on levels of hope, however, with diverse magnitude. The strongest predictors of hope were pathways (the belief in one's ability to overcome difficulties and find many ways to attain a goal), positive emotions, the belief in the benevolence of the world, one's own agency to achieve goals, the belief of luck in life, and to a lesser but still significant extent, the readiness to help other people, and religiosity. However, there were also pronounced differences among some countries. Specifically, the two countries with the highest levels of perceived hope in the study, South Africa and Israel, endorsed different worldviews. Whereas, for the South African sample, hope seemed to be very much anchored in positive emotions, social relationships, the willingness to help other people, religious faith, and the connection to a Higher Power, as well as the general belief in the good, for the Israeli sample individualistic assumptions such as self-worth and belief in luck were stronger predictors. Our findings thus provide support for the notion that context-specific cognitions, affect, and behaviours may influence people's experiences of hope (Averill et al., 1990; Averill & Sundararajan, 2005; Scioli & Biller, 2009).

Fifth, we explored *sources and activities generating hope* across several countries to elucidate the third element of our model, i.e., trust. Analyzing data from 12 countries, we found that several sources and activities contributed to perceived hope, rooted in interpersonal trust and influenced by social attachment and support (Scioli et al., 1997). We referred to this as "trustful hope", which especially comes into play in situations when people cease to be optimistic and cannot foresee a positive outcome anymore, yet, they do not want to give up their hopes (Chap. 6). Based on the results, we identified three groups of countries, which differed with regard to the importance assigned to several hope sources: Social resources and activities such as supporting each other emotionally and talking with family and friends were especially important for people in some Latin countries (Spain, Portugal, and Colombia). People in African countries (Nigeria and South Africa) and India obtained and nurtured hope particularly through religious sources and practices (trusting God, praying, meditating, etc.). Finally, people in more individualistic countries like Switzerland and Czechia primarily relied on self-centered, performance, and mastery-oriented sources and activities, but also acknowledged the importance of external factors such as social support, luck, and inspiring experiences in nature. People in different countries and cultures thus seem to differ in the way they hope and in the activities they perform in order to see their hopes come true. This supports our premise that the universal elements of hope (having a wish, believing in its possibility of being attained, and trust) will play out differently in different contexts and cultures, as reported in existing research (Braun-Lewensohn et al., 2021).

More detailed comparisons between specific countries further expanded our understanding of hope, its correlates, and mechanisms. Comparing samples from *Czechia and Poland*, which experienced similar macro-social changes since the 1980s (Chap. 7), the results indicated that Czech participants generally showed higher levels of hope and other positive indicators than their Polish counterparts. Alarmingly, the youngest respondents in both countries reported lower levels of perceived hope, positive mental health, and satisfaction with the climate and environment, as well as greater loneliness, anxiety, and depression; they also reported more pessimistic expectations for the national economy. Yet, religious participants in both countries exhibited higher levels of perceived hope, which aligns with our premise that hope included spiritual and religious dimensions. In addition to supporting culture-specific manifestations of hope, the findings highlight the importance of examining hope among young adults (Booker et al., 2021), and finding ways to mobilize resources to strengthen hope. The second study compared hope and flourishing among samples from *Spain and South Africa* and revealed that the South African sample experienced higher levels of hope than the Spanish sample, but levels of flourishing were similar (Chap. 8). Both samples believed that taking responsibility for generating hope as individuals was the most important source of hope. Agentic activities such as having a job and motivating friends were strong predictors of hope for both groups. For the South African sample, religious activities were important in generating hope. These results point to the universality of hope in terms of the behavioral dimension (see Chap. 2), but also suggest that hope may be sustained in different ways in different cultural contexts, and that religious/spiritual as well as relational dimensions may serve as resources to strengthen hope (thus reflecting the element of trust in having resources available). This may be particularly important in countries where resources are limited (Counted et al., 2022).

Finally, we reported on the role of hope during the *COVID-19 pandemic*. We also investigated levels of perceived stress, posttraumatic growth, and ways of coping during the pandemic years of 2020 and 2021, reported by participants in 11 countries (Chap. 9). Most reported moderate to high levels of hope, but simultaneously moderate levels of perceived stress characterized by feelings of unpredictability, uncontrollability, and overload. Moreover, despite the crisis, participants reported moderate to high levels of well-being and were able to display positive coping styles such as accepting the new reality by simultaneously adopting a positive stance and actively coping with the challenging situation. Hope and well-being were primarily related to the possibility of reframing negative events in a positive manner, the capacity of accepting and actively coping with everyday challenges, but also to finding relief and comfort in religious faith and practices. In some countries, levels of well-being were also positively related to the availability of social support. These findings align with our proposed hope model, where a wish for a positive outcome to the pandemic was probably sustained by coping behaviors and attitudes (beliefs) with religious faith and social support as resources (trust). Samples from countries characterized as more collectivistic and/or religious (Nigeria, South Africa, India, Portugal) showed higher levels of hope than those from countries seen as more individualistic (Spain, Poland, France, Switzerland). Possibly, with the exception of Australia, participants in countries with higher levels of hope had more relational and spiritual resources to nourish their hopes (Counted et al., 2022).

Overall, the findings in this volume support the premise that hope is multifaceted and culturally influenced, and that an interdisciplinary approach to studying hope can broaden our understanding of this vital resource. It was evident that hope is not only about individual goals, but also about sustained beliefs and actions when it is not certain whether what we are hoping for will be attained. In particular, hope needs to be nourished and nurtured by mobilizing individual and collective resources, which will materialize differently in different cultures and contexts.

10.4 Designing and Implementing Interdisciplinary Interventions

One of the most crucial tasks in the coming years is to design and implement interventions that incorporate insights from several disciplines, fostering hope and encouraging people to act not only to achieve individual goals but also for a better common future of society. For this, Krafft (2022) has developed and implemented a program for students in secondary schools called "Positive Futures—Hope for a Better Life". The program integrates methods and interventions from positive psychology with those of futures studies in education. The program has five basic aims: (1) a change of mindset to recognize and cultivate positive things, experiences, and emotions in life; (2) fostering self-worth and self-esteem by identifying and developing character strengths; (3) developing desirable long-term

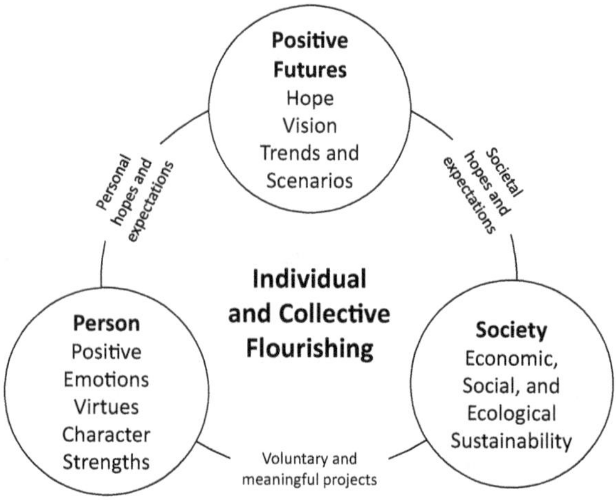

Fig. 10.1 Positive futures. Source: Adapted from Krafft (2022)

future scenarios at the individual and the collective level; (4) learning to hope and to engage together with others, promoting hope through voluntary and meaningful projects; and (5) experiencing the main drivers for a purposeful and thriving life for oneself and the community.

"Positive Futures" combines individual hopes and future expectations with visions of a good life in an economically, socially, and environmentally sustainable world, supporting young people in developing a more fundamental hope for joined happiness and fulfillment. By integrating the basic elements of a flourishing life with the 17 Sustainable Development Goals of the United Nations, the program encourages young people to wish for a better future, to believe that a good life not only for oneself but for all in a healthy planet is possible (although not at all guaranteed), and to trust each other in order to contributing together to its realization. Figure 10.1 presents the integration of the individual and the social level, focusing on visions and hopes for positive futures, and participating in meaningful projects for the common good. At the core of the model resides the belief that the individual can flourish in an environment where all others and the entire nature can flourish too.

Major changes and profound transformations usually cannot take place overnight. They require a long-term vision and common endeavor where the role of individual and collective hope is decisive in persevering and working together. The main task is to guide young people in taking a global perspective and in developing their character strengths, virtues, and potentials to shape a socially and ecologically sustainable world. This does not always mean that everyone must trigger a major social revolution. In one way or another, every person can experience change by acting in the immediate environment (family, social institutions, environmental projects, etc.) through an empathic, caring, and virtuous behavior. In this form, personal well-being and flourishing go hand in hand with a caring social and ecologically sustainable development.

10.5 Future Directions for Research and Practice

This volume is a step forward in broadening our views on hope. Yet, as always, research findings often lead to more *research questions* that need to be answered. First, currently most of our results are descriptive, identifying differences in hope, its correlates and predictors, between samples from various countries. This needs to be further examined to identify possible mechanisms and factors that could explain these differences beyond collectivism/individualism. Could social class, levels of socioeconomic development, or a need to improve existing living conditions contribute to hope in poorer countries? What is the role of religious practices and communities from different cultures in sustaining hope?

Second, qualitative research and mixed-method studies could expand on our broad findings by examining subjective aspects of the proposed model of hope. For example, what do people subjectively perceive as hope resources? How do they actively keep hoping in challenging times? How is hope sustained despite people's endorsements of catastrophic future scenarios? And, can hope be transmitted within a family, from generation to generation?

Since most of the presented studies are correlational studies, more information on the dynamics and the direction of causality of the relations between hope and other investigated variables could be obtained by conducting a longitudinal study that would include personality traits and other psychosocial variables capable of providing a deeper insight into the investigated phenomena.

In addition, the proposed integrated hope model needs to be tested in various contexts and with various groups, using techniques such as structural equation modelling or multilevel analyses. It is further important to examine how to mobilize hope and facilitate action in the context of concerns about climate change and the environment (Kelsey, 2016; Li & Monroe, 2019; Ojala, 2012).

Finally, since hope is about the future, it is particularly important to explore how (and if) this integrated model is relevant to young people. They are the ones who will inherit the future, and it may be useful to extend the Hope Barometer Program to adolescent samples in different countries in the future.

In terms of *practice,* our findings underscored the importance of hope to well-being. The evidence of the protective role of hope in various contexts can be beneficial in clinical settings and in education, public policy, and prevention (both primary, secondary, and tertiary). Fostering a hopeful attitude in vulnerable individuals and assisting them in developing feelings of hope, trust, and a sense of connectedness will help the clients cope with difficult life situations more effectively.

Therefore, developing and evaluating interventions to strengthen hope and hope resources, beyond cognitive-motivational dimensions, is important to support well-being in the face of possible future crises. In particular, there is a need to strengthen hope among youth, who are faced with concerns about the world and environment they will inherit (see also Ojala, 2022). It will further be useful to examine the feasibility and effectiveness of interventions based on our model of hope across different countries and cultures.

10.6 Conclusion

As the world becomes increasingly complex and challenging, our research suggests that there are indeed beacons of hope. These are not only located in the individual, but also in communities of hopers. We have remained hopeful in one of the most challenging times in recent history through mobilizing individual, communal, and spiritual resources. It is our hope that we can continue to refine our understanding of hope and contribute to well-being for all.

References

Averill, J. R., Catlin, G., & Chon, K. K. (1990). *Rules of hope: Recent research in psychology*. Springer.

Averill, J. R., & Sundararajan, L. (2005). Hope as rhetoric: Cultural narratives of wishing and coping. In J. Eliott (Ed.), *Interdisciplinary perspectives on hope* (pp. 133–165). Nova Science.

Booker, J. A., Dunsmore, J. C., & Fivush, R. (2021). Adjustment factors of attachment, hope, and motivation in emerging adult well-being. *Journal of Happiness Studies, 22*(7), 3259–3284. https://doi.org/10.1007/s10902-021-00366-5

Braithwaite, V. (2004). Collective hope. *The Annals of the American Academy of Political and Social Science, 592*(1), 6–15.

Braun-Lewensohn, O., Abu-Kaf, S., & Kalagy, T. (2021). Hope and resilience during a pandemic among three cultural groups in Israel: The second wave of Covid-19. *Frontiers in Psychology, 12*(May 2020), 1–12. https://doi.org/10.3389/fpsyg.2021.637349

Cohn, M. A., & Fredrickson, B. L. (2009). Positive emotions. In S. Lopez & C. R. Snyder (Eds.), *Oxford handbook of positive psychology* (Vol. 2, pp. 13–24).

Counted, V., Pargament, K. I., Bechara, A. O., Joynt, S., & Cowden, R. G. (2022). Hope and well-being in vulnerable contexts during the COVID-19 pandemic: Does religious coping matter? *The Journal of Positive Psychology, 17*(1), 70–81. https://doi.org/10.1080/17439760.2020.1832247

Eckersley, R. (1999). Dreams and expectations: Young people's expected and preferred futures and their significance for education. *Futures, 31*(1), 73–90. https://doi.org/10.1016/S0016-3287(98)00111-6

Eckersley, R., Cahill, H., Wierenga, A., & Wyn, J. (2007). *Generations in dialogue about the future: The hopes and fears of young Australians*. Australian Youth Research Centre.

Gallagher, M. W., Smith, L. J., Richardson, A. L., D'Souza, J. M., & Long, L. J. (2021). Examining the longitudinal effects and potential mechanisms of hope on COVID-19 stress, anxiety, and well-being. *Cognitive Behaviour Therapy, 50*(3), 234–245. https://doi.org/10.1080/16506073.2021.1877341

Jacoby, R., & Goldzweig, G. (2014). *The many faces of hope*. Paper presented at the 6th global conference of hope. Prague, Czech Republic.

Kelsey, E. (2016). Propagating collective hope in the midst of environmental doom and gloom. *Canadian Journal of Environmental Education (CJEE), 21*, 23–40.

Krafft, A. M. (2022). Positive futures and hope for a better life: A transdisciplinary approach for imaging a flourishing and sustainable world. In I. Nasser (Ed.), *Education transformation in Muslim societies–a discourse of hope* (pp. 121–145). Indiana University Press and International Institute of Islamic Thought.

Krafft, A. M., Guse, T., & Maree, D. (2021). Distinguishing perceived hope and dispositional optimism: Theoretical foundations and empirical findings beyond future expectancies and cognition. *Journal of Well-Being Assessment, 4*(3), 217–243. https://doi.org/10.1007/s41543-020-00030-4

Krafft, A. M., Martin-Krumm, C., & Fenouillet, F. (2019). Adaptation, further elaboration, and validation of a scale to measure hope as perceived by people: Discriminant value and predictive utility vis-à-vis dispositional hope. *Assessment, 26*(8), 1594–1609. https://doi.org/10.1177/1073191117700724

Li, C. J., & Monroe, M. C. (2019). Exploring the essential psychological factors in fostering hope concerning climate change. *Environmental Education Research, 25*(6), 936–954. https://doi.org/10.1080/13504622.2017.1367916

Marujo, H. Á., Velez, M. J., Gonçalves, S. P., Neto, L. M., Krafft, A. M., & Casais, M. (2021). The value of hope: Validation of the perceived hope scale in the Portuguese population. *Current Psychology*, 1–9. https://doi.org/10.1007/s12144-021-02115-6

Ojala, M. (2012). Hope and climate change: The importance of hope for environmental engagement among young people. *Environmental Education Research, 18*(5), 625–642. https://doi.org/10.1080/13504622.2011.637157

Ojala, M. (2022). Hope through learning to live with ambivalence: Emerging adults' agency work in the face of sustainability conflicts. In M. Häggström & C. Schmidt (Eds.), *Relational and critical perspectives on education for sustainable development*. Sustainable development goals series. Springer. https://doi.org/10.1007/978-3-030-84510-0_9

Peterson, C., & Seligman, M. E. (2004). *Character strengths and virtues: A handbook and classification* (Vol. 1). Oxford University Press.

Ryff, C. D. (2014). Psychological well-being revisited: Advances in the science and practice of eudaimonia. *Psychotherapy and Psychosomatics, 83*(1), 10–28. https://doi.org/10.1159/000353263

Schwartz, S. H. (2012). An overview of the Schwartz theory of basic values. *Online Readings in Psychology and Culture, 2*(1), 1–20. https://doi.org/10.9707/2307-0919.1116

Scioli, A., & Biller, H. (2009). *Hope in the age of anxiety*. Oxford University Press.

Scioli, A., Chamberlin, C. M., Samor, C. M., Lapointe, A. B., Campbell, T. L., Macleod, A. R., & McLenon, J. (1997). A prospective study of hope, optimism, and health. *Psychological Reports, 81*(3), 723–733. https://doi.org/10.2466/pr0.1997.81.3.723

Slezackova, A., Prošek, T., Malatincová, T., & Krafft, A. M. (2020). Psychometrické vlastnosti české verze Škály prožívané naděje: faktorová struktura a vnitřní konzistence [Psychometric characteristics of the Czech version of the perceived Hope Scale: Factor structure and internal consistency]. *Československá psychologie/Czechoslovak Psychology, 64*(3), 288–305.

Yıldırım, M., & Arslan, G. (2022). Exploring the associations between resilience, dispositional hope, preventive behaviours, subjective well-being, and psychological health among adults during early stage of COVID-19. *Current Psychology, 41*(8), 5712–5722. https://doi.org/10.1007/s12144-020-01177-2

Tharina Guse is a counselling psychologist, professor and Head of the Department of Psychology at the University of Pretoria. Her research focuses are on positive psychology in general, and in particular on psychosocial well-being, positive psychology interventions and psychological strengths such as hope and gratitude. Closely aligned with this broad focus she also conducts research on the application of hypnosis for the promotion of mental health and well-being.

Alena Slezackova, Ph.D., is an Associate Professor of Psychology and a Vice Head of the Dept. of Psychology and Psychosomatics, Faculty of Medicine, Masaryk University, in Brno, Czech Republic. Her scientific interests include mainly hope, mental health, and well-being. She also has a special interest in the research and practice of mindfulness. Alena is a founder and director of the Czech Positive Psychology Centre (CPPC), a member of the Advisory Council of the International Positive Psychology Association (IPPA), and a member of the Executive Board of the European Network for Positive Psychology (ENPP). She has been a member of several international research projects, and she serves on the editorial boards of five academic psychological journals. Alena is the author of the first comprehensive monograph on positive psychology in the Czech language and dozens of scientific publications in positive psychology and health psychology.

Andreas Krafft holds a doctoral degree in Management Sciences at the University of St. Gallen (Switzerland) with special focus on Organizational Psychology, Culture and Development. He has academic specializations in Social Psychology of Organizations, Work and Health Psychology as well as Positive Psychology from the University of Zürich. Andreas is associate researcher for Futures Studies and lecturer at the Institute of Systemic Management and Public Governance at the University of St. Gallen. Furthermore, he teaches at the University of Zürich in the field of Work and Health, at the Master of Applied Positive Psychology at the University of Lisbon, Portugal, as well as at the Master of Futures Studies from the Free University Berlin. He is co-president of swissfuture, the Swiss Society for Futures Studies, member of the executive board of SWIPPA (the Swiss Positive Psychology Association) and of the DACH-PP (German speaking Association of Positive Psychology). Since many years he leads the International Research Network of the Hope Barometer.

CPSIA information can be obtained
at www.ICGtesting.com
Printed in the USA
LVHW060828310523
748263LV00025B/296

9 783031 2441